ILLUSTRATED
CHINESE
MOXIBUSTION

Techniques and Methods

of related interest

Needling Techniques for Acupuncturists
Basic Principles and Techniques
Editor in Chief: Professor Chang Xiaorong
ISBN 978 1 84819 057 3
eISBN 978 0 85701 045 2

Illustrated Treatment for Migraine using Acupuncture, Moxibustion and Tuina Massage
Cui Chengbin and Xing Xiaomin
ISBN 978 1 84819 061 0
eISBN 978 0 85701 057 5

Meridians and Acupoints
Edited by Zhu Bing and Wang Hongcai
Advisor: Cheng Xinnong
ISBN 978 1 84819 037 5
eISBN 978 0 85701 021 6

Acupuncture Therapeutics
Edited by Zhu Bing and Wang Hongcai
Advisor: Cheng Xinnong
ISBN 978 1 84819 039 9
eISBN 978 0 85701 018 6

Case Studies from the Medical Records of Leading Chinese Acupuncture Experts
Zhu Bing and Wang Hongcai
Advisor: Cheng Xinnong
ISBN 978 1 84819 046 7
eISBN 978 0 85701 053 7

Chinese Medical Qigong
Editor in Chief: Tianjun Liu, O.M.D.
Associate Editor in Chief: Kevin W Chen, Ph.D.
ISBN 978 1 84819 023 8
eISBN 978 0 85701 017 9

ILLUSTRATED
CHINESE
MOXIBUSTION
Techniques and Methods

PROFESSOR CHANG XIAORONG, PROFESSOR HONG JING
AND PROFESSOR YI SHOUXIANG

Translated by Henry A. Buchtel V

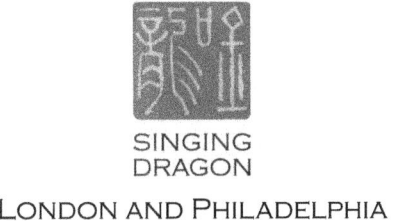

SINGING
DRAGON
LONDON AND PHILADELPHIA

Chief Editors: Chang Xiaorong, Hong Jing, Yi Shouxiang
Deputy Editors: Yue Zenghui, Lin Yaping, Yu Baosheng, Wang Xiaojuan
Chief Reviewers: Yan Jie, Sun Guojie, Wu Huangan
Chief Translator: Henry A. Buchtel V
Associate Translators: Liu Mi, Peng Yan, Lan Lei
English Reviewer: Martin A. Haase
Illustrations: Ai Kun, Yi Zhan
Assistant Editors: Liu Mi, Ai Kun, Wang Dejun, Peng Yan, Yi Zhan, Xie Hua,
Lan Lei, Song Jiong, Peng Fen, Guo Xuan, Zhang Guoshan, Yang Zhou,
Shi Jia, Wen Qiong, Tan Jing, Liu Weiai, Lin Haibo, Xie Wenjuan,
Yang Jingjing, He Yamin, Chen Xuan
Supported by the National Basic Research Program of China

First published in 2012
by Singing Dragon
an imprint of Jessica Kingsley Publishers
116 Pentonville Road
London N1 9JB, UK
and
400 Market Street, Suite 400
Philadelphia, PA 19106, USA

www.singingdragon.com

Library of Congress Cataloguing in Publication Data
A CIP catalogue record for this book is available from the Library of Congress

British Library Cataloguing in Publication Data
A CIP catalogue record for this book is available from the British Library

ISBN 978 1 84819 087 0
eISBN 978 0 85701 070 4

Printed and bound in Great Britain

Contents

Part I Foundation of Moxibustion

Chapter 2 Location and Indications of Commonly Used Points in Moxibustion

Part II Techniques and Methods

Part III Clinical Applications

Preface

Traditional Chinese moxatherapy, part of the field of Acupuncture and Moxibustion, has been held in high regard by physicians in China over many dynasties and occupies an important position in traditional Chinese medicine (TCM) today. Several thousand years of clinical experience have affirmed the ancient saying: 'When acupuncture doesn't work, moxibustion will.' In the theory of moxibustion, the surface of the body is stimulated by heat either produced by certain combustible materials or by applying medicinals directly to the skin. The heat or medicinal stimulation warms and opens the channels thereby expelling cold pathogens; this function can be used to both cure and prevent illness. As a simple, safe and effective treatment method, it is welcomed by patients and physicians alike.

This book presents a comprehensive introduction to Chinese moxatherapy. In three parts and 13 chapters, it covers the history and theory, basic skills and techniques, and clinical applications of moxatherapy. As obtaining a sound understanding of the basic skills and techniques is essential for effective and safe clinical application, these constitute a key aspect of the study of moxatherapy. In this book the illustrations and text present a starting point for learning the clinical skills and techniques needed for application in the clinical setting. This is a highly practical text that is appropriate for students, practitioners and teachers of TCM, both in China and around the world, who wish to quickly and effectively gain a command of moxatherapy. Furthermore, it is an important reference book for those involved in moxatherapy research.

Here, the authors wish to express their gratitude to Zhong Jue, Li Xin, Meng Qing-Ling, and others, who offered support during the editing process. Although this book represents the authors' best efforts, they also extend their thanks to those who provide valuable comments and criticism, in the hope of producing an improved revised edition.

Disclaimer

The more extreme methods described in this book, such as burning and scarring techniques, may not be suitable in the Western clinical setting but are, nonetheless, part of the practice as a whole. These sections have been indicated with an asterisk throughout the book. Readers should always consult a qualified medical practitioner before incorporating any of the therapies mentioned in this book into their treatment plan, whether conventional, complementary or alternative. Neither the author nor the publisher takes any responsibility for any consequences of any decision made as a result of the information contained in this book.

Synopsis

This book presents a comprehensive introduction to Chinese moxatherapy. In three parts and 13 chapters, it covers the history and theory, basic skills and techniques, and clinical applications of moxabustion therapy. In Part I the basic knowledge of moxatherapy, locations and indications for commonly used acupoints, and moxibustion for health cultivation are presented. Part II focuses on the materials, manufacture and operational functions of each type of moxibustion. Part III introduces the clinical applications of moxibustion in the treatment of internal medicine, traumatology, paediatrics, gynaecology, surgery, ear, nose and throat (ENT) and acute diseases. For each condition, the primary patterns, acupoints and moxibustion methods are provided.

PART I

Foundation of Moxibustion

CHAPTER 1

Basic Theory of Moxibustion

1. The Origins and Development of Moxibustion

1.1 THE ORIGINS OF MOXIBUSTION

Moxibustion treatment methods did not arise as a result of subjective imagination or conjecture, but rather developed gradually over hundreds and thousands of years of clinical experience and exploration. The origins of this therapeutic method reach back to the age of primitive society and a description of its earliest form can be found in the chapter *Dao Fa Fang Yi Lun* from the ancient text *Su Wen*: 'The North is where heaven and earth are hidden; it is a land of high mountains, wind, cold and ice. The people of the North love the wild and consume dairy. Cold in the zang organs gives birth to repletion disease; the treatment is moxibustion. Hence, the North is the source of moxibustion.' This text shows that moxibustion was first used in the North, and its use dates from after the discovery of fire by humankind. The discovery of fire was an essential factor in the emergence of moxatherapy. In the harsh environment endured by early humankind, fire was an important weapon against cold and hunger, allowing early man to survive and propagate. Concurrently, it made possible the conditions necessary for the creation of moxibustion. The lives of early humans, a social animal, revolved around fire for cooking and warming properties. In their daily lives they found that discomfort and pain could be relieved or even cured outright by the heat and smoke of fire (Figure 1.1.1).

As humankind developed powers of cognitive thinking and exploration, this unintentional discovery gradually became a method of using heat stimulation to treat disease. Humankind gradually collected experiences that supported certain theories, such as the application of heat to the abdomen to relieve abdominal pain and rumbling caused by exposure to cold, and the use of smoke fumigation of the joints to relieve joint pain due to cold and damp, for example (Figure 1.1.2). What started as accidental success became the intentional and deliberate use of fire to treat and prevent disease; and moxibustion became a stand-alone external treatment method. It was recognized, accepted, and further developed by later generations into the comprehensive treatment modality of today.

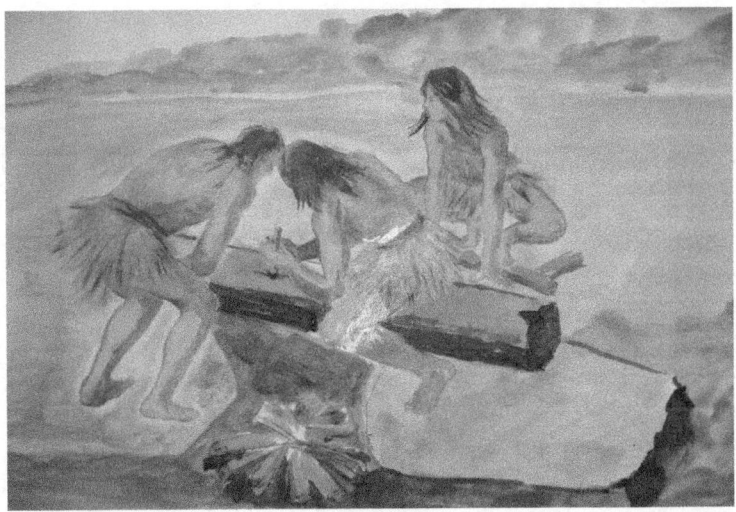

Figure 1.1.1 Primitive Man Relied on Fire for Warmth

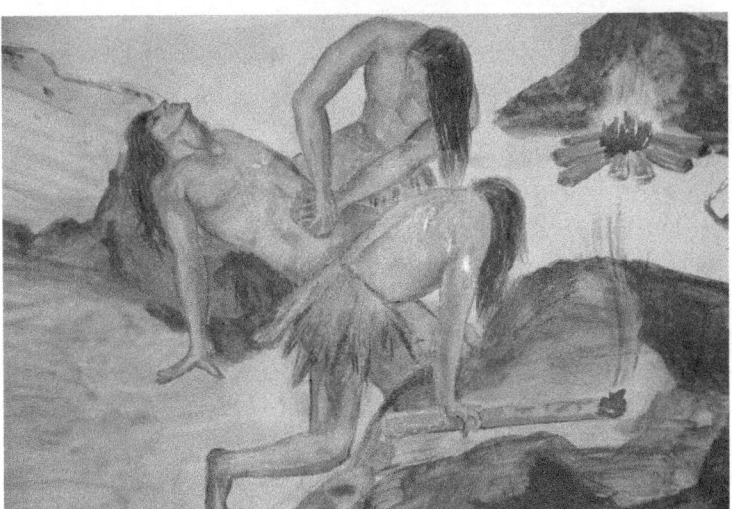

Figure 1.1.2 Application of Heat to Treat Disease

1.2 THE DEVELOPMENT OF MOXATHERAPY

After the appearance of moxibustion, it became widely used and was promoted as a method of medical treatment and health preservation. As the therapy developed over the centuries, the accumulation of experience led to the creation and improvement of medical theory. Among the medical texts excavated from the Han Dynasty tombs at Ma Wang Dui were the two channel vessel texts, the *Yin Yang Shi Yi Mai Jiu Jing* and *Zu Bi Shi Yi Mai Jiu Jing* (*Yin-Yang Eleven Vessel Cauterization Classic* and *Leg-Arm Eleven Vessel Cauterization Classic*) (Figure 1.1.3).

In these texts the pathways, diseases and moxatherapy for each channel vessel are described. In the classic text *Huang Di Nei Jing* (including *Ling Shu* and *Su Wen*), dating from the Warring States period, there are many passages that refer to moxatherapy: the chapter *Yi Fa Fang Yi Lun* of the *Su Wen* asserts that 'In the North [...] cold in the zang organs gives birth to repletion disease; the treatment is moxibustion'; the chapter *Jing Mai Pian* of the *Ling Shu* asserts that 'In the case of fallen [qi], use moxibustion'; furthermore, the chapter *Guan Neng Pian* asserts that 'If acupuncture is not appropriate, moxibustion is recommended.' These quotations illustrate that at that time moxatherapy was already an important and commonly used treatment modality.

During the Spring and Autumn period and Warring States period a new class of physician appeared, known, literally translated, as 'moxa-attack needle-reach'. In *Zuo Zhuan* (*Commentary of Zuo*) a story is recorded about a certain doctor Huan, who in 581 BC was sent from his native country of Tai to attend to the disease of Duke Jing of Jin. Huan stated that 'The disease cannot be treated. It is below the heart and above the diaphragm; it cannot be attacked [with moxa] nor reached [by needle].' The method of 'attacking' referred to in this quotation was moxatherapy, and 'reaching' was acupuncture. In the chapter *Li Lei Pian* from *Mencius* it states that 'treating a disease of seven years requires moxa aged for three years; the careless will not have prepared it, and hence will never be availed of it.' This quotation shows that during the Spring and Autumn and Warring States periods the preparation of mugwort for treating disease already existed.

As society advanced, moxatherapy also developed. During the Eastern Han period the great physician Zhang Zhong Jing (Figure 1.1.4) recorded more than 12 lines regarding moxatherapy in his classic *Shang Han Lun* (*On Cold Damage*). He recorded the contraindicated patterns and moxatherapy methods for certain diseases. The book stated which patterns can be treated with moxa and which should not be, and introduced the viewpoint that 'Yang patterns can be needled; yin patterns can be treated with moxa.'

During the Three Kingdom's period the book *Cao Shi Jiu Jing* (*Cao Family Moxatherapy Classic*) was printed, marking the emergence of the first specialized book on moxatherapy. It summarized the moxatherapy experience from the Qin and Han periods, and did much to promote the development of Chinese moxatherapy; unfortunately the book was lost during the ensuing dynasties.

Although the Jin Dynasty physician Ge Hong is most famous for his alchemy, in his book *Zhou Hou Bei Ji Fang* (*Emergency Formulas to Keep Up One's Sleeve*) he also recorded the use of moxatherapy in the treatment of acute disease patterns such as sudden death (*cu se*), five corpses (*wu hu*), sudden turmoil (cholera) and vomit-dysentery (*tu li*). His wife Bao Gu (Figure 1.1.5) loved the art of medicine and was known to have consummate clinical skills, especially in moxatherapy. She is the first recorded female moxatherapist in Chinese history.

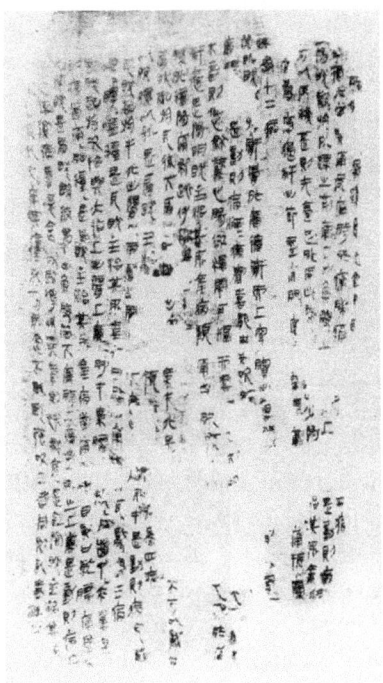

Figure 1.1.3 Yin Yang/Zu Bi Shi Yi Mai Jiu Jing
(Yin-Yang/Leg-Arm Eleven Vessel Cauterization
Classic)

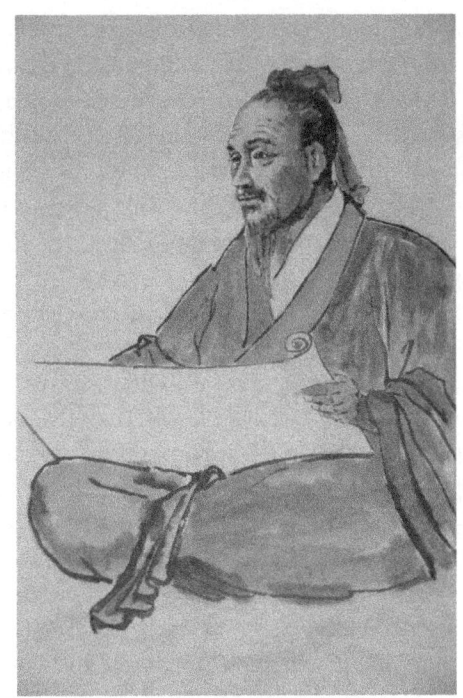

Figure 1.1.4 Zhang Zhongjing

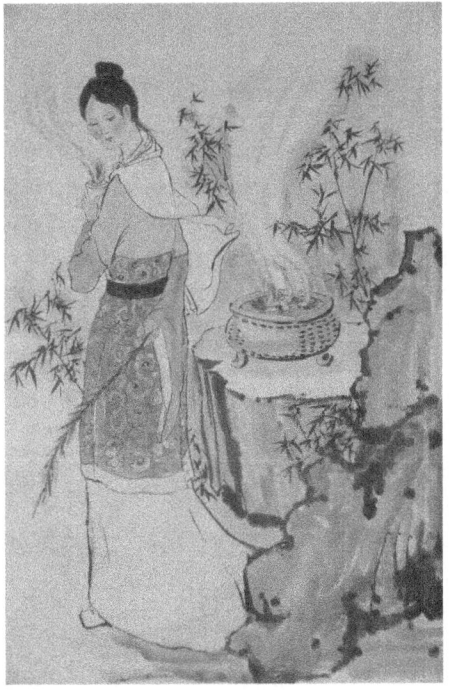

Figure 1.1.5 Bao Gu

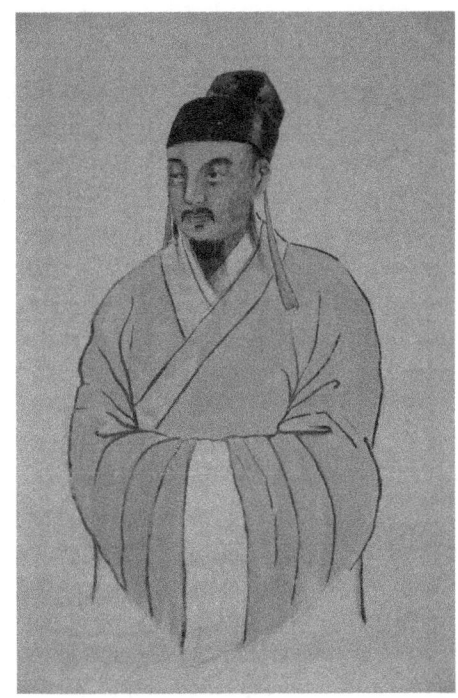

Figure 1.1.6 Sun Simiao

By the Tang Dynasty moxatherapy had developed even further. For example, the famous Tang Dynasty physician Sun Simiao (Figure 1.1.6), in his book *Qian Jin Fang* (*Thousand Pieces of Gold*), recorded a technique to treat ear disease whereby a bamboo or reed tube is inserted into the ear and moxa is burned in the opening. He also asserted that 'without moxibustion one will lack essence: therefore, moxa Zu San Li (ST-36)'; referring to this as 'longevity moxa'. Sun Simiao had clearly recognized the benefits of moxatherapy, its preventative and curative properties, and its ability to strengthen the body and postpone ageing.

The work *Bei Ji Jiu Fa* (*Moxatherapy for Any Emergency*), written during the Song Dynasty, stated: 'In emergencies, moxibustion should be used first.' In the same dynasty there was also a practitioner called Du Cai, who recorded the observation in his book *Bian Que Xin Shu* that using moxa on Guan Yuan (RN-4), Qi Hai (RN-6), and Zhong Wan (RN-12) could lengthen one's lifetime. A major part of the book *Gu Zheng Bing Jiu Fang* (*Moxa Prescriptions for Bone Steaming Disease*) is devoted to the use of moxatherapy in the treatment of consumption; the descriptions in this book made the 'Four Flower Points' (*Si Hua Xue*) moxatherapy technique popular.

During the Song and Yuan dynasties moxatherapy developed considerably. The founder of the Song Dynasty personally applied moxa to his younger brother, and collected and applied it to himself; deeds later praised far and wide. The books *Tai Ping Sheng Hui Fang* (*The Great Peace Sagacious Benevolence Formulary*), *Pu Ji Ben Shi Fang* (*Formulas of Universal Benefit [from My Practice]*) and *Sheng Ji Zong Lu* (*Comprehensive Recording of Sage-like Benefit*) all included extensive content regarding moxatherapy, and resulted in the acceptance of moxatherapy as an emergency treatment method. In the Yuan Dynasty the famous physician Zhu Danxi created the theory of using moxatherapy in the treatment of heat patterns.

During the Ming Dynasty the number of acu-moxatherapists increased greatly. A whole slew of famous works were published in quick succession: *Zhen Jiu Da Cheng* (*The Great Compendium of Acupuncture and Moxibustion*), *Zhen Jiu Da Quan* (*The Compendium of Acupuncture and Moxibustion*), *Zhen Jiu Ji Ying* (*Gathered Blooms of Acupuncture and Moxibustion*), etc. It was at this time that 'Lightning-fire amazing needle', 'Tai Yi amazing needle', and other new techniques of combining moxa with other medicinals emerged. At the same time techniques such as Sang Zhi (mulberry twig) moxa, juncibustion (lantern-fire moxa), Yang Sui (yang-flint) moxa and others also made a contribution to enriching the field of moxatherapy.

During the Qing Dynasty there was still a certain amount of creativity and development. *Shen Jiu Jing Lun*, a moxatherapy monograph published during this period, represented a new high point in the development of the field. However, the weakening of the Qing government and the encroachment of Western ideas at the end of the Qing Dynasty devastated the practice and development of moxatherapy, and it followed its sister fields of acupuncture and herbal medicine to the brink of extinction.

After the birth of postmodern China, moxatherapy and its fellow fields achieved significant redevelopment. Following the advancement of scientific techniques, the millennia old therapeutic technique increasingly showed wide promise and future potential. The authors firmly believe that moxatherapy has the capacity to contribute greatly to the health of peoples throughout the world, in its role as both prevention and treatment, by achieving sustainable, affordable and effective results.

2. The Concept of Moxatherapy

Moxatherapy is a form of external therapy making use of moxa as the primary material to heat, burn and/or fumigate either acupoints or specific areas on the surface of the body. Utilizing the functions of the channels and acupoints, moxa warms and opens the channels and network vessels, assists right qi, expels pathogenic qi and regulates the body's physiological functions; thus treating disease and cultivating health. Moxatherapy has been valued by physicians throughout the ages for its simplicity, inexpensiveness, efficacy and lack of side effects. This therapeutic method has been constantly developing and improving, and is now a comprehensive system of therapy that includes basic theory, knowledge and skills – the field of Moxatherapy.

3. The Basics of Moxatherapy

The use of moxatherapy in the treatment of disease has a long history. What started as the simple use of moxa later evolved into numerous and diverse methods. Until recently, the most prominent method used the herb Ai Ye (moxa; mugwort; Artemisiae Argyi Folium) as the primary combustible material and is, this, known as moxibustion. Methods using materials other than Ai Ye are referred to as non-moxa moxibustion. There is a further type of moxatherapy called 'special' moxibustion. So, presently there are three general methods: moxibustion, non-moxa moxibustion and 'special' moxibustion. Moxibustion includes moxa cones, moxa poles, warm needle moxa and gentle moxa. Non-moxa moxibustion includes non-burning medicinal moxa and burning medicinal moxa. 'Special' moxibustion includes medicinal steam moxa, freezing moxa, and Zhuang-style thread moxa.

4. Specific Characteristics and Range of Application of Moxatherapy

4.1 SPECIFIC CHARACTERISTICS

As moxatherapy is a part of the general field of traditional Chinese medicine, it shares with other treatment methods the overall function of both treating and preventing disease. Concurrently, as a special part of Chinese medicine, it also has its own unique characteristics, which can be summarized by the points below.

Wide Range of Application

Moxatherapy is applicable to patterns in the majority of medical departments. Common diseases in the internal, paediatric, gynaecology, andrology, dermatology, surgical, traumatology, oculopathy, and ENT departments can all be treated using this method. In addition to treating disease, moxatherapy can also promote right qi, strengthen the body's immune system, and bring about improvements in general health and disease prevention.

Experiential Results

Extensive clinical experience shows that moxatherapy provides rapid and strong clinical results, and can also make up for shortcomings in acupuncture and herbal therapy treatments. When used in the treatment of diseases within its range of application, whether cosmetic or health-related, moxatherapy achieves good results, sometimes with only one treatment. With patience and persistence, even chronic long-term diseases can be treated effectively.

Convenient and Timely

Moxatherapy is not limited to use in the hospital, as it can, to some extent, be conducted by patients in their own home. This allows for early treatment, which is considered most valuable by the principles of Chinese medicine. The use of moxa poles is very convenient; it is only necessary to indicate the area and time of application for the patient to perform effective treatment themselves, particularly as the temperature can be controlled easily. For patients with chronic gastroenteritis and neurasthenia, for example, daily visits to the hospital may be inconvenient, however, after learning how to apply moxa themselves, patients can carry out regular treatments in the comfort of their own home, achieving even better results.

Simple and Easy to Learn

Moxatherapy has the advantage of being simple, easy to learn and relatively straight forward to apply. For these reasons, para-professionals may be able to learn and apply it with excellent results.

Safe and Economical

Moxatherapy does not have any known side effects and is considered to be even safer than acupuncture. Complications such as stuck, bent or broken needles or needle-related fainting will not occur. The Scarring Moxa technique causes a moxa sore; however, this sore is a desired result as it increases the treatment efficacy and the treatment method is, nonetheless, safe and reliable.* Besides the safety aspect of moxatherapy, it is also economical. The only material required is the herb Ai Ye (mugwort; moxa; Artemisiae Argyi Folium), which grows widely and is easy to harvest. After it is processed into moxa cones and poles, it only needs to be ignited to commence treatment.

4.2 RANGE OF APPLICATION

Moxatherapy is indicated in the case of cold patterns, heat patterns, repletion and deficiency. Though presently it is used most often in the case of cold patterns, chronic diseases and all long-term yang-deficiency conditions, it is also applicable for a few repletion-heat patterns. Irrespective of the presenting disease it is being used for, medical providers must always carefully examine the disease-state and choose the most appropriate acupoints and moxa method. In this way a multitude of different diseases can be treated effectively with moxatherapy. Generally speaking, the indications for moxatherapy are very broad. To summarize, the indications are as follows:

- Externally contracted external patterns.

- Cough and phlegm panting.

- Expectoration of blood and nosebleed.

- Spleen and kidney deficiency.

- Qi stagnation and abdominal masses.

- Wind-cold-damp impediment.

- Upper body exuberance and lower body vacuity.

- Reverse-flow qi desertion pattern (loss of consciousness with extreme cold of the extremities).

- Gynaecological disease.

- Stubborn lichen swellings and sores.

- Scrofula, swelling and tumours.

5. Contraindications and Cautions

5.1 CONTRAINDICATIONS

Contraindicated Areas

In ancient texts there are many recordings of areas contraindicated for the application of moxatherapy. In the work *Zhen Jiu Jia Yi Jing* (*The Systematized Canon of Acupuncture and Moxibustion*), 24 acupoints are listed; in *Yi Zong Jin Jian* (*The Golden Mirror of Medicine*) there are 47 contraindicated acupoints; in *Zhen Jiu Da Cheng* there are 45 points; and 49 are recorded in *Zhen Jiu Ji Cheng* such as Nao Hu (DU-17), Feng Fu (DU-16), Ya Men (DU-15), Wu Chu (BL-5), Cheng Guang (BL-6), Ji Zhong (DU-6), Xin Shu (BL-15), Bai Huan Shu (BL-30), Si Zhu Kong (TH-23), Cheng Qi (ST-1), Ren Ying (ST-9), Ru Zhong (ST-17), Yuan Ye (GB-22), Jiu Wei (RN-15), Jing Qu (LU-8), Tian Fu (LU-3), Yin Shi (ST-33), Fu Tu (ST-32), Di Wu Hui (GB-42), Xi Yang Guan (GB-33), Ying Xiang (CO-20), Di Cang (ST-4), Shao Fu (HT-8), Zu Tong Gu (BL-66), Tian Zhu (BL-10), Tou Lin Qi (GB-15), Tou Wei (ST-8), Cuan Zhu (BL-2), Jing Ming (BL-1), Xia Guan (ST-7), Zhou Rong (SP-20), Fu Ai (SP-16), Jian Zhen (SI-9), Yang Chi (TH-4), Zhong Chong (PC-9), Shao Shang (LU-11), Yu Ji (LU-10), Yin Bai (SP-1), Lou Gu (SP-7), Yin Ling Quan (SP-9), Tiao Kou (ST-38), Du Bi (ST-35), Shan Mai (BL-62), Wei Zhong (BL-40), Su Liao (DU-25), Ju Liao (GB-29), He Liao (LI-19), Quan Liao (SI-18), Tian You (TH-16), Bi Guan (ST-31), Cheng Fu (BL-36). The majority of these points are distributed on the head or face, near important organs and blood vessels, and in areas where the skin is thin or where sinews and muscles are concentrated. For these reasons, moxa of these areas should be avoided, especially when using the Scarring Moxa method.* Moxa should not be applied to the lower abdomen, lumbar region, breasts and genitals of pregnant women. These contraindications have developed from the valuable experience and collective wisdom of the ancients and should not be overlooked.

Contraindicated Disease Patterns

As moxibustion provides heat stimulation and heat can injure yin, patterns involving yin vacuity and yang hyperactivity or internal accumulation of pathogenic heat should not receive moxatherapy, according to the theory of traditional Chinese medicine. Examples include yin vacuity with internal heat, expectoration and ejection of blood, profuse dreaming and seminal emission, wind strike (stroke) block pattern, high fever with clouded spirit, etc. From the perspective of Western medicine, such as high fever, hypertensive crises, late stage tuberculosis, massive hemoptysis, vomiting, severe anaemia, acute infectious disease and skin boils with fever should not receive moxatherapy. In addition, moxatherapy should not be applied to the abdomen and lumbar region of pregnant women or in cases of organic heart disease with cardiac dysfunction and schizophrenia.

Inappropriate use of moxa for heat diseases can injure yin-blood. Contraindicated pulse and tongue signs are: surging, large, string-like, rapid and replete pulses, and bright crimson or rough yellow tongue and coating. These signs indicate patterns of yin fluid depletion and yang heat excess. Application of moxatherapy demands careful examination of the clinical signs and customization of the treatment according to the pattern.

Contraindicated Time Periods

Times when it is not appropriate to apply moxibustion include when the patient is quite hungry, full, tired, intoxicated, thirsty, in a state of shock, terror or rage, or sweating profusely. Patients in an agitated emotional state or women during menstruation should also not receive moxa, but this does not preclude curing heavy bleeding. In clinical practice, these temporary contraindicated conditions should receive special attention in order to avoid moxa-sickness and other accidental injury.

5.2 CAUTIONS

The practitioner or individual carrying out moxibustion should be focused and perform all procedures with care. The requirements of moxibustion should be explained to the patient so as to avoid unnecessary concern and to achieve their full cooperation. If it is necessary to use scarring moxa, the patient's agreement must be obtained prior to treatment.

1. An appropriate posture is important during moxibustion treatment. The patient's posture should be symmetrical and comfortable in order to facilitate the correct location of acupoints, the placement of moxa cones and the application of moxa.

2. The standards for quantification of the amount of moxa are the size and number of moxa cones. Generally speaking, early stages of disease and strong patients are treated with a higher number of larger cones; late stages of disease and weaker patients are given smaller and fewer cones. The number and size should also be adjusted according to the characteristics of the area of application: cones on the head, face and chest should not be too big nor too numerous; cones on the lumbar region and abdomen can be large and multitudinous; areas on the limbs where the skin is thin and where there is a high concentration of sinew and proximity to bone are not suitable for frequent or excessive moxatherapy. In the case of sunken and intractable cold and yang qi on the verge of desertion (at this stage the patient

will be almost unconscious and their limbs will be ice cold), efficacy will only be achieved by using a multitude of large cones; in the case of externally contracted wind-cold or welling, flat abscesses and impediment pain, it is important to keep the amount appropriate to avoid causing internal depression of pathogenic heat, resulting in harm.

3. The indications for moxa treatment are very broad, but one should keep in mind that although it boosts yang, at the same time it can also injure yin. In the case of patterns that belong to yin vacuity and yang hyperactivity, pathogenic repletion internal block, and exuberant toxic heat, moxa should be used with caution.

4. When performing moxibustion, areas such as the face, five sensory organs and large blood vessels should not receive direct moxa, and the abdomen and lumbar region of pregnant women should be avoided.

5. When performing moxibustion or using the warm needle moxa method, care should be taken that a burning ember does not fall onto the skin or other surfaces. During moxibustion one should be aware of the patient's response to the heat stimulation, and adjust the distance between the moxa and surface of the skin accordingly. One should develop a good understanding of the amount of moxa to use, in order to avoid over-moxibustion and burning. In the event that blistering occurs after moxibustion, as long as the blisters are not broken they can be left to recede naturally. If the blisters are too large, they can be drained by puncturing the lower side of the blister with a sterilized needle; followed by applying Long Dan Zi medicated water.

6. Moxibustion facilities should have good airflow of fresh air to avoid excessively thick smoke and poor air quality, which can harm the body.

6. Moxibustion Supplementing and Draining

6.1 MOXIBUSTION SUPPLEMENTING

After lighting the moxa, do not blow on the ember, but rather let it slowly heat up and wait for it to extinguish naturally. The strength of the heat is gentle and long lasting, and can be applied multiple times. After moxibustion use the hand to press on the area of application, causing the moxa-qi to concentrate and not be dispersed. If performing pole moxa, light pecking sparrow moxa may be used on each acupoint for 0.5–2 minutes for each point. Another option is gentle moxa on each acupoint for 3–5 minutes. These methods promote the body's physiological functioning and eliminate excessive inhibition of the nervous system, bringing about a normal state of excitation.

6.2 MOXIBUSTION DRAINING

After igniting the moxa, blow the ember until it is burning vigorously. Ignite and extinguish quickly, and once the patient feels a sensation of burning, quickly replace the moxa cone and continue. The treatment is relatively short, and the number of cones used is relatively few. After moxibustion do not press the acupoint in order to allow the pathogenic qi at the acupoint to disperse. If using pole moxa, one could choose the gentle moxa or circling moxa, and stimulate each acupoint strongly for 10 minutes or more to achieve calming of the acupoints and promote normal inhibition.

7. Postures and Order of Execution for Moxatherapy

7.1 APPROPRIATE POSTURE FOR PERFORMING MOXIBUSTION

The physical posture of the patient should be carefully chosen in order to make the process of locating acupoints and carrying out moxibustion safe, convenient and accurate. The patient should feel comfortable and at ease, and should be able to maintain the position throughout the entire process, or, according to the needs of the treatment, make appropriate changes in posture. Commonly used postures include: supine (Figure 1.7.1 A), prone (Figure 1.7.1 B), lateral (Figure 1.7.1 C), supine supported sitting (Figure 1.7.1 D), prone supported sitting (Figure 1.7.1 E), supported cupped arms (Figure 1.7.1 F), supported prone arms (Figure 1.7.1 G), supported supine arms (Figure 1.7.1 H), prone sitting (Figure 1.7.1 I), standing (Figure 1.7.1 J), and sitting (Figure 1.7.1 K). The overall requirements allow for a natural posture, exposed acupoints, stability in placing moxa cones and convenient operations.

7.2 THE ORDER OF EXECUTION OF MOXIBUSTION

The usual order of performing moxibustion in the clinical setting is as follows: upper body → lower body → back → abdomen → head → limbs. First select yang channels, then select yin channels. The number of moxa cones used during course of treatments starts low and then increases, and the moxa cones start small and gradually increase in size. Carrying out the procedure in this order allows you to encourage yin from yang while not being damaged by an exuberance of yang. If one does not follow this progression, and first performs moxa on the lower body and then on the head, the patient may experience baking heat in their head and face as well as dry mouth and throat.

Of course, when performing moxibustion, one ought to be flexible in customizing the treatment for different patients and conditions. For example, when treating anal prolapse, one may first moxa Chang Qiang (DU-1) in order to cause the intestine to retreat, then moxa Bai Hui (DU-20) to encourage upward movement.

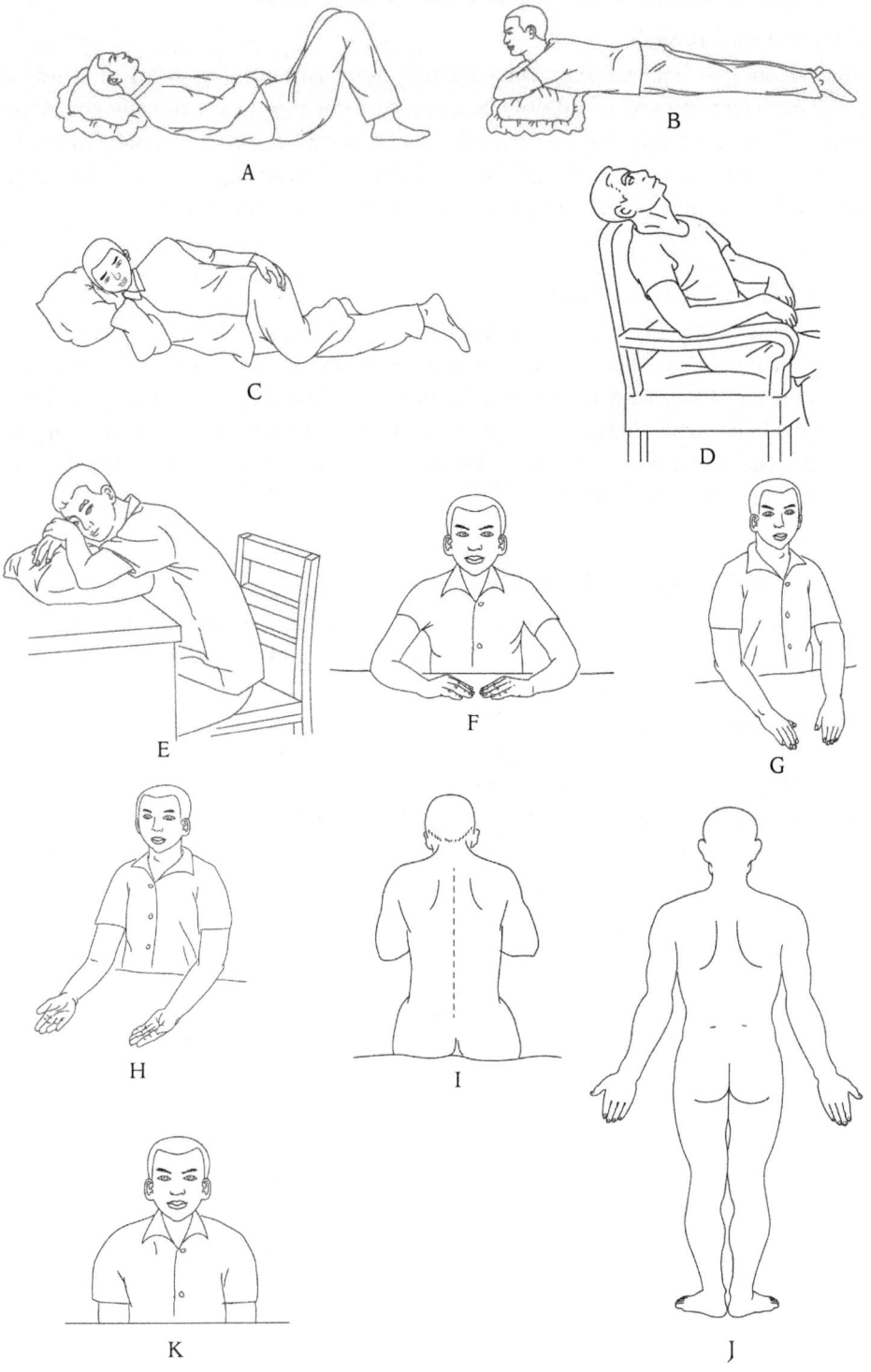

Figure 1.7.1 Posture Diagram

8. Managing Moxa Sores and Post-Moxa Care

8.1 MANAGING MOXA SORES

Ancient practitioners believed that using scarring moxa and creating moxa sores was a necessity; treatment efficacy would only be achieved if the moxa cone directly contacted the skin and created a sore. However, it is currently considered not necessary to create moxa sores in order to achieve the goal of treatment; non-scarring moxa, indirect moxa methods and gentle pole moxa, for example, also achieve excellent results.

Causative Factors for Moxa Sores

Moxa-sores are caused by blisters that form after moxibustion. This may occur in the following circumstances: when the moxa cone is not compacted tightly enough, causing a loose portion of burning cone to fall onto the skin; when the cones are too large and too many are used; and when blisters are punctured and become infected. However, a moxa sore will present only if puss forms in the blisters, whereby the formation of pus is due to breaking or infection of the blister.

Prevention and Treatment of Moxa Sores

The first requirement is that moxa cones are tightly compacted to prevent large burning moxa cones from directly contacting the skin. Secondly, control the size and number of moxa cones to prevent burning and blistering and, finally, after blisters are caused, keep the area clean. Small blisters can heal naturally, but they must not be scratched even if they are itchy. If the blisters are large, a sterilized needle can be used to drain the liquid, then the blister can be covered with a cloth bandage or mild medicated plaster. If the blister is accidentally broken it should be sterilized then tightly wrapped; this will prevent suppuration and festering. If the heat of the moxa is too intense and moxa sores are created, the following treatment should be performed:

1. Protect the Sore: Besides draining liquid as described above, the moxa sore must also be protected to prevent infection. An appropriate amount of red-skinned scallion and mint can be decocted and used to wash the area around the sore. Yu Hong Gao (Jade and Red Paste) can be used to encourage scab formation, allowing it to heal naturally.

2. Resist Infection: If the moxa sore becomes infected and suppurative, herbs with antibacterial properties should be used. If after the sore heals the skin is still dark and does not improve, the tender skin of Tao Zhi (peach twigs; Persicae Fructus) can be decocted and used while warm to wash the area. If the moxa sore is unbearably painful, then appropriate amounts of Tao Zhi (Persicae Fructus), Liu Zhi (Salicis Ramulus), Yan Sui (Coriandri Herba cum Radice) and Huang Lian (Coptidis Rhizoma) can be decocted and used to wash the area, immediately stopping the pain. If the moxa sore fails to close, it is usually because of qi vacuity, in which case Nei Tuo Huang Lian Wan (Internal Drawing Coptic Balls) should be taken: 48g of Huang Qi (Astragali Radix), 12g of Dang Gui (Angelicae Sinensis Radix), and 6g each of Rou Gui (Cinnamomi Cortex), Mu Xiang (Aucklandiae Radix), Ru Xiang

(Olibanum) and Chen Xiang (Aquilariae Lignum Resinatum). During hot weather, if there is excessive secretion of liquids, a paper towel or cloth bandage may be used to dry them; do not wash with cold water. During cold weather it is difficult for granulation to occur, scallion decoction can be used to clean the area around the sore to assist the action of medicinal paste. When the scab detaches from the moxa sore, besides using decoctions of peach twigs and willow twig to wash the area, it ought also to be protected from exposure to wind and cold.

8.2 POST-MOXA CARE

Scarring cone moxa has an effect on essence, blood and fluids, so it is important to emphasize post-moxibustion care. Certain individuals with weak constitutions may experience mild heat-effusion, a dry mouth, fatigue and other discomforts. It is not necessary to cease moxatherapy, as these will disappear with continued treatment. If this discomfort becomes more pronounced, and symptoms such as dry mouth, dark yellow urine, and constipation occur, it is a sign that the moxa has caused injury to the body's yin. To eliminate these symptoms the patient can be prescribed Jia Wei Zeng Ye Tang (Supplemented Humor-increasing Decoction): 15g each of Shen Di Huang (Rehmanniae Radix Exsiccata seu Recens), Mai Dong (Ophiopogonis Radix), Xuan Shen (Scrophulariae Radix), and Rou Cong Rong (Cistanches Herba) (decoct and take once per day). Other methods of moxibustion rarely result in such discomfort, and therefore do not require any special post-treatment care.

9. Moxibustion Sensation and Moxibustion Quantification

9.1 MOXIBUSTION SENSATION

Moxibustion sensation refers to the subjective sensations experienced by the patient during moxibustion. Moxibustion achieves its curative and preventative effects through directly or indirectly providing an appropriate level of heat stimulation to the surface of the body. For this reason, with the exception of scarring moxibustion, the primary subjective sensation experienced during moxibustion is a feeling of warmth or burning on the surface of and below the skin. In addition, the sensation of heat may be experienced at a deep level, remain for a long time or travel along channel pathways.

9.2 MOXIBUSTION QUANTIFICATION

In ancient times, the quantification aspect of moxibustion therapy was considered to be very important. In Qian Jin Fang it is recorded: 'On the limbs, moxibustion should be light and not carried out for too long. On the chest, back and abdomen, moxibustion should be stronger, but on the lower back and spine moxa should be applied less.' Wai Tai Mi Yao asserts that: 'The elderly and infirm should receive less moxatherapy, and those with strong constitutions should receive more moxatherapy.' Bian Que Xin Shu states that 'Severe diseases receive 100 cones […] and for minor disease less than 3, 5, or 7 cones.' From these examples it can be seen that determining the amount of moxibustion performed depends on, for example, the patient's constitution, age, area receiving treatment and disease condition. Clinically, the unit by which moxibustion is quantified is the size and amount of moxa cones. The length of the course of moxibustion treatment is another important aspect: a course of treatment in the case of acute disease is shorter (sometimes only 1–2 treatments), while chronic conditions require a longer treatment course (from several months to more than one year). Generally speaking, at the beginning of a course of treatment, moxibustion is performed once every day; after 3 treatments, the frequency is adjusted to once every 2–3 days. In acute cases 2–3 treatment sessions can be performed per day, while in chronic cases requiring long-term treatment, one treatment can be performed every 2–3 days.

10. Moxibustion Treatment Principles

10.1 Root and Branch, Moderate and Acute

The concepts of root and branch, moderate and acute, are relative, not absolute. In the occurrence and development of disease, root, branch, moderate and acute are complex and changeable. According to the principle of 'striving for the root in the treatment of disease' found in *Huang Di Nei Jing*, combined with the summarization of clinical practice and experience, the following four points regarding the usage of root, branch, moderate and acute can be made:

1. Treat the Root: Treatment of disease should be directed at the root of the disease. Clinical signs and symptoms are only the external phenomena reflecting the disease, and through identification of patterns, starting with analysis of the exterior and then the interior, from phenomena to basic nature, the cause, location and mechanism of the disease can be identified and concluded as a certain pattern type. This pattern type substantially summarizes the basic nature of the disease. The next step is to determine a treatment for this specific pattern type to achieve the goal of treating the root.

2. In Acute Conditions, Treat the Branch: In certain circumstances, the root and branch are complicated pathomechanically, and the signs and symptoms manifest as the branch being more acute than the root. If not dealt with promptly, the branch manifestation can develop into a severe and dangerous disease pattern. In this case the process of treatment determination should be done according to the pathomechanism, and the branch should be treated before the root.

3. In Moderate Conditions, Treat the Root: Generally speaking, when the disease condition is stable, unstable but not dangerous or in the case of dual disease of branch and root, after the branch disease has been relieved through treatment, the principle of 'in moderate conditions, treat the root' can be applied.

4. Treat Both Branch and Root: When the branch and root disease are both moderate or both acute, both branch and root should be treated.

10.2 Supplement Vacuity and Drain Repletion

'Supplement vacuity and drain repletion' is the basic principle that guides moxibustion therapy. 'Vacuity' refers to the condition of vacuity of right qi; 'repletion' means that pathogenic qi is abnormally strong. Supplementing vacuity indicates supporting right qi, strengthening internal organ function and supplementing and boosting yin, yang, qi and blood, with the goal of resisting disease. Draining repletion refers to expelling pathogenic qi, to allow right qi to recover. 'Supplementing vacuity' and 'draining repletion' in moxibustion therapy means using methods of moxibustion to stimulate the body's own regulatory functions, creating the effects of supplementation and draining, thereby supporting right and expelling pathogens.

Supplementation and drainage are achieved through choosing different acupoints and different methods of operation. Supplementation of vacuity by choosing different acupoints is primarily achieved through the use of acupoint combination methods such as supplementing the same channel, supplementing the exterior-interior-related channel, and supplementing the mother to feed the child. Choice of acupoint combinations for drainage of repletion is primarily achieved through draining the same channel, exterior-interior-related channel, and following the principle of draining the child in repletion. The choice of method can also be used to differentiate between supplementation and drainage. In supplementation, the burning ember is left to expire completely, allowing the heat to slowly penetrate to a deep layer in order to supplement vacuity and support emaciation, warm yang and supplement centre qi. In drainage the ember should be blown so it burns quickly, and the moxa should be swept away before it burns down to the surface of the skin; the heat should be urgent and strong to achieve the effects of dissipating and dispersing.

10.3 Act According to Time, Place and Person

These three principles refer to enacting an appropriate treatment method according to the season (and time), geographic location and individual.

1. Act According to Time: The special characteristics of different seasons and times (namely the 12 earthly branches) determine the treatment method. The different climate in each of the four seasons initiates a certain effect on physiological functions and pathological changes. In a single day, the strength and weakness of the qi and blood of each channel will vary. The influence of changes in season and time lead to differences in acupoint and method choice. Besides these, one ought also to understand the most effective time for treatment; for example, treatment of menstrual pain is usually carried out before menstruation begins.

2. Act According to Place: The treatment should take into consideration the special characteristics of different geographical environments. Just as there are differences among geographical environments, climates, living habits and customs; differences also exist in human physiological activity and pathological characteristics. The method of treatment should take these into consideration.

3. Act According to Person: Factors such as sex, age and constitution of the patient all require special consideration when determining treatment. Men and women have different physiological characteristics, which are especially apparent when dealing with menstruation, pregnancy and postpartum conditions. Treatment should also take into consideration the different physiological functions of different age groups.

11. Primary Therapeutic Effects of Moxibustion

11.1 COURSE WIND AND RESOLVE THE EXTERIOR, WARM AND DISSIPATE COLD PATHOGEN

Due to the warming and fumigating properties of moxibustion, it has the function of warming and dissipating cold pathogens. Cold includes both externally contracted cold pathogen and vacuity cold of the centre burner. In Chinese medicine 'externally contracted cold pathogen' refers to symptoms such as an aversion to and fear of cold, cold limbs, cold pain, a preference for warmth and lying in the foetal position, caused by exposure to cold or by over consumption of raw or cold foods. Vacuity cold of the centre burner is usually caused by internal injury and enduring illness causing injury and taxation of yang qi. This is observable in symptoms such as cold limbs and lying in the foetal position, an absence of thirst, clear and thin phlegm, drool, mucus, clear and excessive urine, thin and loose stools. Moxibustion can dispel cold pathogens, return yang qi, cause cold pathogens to dissipate, and bring warmth back to the limbs. According to the viewpoint of modern medicine, the heat characteristic of moxibustion can cause vasodilation of local capillary blood vessels, lead to tissue hyperaemia and increase the speed of blood flow and metabolism, improving areas that lack blood, oxygen and nutrition. This results in the function of warming and dissipating cold pathogens. This effect can be relied upon to treat symptoms such as vomiting, abdominal pain, diarrhoea, which are caused by externally contracted wind-cold exterior pattern and centre burner vacuity cold.

11.2 WARM AND FREE CHANNELS AND COLLATERALS, QUICKEN BLOOD AND EXPEL IMPEDIMENT

It is believed in Chinese medicine that qi, blood and fluids are the basic materials for human life, and that they circulate throughout the entire body. The paths that these materials follow around the body are the channels, and if these channels are blocked or inhibited the result will be limb pain or dysfunction, or irregular internal organ qi dynamics, which lead to disease. Obstruction of the channels is often due to cold pathogens settling in the channels, inhibition of qi dynamics, or injury to the channels. This can manifest as dysfunction of limb movement, joint pain, headache, lower backache, abdominal pain and painful menstruation, as well as stroke paralysis and facial paralysis (Bell's Palsy). When moxibustion is performed on acupoints, it has the effect of warming and freeing the channels. The viewpoint of modern medicine is that moxibustion speeds up metabolism of local tissues, speeding up pain mechanisms causing products of inflammation and discharging them out of the body. At the same time, moxibustion regulates the excitability of nerves, inhibiting over-excited nerves and exciting functionally decreased nerves. This brings about a cessation of pain and improvements in nerve palsy and limb paralysis.

11.3 REINFORCE YANG AND STEM QI DESERTION, LIFT YANG AND RAISE PROLAPSE

Yin and Yang represent the root of human life. Yang debilitation leads to yin exuberance, and yin exuberance manifests as cold, reversal or even verging on desertion. Conditions such as enduring illness, a weak constitution or fulminant desertion (sudden loss of consciousness) of qi and blood are common. These result in insecurity of defensive yang, insecurity of the interstices and a tendency towards wind damage and common cold. In extreme cases sinking of central qi, organ prolapse or extreme yang debilitation, separation of yin and yang, with the signs and symptoms of a sombre white facial complexion, reversal cold of the limbs, copious sweating and a drop in blood pressure. The heat of moxibustion can warm, supplement and support yang qi, and treat vacuity qi desertion. From the perspective of modern medicine, moxibustion can regulate the body's stress levels and raise tolerance, regulating various glandular functions and maintaining the organism's physiological functionality. For these reasons, moxibustion can treat chronic diarrhoea and dysentery, seminal emissions, impotence, and vacuity qi desertion, resulting from spleen and kidney yang vacuity, as well as organ prolapse, flooding and spotting, caused by sinking of centre qi.

11.4 DISPERSE STASIS AND DISSIPATE KNOTS, DRAW OUT TOXINS AND DRAIN HEAT

With regards to stasis and knots, Chinese medicine believes that they are caused by coagulation of cold or poor movement of qi and blood, resulting in phlegm-damp obstruction or blood stasis. This manifests as welling or flat abscesses, lumps or blood stasis. Moxibustion can free and regulate the qi dynamic, and harmonize and disinhibit construction and defence, allowing stasis and knots to naturally dissipate. For this reason, in clinical practice moxibustion is often used for the treatment of diseases involving qi and blood stagnation, such as early mammary welling abscess, scrofula and goitre. According to modern medical research, moxibustion can cause an increase in neutrocytes and phagocytic function, and a decrease in inflammatory exudation. For these reasons moxibustion is able to dissipate congealed cold, disperse swelling, disperse welling and flat abscesses, either speeding the ulceration of suppurative sores or dispelling putridity and engendering flesh in the case of qi vacuity sores that fail to close. In this way, moxibustion achieves the effects of dispersing stasis and dissipating binds, quickening blood and ceasing pain.

11.5 PREVENT DISEASE, IMPROVE HEALTH AND PROLONG LIFE

In *Bian Que Xin Shu* it says, 'In times of health, moxibustion of Guan Yuan (RN-4), Qi Hai (RN-6), Ming Men (DU-4), and Zhong Wan (RN-12), will guarantee a hundred or more years of life.' This quotation describes the disease prevention and health improving effects of moxibustion. Performing moxibustion when there is no disease can stimulate right qi, strengthen the ability to resist disease, restore energy and allow longevity without debilitation. Modern medical research points out that moxibustion of Zu San Li (ST-36), Bai Hui (DU-20), for example, can reduce blood coagulation and lower blood lipids and cholesterol. From this we can see why performing moxibustion in times of health can strengthen disease resistance, increase energy levels and prolong life.

12. Point Selection Principles and Combined Point Prescriptions

Moxibustion prescriptions are formed under the guidance of the theories of traditional Chinese medicine (TCM), especially those of the channel and collateral doctrine. According to the principles for point selection and methods of combining points, acupoints are chosen and combined to form a treatment strategy. As acupoints are the basic element in moxatherapy prescriptions, the precise and appropriate selection of acupoints will directly influence the treatment efficacy. The creation of point prescriptions should be done in accordance with the basic point selection principles and methods of combining points.

12.1 POINT SELECTION PRINCIPLES

The principles for selection of points are the basic rules to be followed when choosing which points to direct treatment at when performing moxatherapy. They include selection of local points, distal points, points according to pattern, and selection of points according to signs and symptoms. The principles for selection of local and distal points are based primarily on the area of pathology, while the selection of points according to pattern and signs and symptoms is based on analysis of the manifestation of pathology.

1. Selection of Local Points: This is a method of choosing points that are at or near to the area of pathological change, and is a reflection of the local therapeutic response characteristic of acupoints. It is usually used in the case of obvious local symptoms, such as choosing Zhong Wan (RN-12) to treat stomach pain, Ting Gong (SI-19) to treat tinnitus, and Xia Che (ST-6) and Di Cang (ST-4) to treat facial paralysis.

2. Selection of Distal Points: This is a method of choosing points that are distant from the area of pathological change, but that are located on the channel or collateral that the area is associated with. This is a reflection of the rule that 'if the channel reaches an area, the channel is the primary treatment choice'. For example, in the case of stomach pain, Zu San Li (ST-36), on the Foot-Yangming Stomach channel, will be chosen; Nei Ting (ST-44), also on the Foot-Yangming Stomach channel, is chosen for treating toothache in the upper jaw; while the point He Gu (LI-4) on the Hand-Yangming Large Intestine channel is chosen for treating lower jaw toothache.

3. Selection of Points According to Pattern: This method of point selection is carried out according to the patient's syndromes, cause of disease and pathomechanism; after analysis the points selected are based on the resulting pattern. In clinical practice there are some disease patterns such as heat effusion, profuse sweating, night sweating, vacuity qi desertion, tugging wind and stupor that do not have an obvious limited area of pathological change, but rather are generalized conditions. Additionally, some internal organ disease patterns require point selection based on organ pattern identification. In these cases the method of selecting points according to pattern is used, for example: Shen Shu (BL-23) and Tai Xi (KI-3) for vacuity heat caused by deficiency of kidney yin; Tai Chong (LR-3) and Xing Jian (LR-2) for headache caused by ascendant liver yang. Besides this, in the case of diseases in which there is an obvious area of pathological change, basing selection of points

on the cause and mechanism of disease is the realization of the principle of 'treating the root'. For example, toothache can be divided into wind-fire toothache, stomach fire toothache and kidney vacuity toothache depending on the cause of disease; Feng Chi (GB-20) and Wai Guan (SJ-5) are chosen for wind-fire toothache, Nei Ting (ST-44) and Er Jian (LI-2) are chosen for stomach-fire toothache, and Tai Xi (KI-3) and Xing Jian (LR-2) are chosen for kidney vacuity toothache.

4. Selection of Points According to Signs and Symptoms: This principle, also known as 'selection of points based on experience', is based on specific therapeutic characteristics of certain acupoints. For example, Ding Chuan (M-BW-1) is selected for treatment of asthma, Si Feng (M-UE-9) is for child gan accumulation (spleen vacuity with food accumulation) and Yao Tong (N-UE-19) is for lower back pain. This is the treatment characteristic of the majority of extra points.

12.2 METHODS FOR POINT COMBINATION

This is a method for choosing combinations of points with similar indications, or that have a synergistic function in treating disease. It is guided by the point selection principles, and is done in accordance with the area, cause and mechanism of the disease being treated. A variety of different methods are used in clinical practice, and they can be divided into two general categories: point combination according to location and point combination according to channel.

1. Point Combination According to Location: This point combination method selects acupoints from different regions of distribution to deliver combined effects. It includes local and distal point combination, upper and lower point combination, front and back point combination, and left and right point combination.

   ◦ Local and Distal Point Combination: In this method, point combination is based on the area of pathological change. Points local and distal to the disease are combined into one treatment. This method is the most commonly used in clinical practice. For example, when treating toothache, the local point Xia Che (ST-6) will be combined with the distal points He Gu (LI-4) and Nei Ting (ST-44); for lower back pain local Jia Ji Xue (M-BW-35) are combined with the distal points Cheng Shan (BL-57) and Kun Lun (BL-60).

   ◦ Upper and Lower Point Combination: This is also a common method in clinical practice, and involves classifying all acupoints as either above or below the waist or on the upper or lower limbs, then combining points from each group. For example, in the treatment of epigastric pain the upper point of Nei Guan (PC-6) is combined with the lower point Zu San Li (ST-36); when treating head and neck ache and stiffness the upper point Da Zhui (DU-14) is combined with the lower point Kun Lun (BL-60); in uterine prolapse Bai Hui (DU-20) is combined with San Yin Jiao (SP-6). Combining the confluence points of the eight vessels is also associated with this method.

   ◦ Front and Back Point Combination: In this method acupoints that are on the front of the body and those on the back are combined. The points chosen are primarily those on the chest, abdomen and the upper and lower back. This method is often used in treating organ diseases, for example: in treating bladder disease, the front points Shui Dao (ST-28) or Zhong Ji (RN-3) are combined with the back points Pang Guang Shu (BL-28) or Zhi Bian (BL-54); in treating lung disease the front point Zhong Fu (LU-1) is combined with the back point Fei Shu (BL-13); in treating epigastric pain the front point Zhong Wan (RN-12) and the back point Wei Shu (BL-21) are chosen. The common clinical use of transport and alarm point combinations is associated with this method.

◦ Left and Right Point Combination: In this method points on the right and left sides of the body are combined in treatment. This method is summarized based on the symmetrical distribution of the 12 channels and the left-right intersection of certain channels. For example, in treating stomach pain, bilateral Zu San Li (ST-36) and Liang Qiu (ST-34) are chosen. However, combining left and right points does not only mean choosing symmetrical points, for example in treating left-side hemi lateral headache, Tai Yang (M-HN-9) and Tou Wei (ST-8) on the affected side are combined with Wai Guan (SJ-5) and Zu Lin Qi (GB-41) on the opposite side; in paralysis of the left side of the face, Tai Yang (M-HN-9), Xia Che (ST-6) and Di Cang (ST-4) on the affected side are combined with He Gu (LI-4) on the opposite side. Besides this, the point selection principles of 'when the disease is on the left, choose the right' and 'when the disease is on the right, choose the left' are also associated with this method.

2. Point Combination According to Channel: In this method, the combinations of points is based on the relationship between channel. The different methods include same channel point combination, interior-exterior channel point combination, same-name channel point combination, and mother-child point combination.

◦ Same Channel Point Combination: In the case of pathology of a particular organ or channel, points on that organ's channel or on the affected channel itself are chosen to form a treatment. For example: for toothache caused by stomach fire traveling up the channel and harassing the upper body, points on the Foot-Yangming Stomach channel such as Xia Che (ST-6) (local) and Nei Ting (ST-44) (distal; brook point) are chosen; in the case of posterior headache, the local points Nao Hu (DU-17) and Tian Zhu (BL-10) are combined with the distal channel point Kun Lun (BL-60).

◦ Interior-Exterior Channel Point Combination: In this case, the yin-yang and interior-exterior relationship between organs and channels are used as the basis for point combinations. When pathology occurs in a certain organ or channel, points from that channel can be combined with points from its interior-exterior-related channel. For example, in the case of common cold and cough due to wind-heat assailing the lung, Chi Ze (LU-5) on the lung channel and Qu Chi (LI-11) and He Gu (LI-4) from the large intestine channel are chosen.

◦ Same-Name Channel Point Combination: Based on the theory of combining 'same qi-mutual flow' points on the hand and foot channels with the same name. For example, in the case of Yangming headache He Gu (LI-4) (Hand-Yangming) and Nei Ting (ST-44) (Foot-Yangming) are combined; in the case of Shaoyang type scapulo-humeral periarthritis Jian Liao (SJ-14) (Hand-Shaoyang) and Yang Ling Quan (GB-34) (Foot-Shaoyang) are combined.

○   Mother-Child Channel Point Combination: Based on the theory of 'in vacuity, supplement the mother' and 'in repletion, drain the child', the five phase association of organs and channels are used to make point combinations. For example, in the case of lung vacuity cough, besides points on the lung channel like Fei Shu (BL-13), points on the spleen and stomach channels like Tai Bai (SP-3) and Zu San Li (ST-36) are chosen.

CHAPTER 2

Location and Indications of Commonly Used Points in Moxibustion

1. Points of the 14 Channels

1.1 POINTS OF THE LUNG CHANNEL OF HAND-TAIYIN, LU

Name of point	Location	Indications
Zhong Fu (LU-1)	On the anterior thoracic region, 6 *cun* lateral to the anterior midline, 1 *cun* inferior to Yun Men (LU-2), level with the first intercostal space.	• Lung disease • Pain in the shoulder and back
Chi Ze (LU-5)	At the anconal crease, in the radial depression of the biceps tendon.	• Lung disease • Pain and constriction in the elbow and arm • Acute vomiting and diarrhoea, heatstroke, febrile convulsions
Kong Zui (LU-6)	On the radial side of palmar forearm, on the line connecting Chi Ze (LU-5) and Tai Yuan (LU-9), 7 *cun* superior to the carpal crease.	• Lung conditions such as haemoptysis, cough, asthma, sore throat • Pain in the elbow and arm
Lie Que (LU-7)	On the radial side of forearm superior to the styloid process of radius, 1.5 *cun* superior to the carpal crease between the brachioradialis and the tendon of abductor pollicis longus.	• Lung disease • Head and neck conditions
Tai Yuan (LU-9)	On the radial side of palmar wrist crease, over the radial artery.	• Cough, asthma • Pulseless disease • Pain in the wrist and arm
Yu Ji (LU-10)	In the depression proximal to the first metacarpophalangeal joint of the thumb, on the midpoint of the first metacarpal bone, at the border between the red and white flesh.	• Cough, haemoptysis • Dry and sore throat, aphonia • Malnutrition and indigestion syndrome in children
Shao Shang (LU-11)	On the radial side of phalangette of the thumb, approximately 0.1 *cun* from the corner of the fingernail.	• Sore throat, epistaxis • Fever, coma, mania

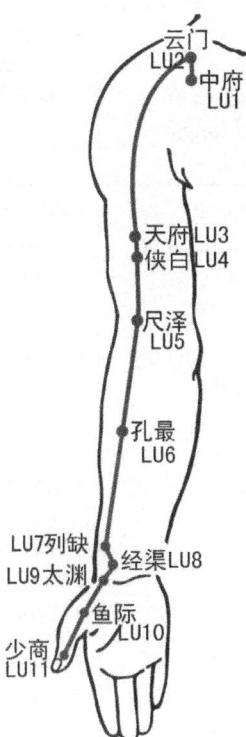

Figure 2.1.1 General Chart of Points of the Lung Channel of Hand-Taiyin

1.2 POINTS OF THE LARGE INTESTINE CHANNEL OF HAND-YANGMING, LI

Name of point	Location	Indications
Shang Yang (LI-1)	On the radial side of the phalanx of the index finger, approximately 0.1 *cun* from the corner of the fingernail.	• Toothache, sore throat • Heat syndrome, emergency
Er Jian (LI-2)	With a loose fist, in the depression distal to the radial side of the second metacarpophalangeal joint of the index finger.	• Epistaxis, toothache • Fever
San Jian (LI-3)	With a loose fist, in the depression proximal to the radial side of the second metacarpophalangeal joint of the index finger.	• Toothache, sore throat • Abdominal distension, abdominal pain, borborygmus, diarrhoea
He Gu (LI-4)	On the dorsum of the hand, between the first and the second metacarpal bones, on the radial side of the midpoint of the second metacarpal bone.	• Conditions of the head, face and the five sense organs • Exterior syndrome • Amenorrhoea, prolonged labour

Yang Xi (LI-5)	At the radial side of the dorsal wrist crease, in the depression appearing between the tendons of extensor pollicis brevis and longus when the thumb is extended.	• Pain in the wrist • Headache, bloodshot eyes, deafness, toothache
Shou San Li (LI-10)	On the radial side of the dorsal forearm, on the line connecting Yang Xi (LI-5) with Qu Chi (LI-11), 2 *cun* inferior to the cubital crease.	• Myasthenia and paralysis of the arms • Abdominal pain and distension • Toothache, swollen cheeks
Qu Chi (LI-11)	With the elbow flexed, at the lateral end of the cubital crease, at the midpoint of the line connecting Chi Ze (LU-5) and the lateral epicondyle of the humerus.	• Pain in the arm, paralysis of the arms • Fever • Hypertension • Mania • Abdominal pain, vomiting and diarrhoea • Sore throat, toothache, bloodshot and painful eyes • Urticaria, eczema, scrofula
Bi Nao (LI-14)	On the lateral aspect of the arm, at the distal end of the deltoid, on the line connecting Qu Chi (LI-11) with Jian Yu (LI-15), 7 *cun* superior to Qu Chi (LI-11).	• Pain in the shoulder and the arm, paralysis of the arms • Restriction of the neck • Scrofula • Eye disease
Jian Yu (LI-15)	On the shoulder, at the superior border of the deltoid, in the lower anteroinferior depression of the acromion when the arm is abducted or stretched forward.	• Pain and constriction in the shoulder and the arm, paralysis of the arms • Urticaria
Ying Xiang (LI-20)	Level with the midpoint of the lateral border of the alanasi, in the nasolabial sulcus.	• Nasal congestion, epistaxis, a deviated mouth, facial itchiness • Biliary ascariasis

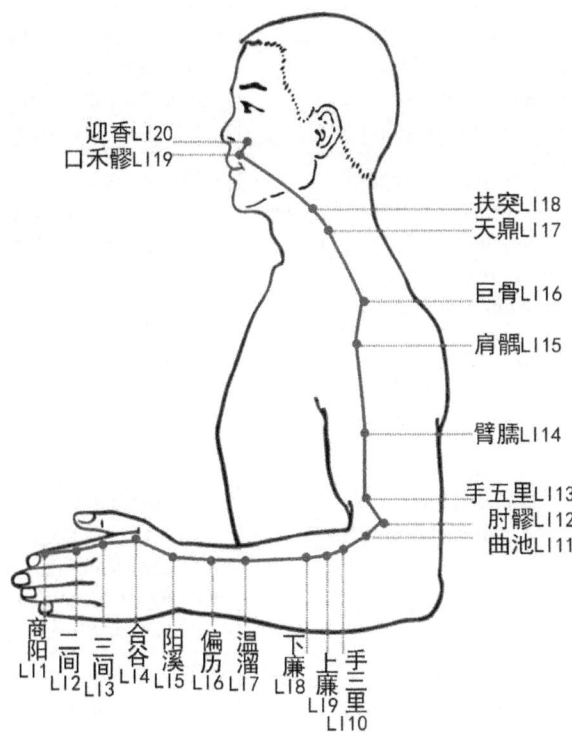

Figure 2.1.2 General Chart of Points of the Large Intestine Channel of Hand-Yangming

1.3 POINTS OF THE STOMACH CHANNEL OF FOOT-YANGMING, ST

Name of point	Location	Indications
Cheng Qi (ST-1)	On the face, directly inferior to the pupil, between the eyeball and the infraorbital margin.	• Twitching of the eyelid, acrimation upon exposure to wind, bloodshot and painful eyes, night blindness • Deviated mouth and eye, facial spasm
Si Bai (ST-2)	On the face, directly inferior to the pupil, in the depression of the infraorbital foramen.	• Bloodshot, painful and itching eyes, nebula or macule of the cornea, twitching of the eyelids • Deviated mouth and eye, facial spasm • Headache, dizziness
Jia Che (ST-6)	On the cheek, one finger's breadth (middle finger) anterosuperior to the angle of mandible, in the depression where the masseter muscle is prominent.	• Deviated mouth, toothache, swollen cheek, trismus

Ru Zhong (ST-17)	In the anterior thoracic region, in the fourth intercostal space, at the centre of the nipple, 4 *cun* lateral to the anterior midline.	• Acupuncture and moxibustion are contraindicated on this point; it is used only as a mark for locating points on the chest and abdomen
Ru Gen (ST-18)	In the anterior thoracic region, directly inferior to the nipple and at the root segment of the nipple, in the fifth intercostal space, 4 *cun* lateral to the anterior midline.	• Mammary abscess, insufficiency of lactation • Cough, asthma, hiccups • Thoracalgia
Liang Men (ST-21)	On the upper abdomen, 4 *cun* superior to the centre of the umbilicus, 2 *cun* lateral to the anterior midline.	• Acute stomach ache • Swollen and painful knees, paralysis of the legs • Mammary abscess
Tian Shu (ST-25)	On the middle abdomen, 2 *cun* lateral to the centre of umbilicus.	• Abdominal distension, borborygmus, pain around the umbilicus, constipation, diarrhoea, dysentery • Irregular menstruation, dysmenorrhoea
Gui Lai (ST-29)	On the lower abdomen, 4 *cun* inferior to the centre of the umbilicus, 2 *cun* lateral to the anterior midline.	• Abdominal pain, hernia • Irregular menstruation, leucorrhoea, prolapse of the uterus
Fu Tu (ST-32)	On the anterior aspect of the thigh, on the line connecting the lateral end of the base of the patella with the anterior superior iliac spine, 6 *cun* superior to the base of the patella.	• Lumbago and cold knees, paralysis of the legs • Hernia • Dermatophytosis
Liang Qiu (ST-34)	With the knee bent, on the anterior aspect of the thigh, on the line connecting the lateral end of the base of the patella with the anterior superior iliac spine, 2 *cun* superior to the base of the patella.	• Acute stomach ache • Swelling and pain in knees, paralysis of the legs • Mammary abscess
Du Bi (ST-35)	With the knee bent, on the anterior aspect of the knee, in the depression lateral to the patellar ligament.	• Knee pain, paralysis of the legs, disadvantage in flexion and extension, dermatophytosis
Zu San Li (ST-36)	On the anterior aspect of crus, 3 *cun* inferior to Du Bi (ST-35), one finger's breadth (middle finger) lateral to the anterior border of tibia.	• Stomach ache, vomiting, dysphagia, abdominal distension, diarrhoea, dysentery, constipation • Mammary abscess, periappendicular abscess • Paralysis and pain in the legs, oedema • Mania, dermatophytosis • Consumptive disease with marked emaciation, it is an important point for general health care

Shang Ju Xu (ST-37)	On the anterior aspect of crus, 6 *cun* inferior to Du Bi (ST-35), one finger's breadth (middle finger) lateral to the anterior border of tibia.	• Borborygmus, abdominal pain, diarrhoea, constipation, periappendicular abscess • Atrophy and paralysis of the legs and knees, dermatophytosis
Xia Ju Xu (ST-39)	On the anterior aspect of crus, 9 *cun* inferior to Du Bi (ST-35), one finger's breadth (middle finger) lateral to the anterior border of tibia.	• Lower abdominal pain, diarrhoea, dysentery • Atrophy and paralysis of the legs and knees • Mammary abscess
Feng Long (ST-40)	On the anterolateral aspect of the crus, 8 *cun* superior to the prominence of the lateral malleolus, lateral to Tiao Kou (ST-38), two fingers' breadths (middle finger) lateral to the anterior border of the tibia.	• Headache, dizziness • Mania • Cough with copious phlegm • Atrophy and paralysis of the legs and knees • Abdominal distension, constipation
Jie Xi (ST-41)	In the depression at the midpoint of the transverse crease of the malleolus joint, between the tendons of extensor hallucis longus and extensor digitorum longus.	• Atrophy and paralysis of the legs and knees, ankle disease, foot drop • Headache, dizziness • Mania • Abdominal distension, constipation
Chong Yang (ST-42)	At the highest point of the dorsum of the foot, between the tendons of extensor hallucis longus and extensor digitorum longus, over the dorsalis pedis artery.	• Stomach ache • Deviated mouth and eye • Mania and epilepsy • Atrophy and myasthenia of the legs
Xian Gu (ST-43)	On the dorsum of the foot, in the depression proximal to the metatarsophalangeal joint between the second and third metatarsal bones.	• Oedema of the face • Swelling and pain of the dorsum of the foot • Borborygmus, abdominal pain
Nei Ting (ST-44)	On the dorsum of the foot, between the second and third toes, posterior to the web margin, at the border between the red and white flesh.	• Toothache, sore throat, a deviated mouth, epistaxis • Fever • Stomach disease with sour regurgitation, abdominal distension, diarrhoea, dysentery, constipation • Swelling and pain of the dorsum of the foot
Li Dui (ST-45)	On the second toe, lateral to the distal phalanx, 0.1 *cun* proximal-lateral to the corner of the second toenail.	• Epistaxis, toothache, sore throat • Fever • Dreaminess, mania

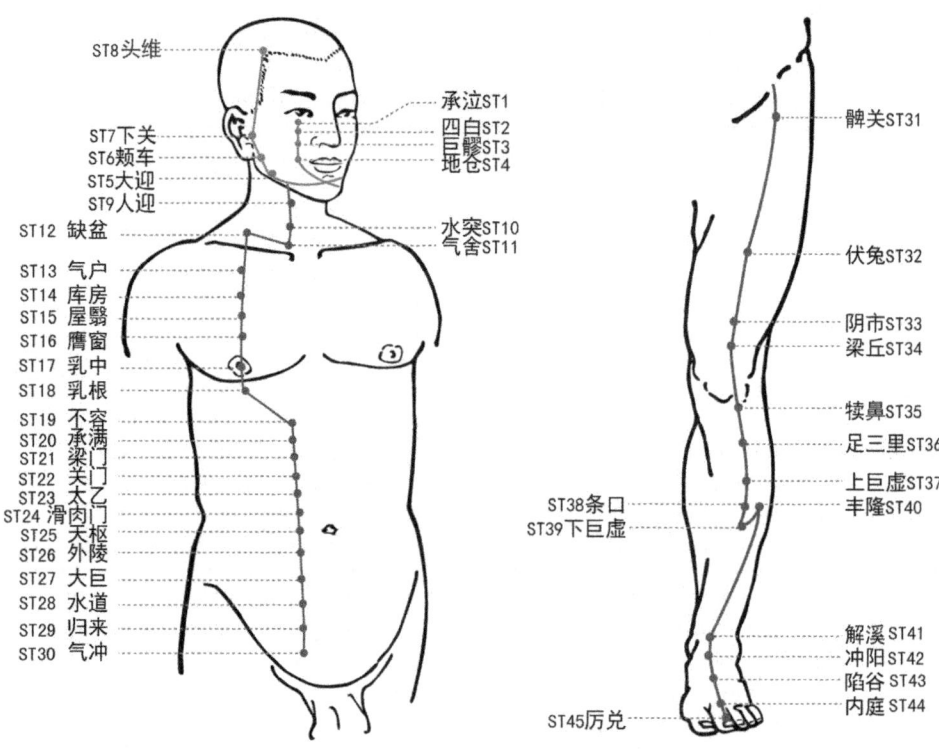

Figure 2.1.3 General Chart of Points of the Stomach Channel of Foot-Yangming

1.4 Points of the Spleen Channel of Foot-Taiyin, SP

Name of point	Location	Indications
Yin Bai (SP-1)	On the big toe, medial to the distal phalanx, 0.1 *cun* proximal-medial to the corner of the toenail.	• Menorrhagia and metrostaxis • Hematochezia, haematuria • Mania, dreaminess • Infantile convulsions • Abdominal distension
Da Du (SP-2)	On the medial aspect of the foot, in the depression distal to the first metatarsophalangeal joint, at the border between the red and white flesh.	• Abdominal distension, stomach ache, vomiting, diarrhoea, constipation • Fever
Tai Bai (SP-3)	On the medial aspect of the foot, in the depression proximal to the first metatarsophalangeal joint, at the border between the red and white flesh.	• Borborygmus, abdominal distension, diarrhoea, stomach ache, constipation • Heaviness of the body and painful extremities • Haemorrhoids and anal fistula

Gong Sun (SP-4)	On the medial aspect of the foot, anteroinferior to the base of the first metatarsal bone, at the border between the red and white flesh.	• Stomach ache, vomiting, abdominal pain, diarrhoea, dysentery • Upset insomnia, mania • Reflux of gas to the heart
San Yin Jiao (SP-6)	On the tibial aspect of the crus, 3 *cun* superior to the prominence of the medial malleolus, posterior to the medial border of the tibia.	• Borborygmus, abdominal distension, diarrhoea • Irregular menstruation, abnormal vaginal discharge, prolapse of the uterus, sterility, prolonged labour • Spermatorrhoea, impotence, urorrhoea hernia • Insomnia • Atrophy and paralysis of the legs, dermatophytosis
Yin Ling Quan (SP-9)	On the tibial aspect of the crus, in the posteroinferior depression of the medial condyle of the tibia.	• Abdominal distension, diarrhoea, oedema, jaundice, dysuria or uroclepsia • Knee pain
Xue Hai (SP-10)	With the knee bent, on the medial aspect of the thigh, 2 *cun* superior to the medial end of the base of the patella, on the bulge of the medial end of quadriceps femoris.	• Irregular menstruation, metrorrhagia and metrostaxis, amenorrhoea • Urticaria, eczema, erysipelas
Da Bao (SP-21)	In the lateral thoracic region, on the midaxillary line, in the sixth intercostal space.	• Asthma • Pain in the chest and hypochondrium • Body pain • Myasthenia of the limbs

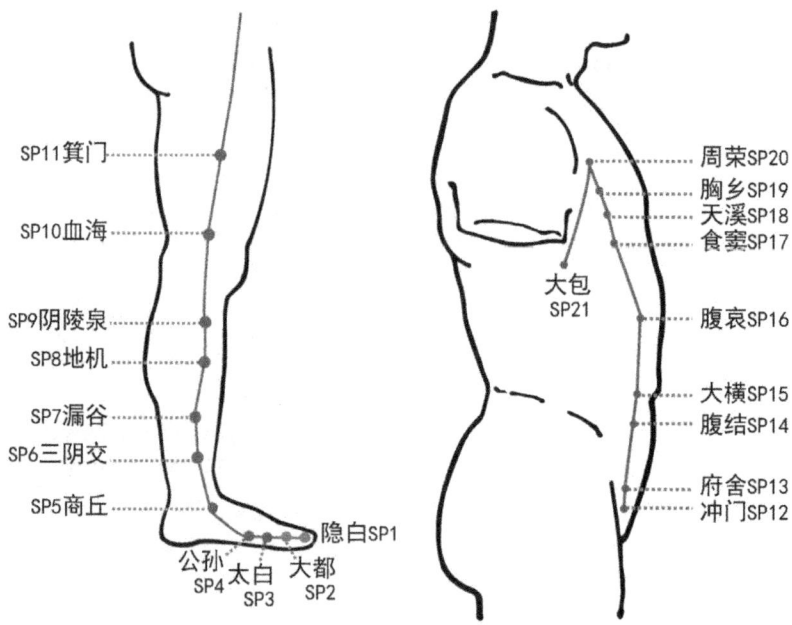

Figure 2.1.4 General Chart of Points of the Spleen Channel of Foot-Taiyin

1.5 Points of the Heart Channel of Hand-Shaoyin, HT

Name of point	Location	Indications
Shao Hai (HT-3)	With the elbow bent, at the midpoint of the medial end of the cubital crease and the medial epicondyle of the humerus.	• Cardiodynia, hysteria, mental conditions • Pain and constriction of the elbow and arm • Pain in the head and neck, pain in the armpit and hypochondrium • Scrofula
Tong Li (HT-5)	On the palmar aspect of the forearm, just radial to the flexor carpi ulnaris tendon, 1 *cun* proximal to the palmar wrist crease.	• Palpitations, haematemesis • Sudden loss of voice, aphasia with a stiff tongue • Pain in the wrist and arm
Yin Xi (HT-6)	On the palmar aspect of the forearm, just radial to the flexor carpi ulnaris tendon, 0.5 *cun* proximal to the palmar wrist crease.	• Cardiodynia, palpitations with fear • Bone-steaming night sweating • Haematemesis, hemorrhinia

Shen Men (HT-7)	At the ulnar end of palmar wrist crease, at the radial depression of the flexor carpi ulnaris tendon.	• Heart disease, irritability, palpitations with fear, severe palpitations, forgetfulness, insomnia, epilepsy • Hypertension • Pain in the chest and hypochondrium
Shao Chong (HT-9)	On the little finger, radial to the distal phalanx, 0.1 *cun* proximal-lateral to the radial corner of the little fingernail.	• Palpitations, cardiodynia, mania, coma • Fever • Pain in the chest and hypochondrium

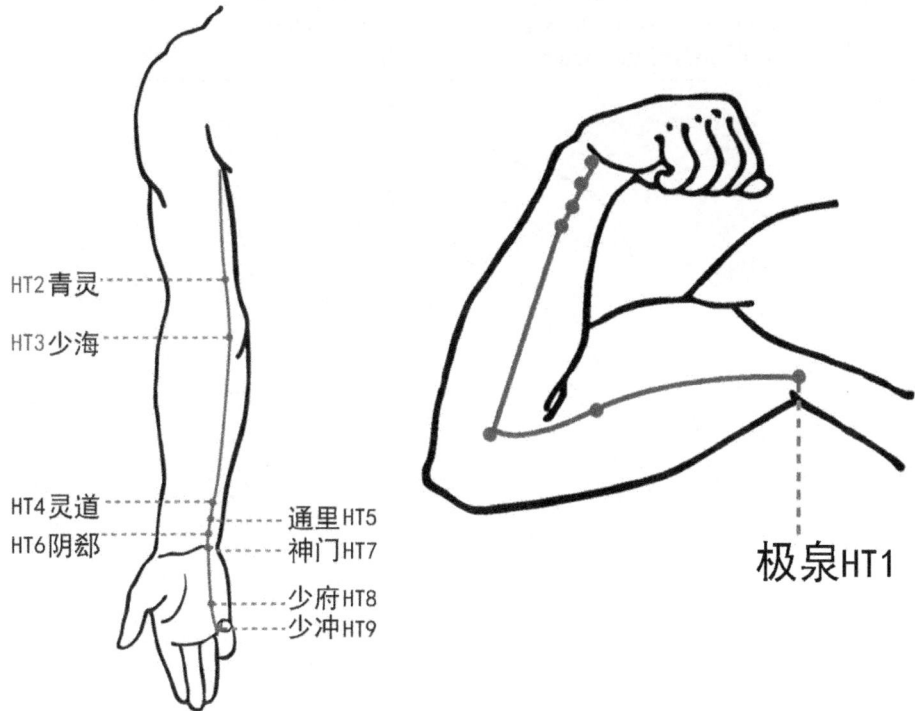

Figure 2.1.5 General Chart of Points of the Heart Channel of Hand-Shaoyin

1.6 Points of the Small Intestine Channel of Hand-Taiyang, SI

Name of point	Location	Indication
Shao Ze (SI-1)	On the little finger, on the ulnar of the distal phalanx, 0.1 *cun* proximal-medial to the ulnar corner of the little fingernail.	• Acute mastitis, hypogalactia • Coma, fever • Headache, nebula or macule of the cornea, sore throat

Hou Xi (SI-3)	On the ulnar side of the palm; when making a loose fist, at the border between the red and white flesh at the end of metacarpophalangeal transverse crease proximal to the fifth metacarpophalangeal joint.	• Stiff and painful head and neck; lumbar and back pain, pain and restriction of the fingers, elbow and arm • Bloodshot eyes, deafness, sore throat • Mania • Malaria
Yang Lao (SI-6)	On the ulnar dorsal forearm, in the radial depression proximal to the head of the ulnar bone.	• Blurred eyes • Soreness of the shoulder, back, elbow and arm
Ting Gong (SI-19)	On the face, anterior to the tragus, posterior to the condylar process of the mandible, in the depression when opening the mouth.	• Tinnitus, deafness, purulent ear conditions • Toothache

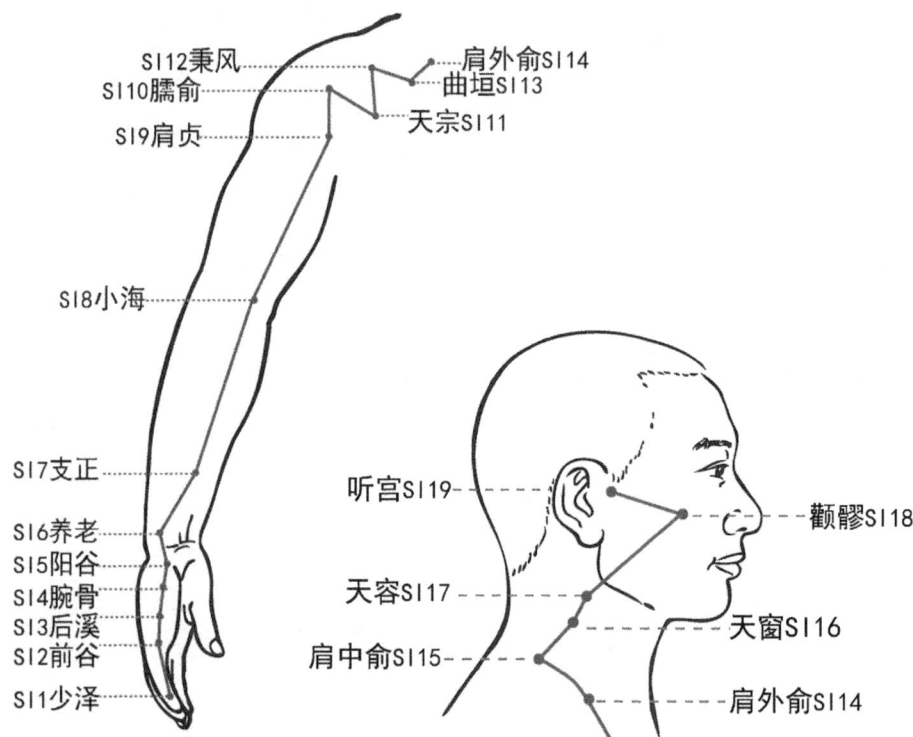

Figure 2.1.6 General Chart of Points of the Small Intestine Channel of Hand-Taiyang

1.7 POINTS OF THE BLADDER CHANNEL OF FOOT-TAIYANG, BL

Name of point	Location	Indications
Jing Ming (BL-1)	On the face, in the depression just superior to the inner canthus of the eye.	• Bloodshot and swollen eyes, dizziness, shortsightedness • Acute lumbar sprain • Tachycardia
Tian Zhu (BL-10)	On the neck, in the depression of the posterior hairline lateral to the trapezius, 1.3 *cun* lateral to the centre of the posterior hairline.	• Pain in the posterior head, stiff neck, pain in the shoulder and back, lumbago • Nasal congestion • Mania, epilepsy, fever
Da Zhu (BL-11)	On the back, level with the inferior border of the spinous process of the first thoracic vertebra (T1), 1.5 *cun* lateral to the posterior midline.	• Cough • Stiff neck, pain in the shoulder and back
Feng Men (BL-12)	On the back, level with the inferior border of the spinous process of the second thoracic vertebra (T2), 1.5 *cun* lateral to the posterior midline.	• Cold, cough, fever, headache • Stiff neck, pain in the chest and back
Fei Shu (BL-13)	On the back, level with the inferior border of the spinous process of the third thoracic vertebra (T3), 1.5 *cun* lateral to the posterior midline.	• Lung conditions such as cough, asthma, emptysis • Bone-steaming tidal fever, night sweating
Xin Shu (BL-15)	On the back, level with the inferior border of the spinous process of the fifth thoracic vertebra (T5), 1.5 *cun* lateral to the posterior midline.	• Cardiodynia, palpitations with fear, insomnia, forgetfulness, epilepsy • Cough, hematemesis.
Du Shu (BL-16)	On the back, level with the inferior border of the spinous process of the sixth thoracic vertebra (T6), 1.5 *cun* lateral to the posterior midline.	• Cardiodynia, oppression in the chest • Cold, fever and asthma
Ge Shu (BL-17)	On the back, level with the inferior border of the spinous process of the seventh thoracic vertebra (T7), 1.5 *cun* lateral to the posterior midline.	• Qi counterflow syndrome such as vomiting, hiccups, asthma, hematemesis • Anaemia • Urticaria, skin itch • Tidal fever, night sweating
Gan Shu (BL-18)	On the back, level with the inferior border of the spinous process of the ninth thoracic vertebra (T9), 1.5 *cun* lateral to the posterior midline.	• Jaundice, distending pain in the chest and ribs, eye disease • Mania, epilepsy • Back pain

Dan Shu (BL-19)	On the back, level with the inferior border of the spinous process of the tenth thoracic vertebra (T10), 1.5 *cun* lateral to the posterior midline.	• Hepatobiliary diseases such as jaundice, a bitter taste in the mouth, hypochondriac pain • Phthisis, tidal fever
Pi Shu (BL-20)	On the back, level with the inferior border of the spinous process of the eleventh thoracic vertebra (T11), 1.5 *cun* lateral to the posterior midline.	• Diseases of spleen and stomach and intestines such as abdominal distension, diarrhoea, vomiting, dysentery, hematochezia • Back pain
Wei Shu (BL-21)	On the back, level with the inferior border of the spinous process of the twelfth thoracic vertebra (T12), 1.5 *cun* lateral to the posterior midline.	• Diseases of spleen and stomach such as stomach ache, vomiting, abdominal distension, borborygmus • Back pain
San Jiao Shu (BL-22)	In the lumbar region, level with the inferior border of the spinous process of the first lumbar vertebra (L1), 1.5 *cun* lateral to the posterior midline.	• Diseases of spleen and stomach such as borborygmus, abdominal distension, diarrhoea, oedema • Stiff and painful waist and back
Shen Shu (BL-23)	In the lumbar region, level with the inferior border of the spinous process of the second lumbar vertebra (L2), 1.5 *cun* lateral to the posterior midline.	• Lumbago • Urogenital system conditions such as urorrhoea, spermatorrhoea, impotence, irregular menstruation, abnormal vaginal discharge • Tinnitus, deafness
Qi Hai Shu (BL-24)	In the lumbar region, level with the inferior border of the spinous process of the third lumbar vertebra (L3), 1.5 *cun* lateral to the posterior midline.	• Borborygmus abdominal distension • Dysmenorrhoea, lumbago
Da Chang Shu (BL-25)	In the lumbar region, level with the inferior border of the spinous process of the fourth lumbar vertebra (L4), 1.5 *cun* lateral to the posterior midline.	• Lumbar and back pain; abdominal distension, diarrhoea, constipation
Guan Yuan Shu (BL-26)	In the lumbar region, level with the inferior border of the spinous process of the fifth lumbar vertebra (L5), 1.5 *cun* lateral to the posterior midline.	• Abdominal distension, diarrhoea • Lumbosacral pain • Frequent urination or dysuria, urorrhoea
Xiao Chang Shu (BL-27)	In the sacral region, 1.5 *cun* lateral to the median sacral crest, level with the first posterior sacral foramen.	• Urogenital system conditions such as spermatorrhoea, urorrhoea, hematuria, urodynia, abnormal vaginal discharge • Diarrhoea, dysentery • Lumbosacral pain
Pang Guang Shu (BL-28)	In the sacral region, 1.5 *cun* lateral to the median sacral crest, level with the second posterior sacral foramen.	• Functional disorders of the bladder such as dysuria, urorrhoea • Lumbosacral pain • Diarrhoea, constipation

Shang Liao (BL-31)	In the sacral region, between the posterosuperior iliac spine and the posterior midline, in the first posterior sacral foramen.	• Constipation and dysuria • Gynaecological conditions such as irregular menstruation, abnormal vaginal discharge, prolapse of the uterus • Spermatorrhoea, impotence • Lumbosacral pain
Ci Liao (BL-32)	In the sacral region, inferior to the posterosuperior iliac spine, in the second posterior sacral foramen.	• Gynaecological conditions such as irregular menstruation, dysmenorrhoea, abnormal vaginal discharge • Dysuria • Spermatorrhoea • Hernia • Lumbosacral pain, atrophy and paralysis of the legs
Zhong Liao (BL-33)	In the sacral region, inferior to Ci Liao (BL-32), in the third posterior sacral foramen.	• Constipation, diarrhoea • Dysuria • Irregular menstruation, abnormal vaginal discharge • Lumbosacral pain
Xia Liao (BL-34)	In the sacral region, inferomedial to Zhong Liao (BL-33), in the fourth posterior sacral foramen.	• Abdominal pain, constipation • Dysuria • Abnormal vaginal discharge • Lumbosacral pain
Wei Yang (BL-39)	On the lateral end of the popliteal crease, just medial to the biceps femoris tendon.	• Abdominal distension, dysuria • Stiff and painful loin, pain and constriction in the legs and feet
Wei Zhong (BL-40)	At the midpoint of the popliteal crease, between the biceps femoris tendon and the semitendinosus tendon.	• Diseases of the waist and lower limbs such as lumbar and back pain, atrophy and paralysis of the legs • Abdominal pain, acute vomiting and diarrhoea • Dysuria, urorrhoea, erysipelas
Gao Huang (BL-43)	On the back, level with the inferior border of the spinous process of the fourth thoracic vertebra (T4), 3 *cun* lateral to the posterior midline.	• Deficiency syndrome of lung disease such as cough, asthma, phthisis • Scapular pain • Deficiency syndrome such as forgetfulness, night sweating, spermatorrhoea
Zhi Shi (BL-52)	In the lumbar region, level with the inferior border of the spinous process of the second lumbar vertebra (L2), 3 *cun* lateral to the posterior midline.	• Kidney deficiency diseases and syndrome such as spermatorrhoea, impotence • Dysuria • Stiff and painful loins

Bao Huang (BL-53)	In the buttock region, level with the second posterior sacral foramen, 3 *cun* lateral to the median sacral crest.	• Borborygmus, abdominal distension, constipation • Anuria and dysuria • Stiff and painful loins
Cheng Shan (BL-57)	In the centre of posterior aspect of the crus, between Wei Zhong (BL-40) and Kun Lun (BL-60), in the triangle depression below the bellies of the gastrocnemius when the foot is flexed.	• Contraction and pain in the waist and leg • Haemorrhoids, constipation
Kun Lun (BL-60)	On the posterolateral aspect of the malleolus, in the depression between the prominence of the lateral malleolus and the calcaneal tendon.	• Pain in the posterior head, stiff neck, lumbosacral pain, swelling and pain of the ankle • Epilepsy • Prolonged labour
Shen Mai (BL-62)	On the lateral aspect of the foot, directly in the depression inferior to the lateral malleolus.	• Headache, dizziness • Mental diseases such as mania, epilepsy, insomnia • Sore lumbar and leg
Zhi Yin (BL-67)	On the little toe, lateral to the distal phalanx, 0.1 *cun* proximal to the lateral corner of the toenail.	• Malposition, prolonged labour • Headache, eye pain, nasal congestion, hemorrhinia

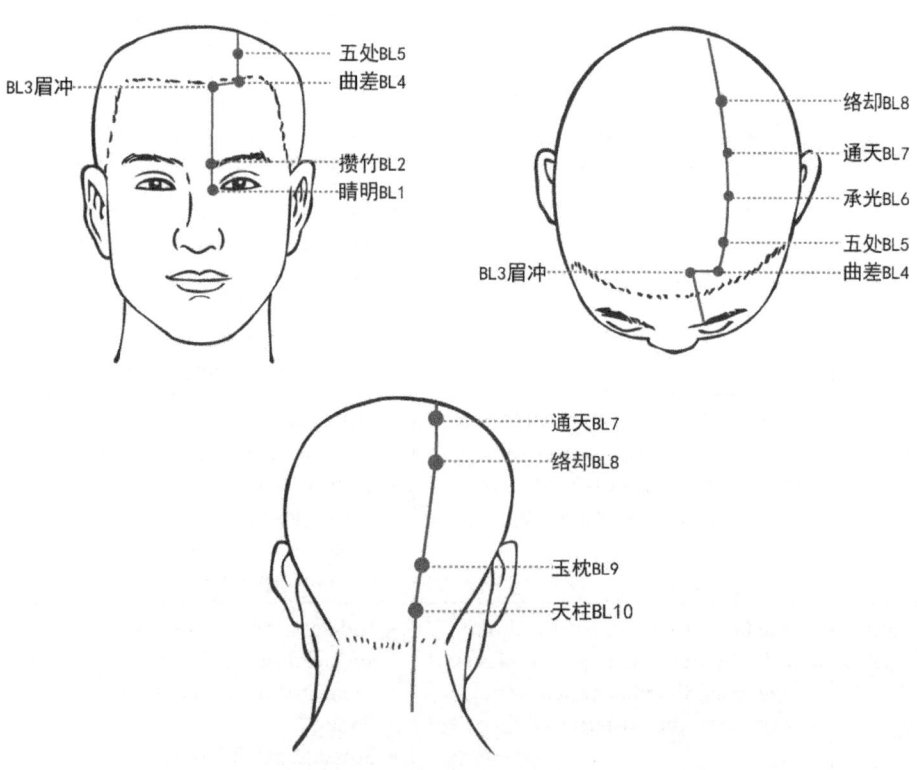

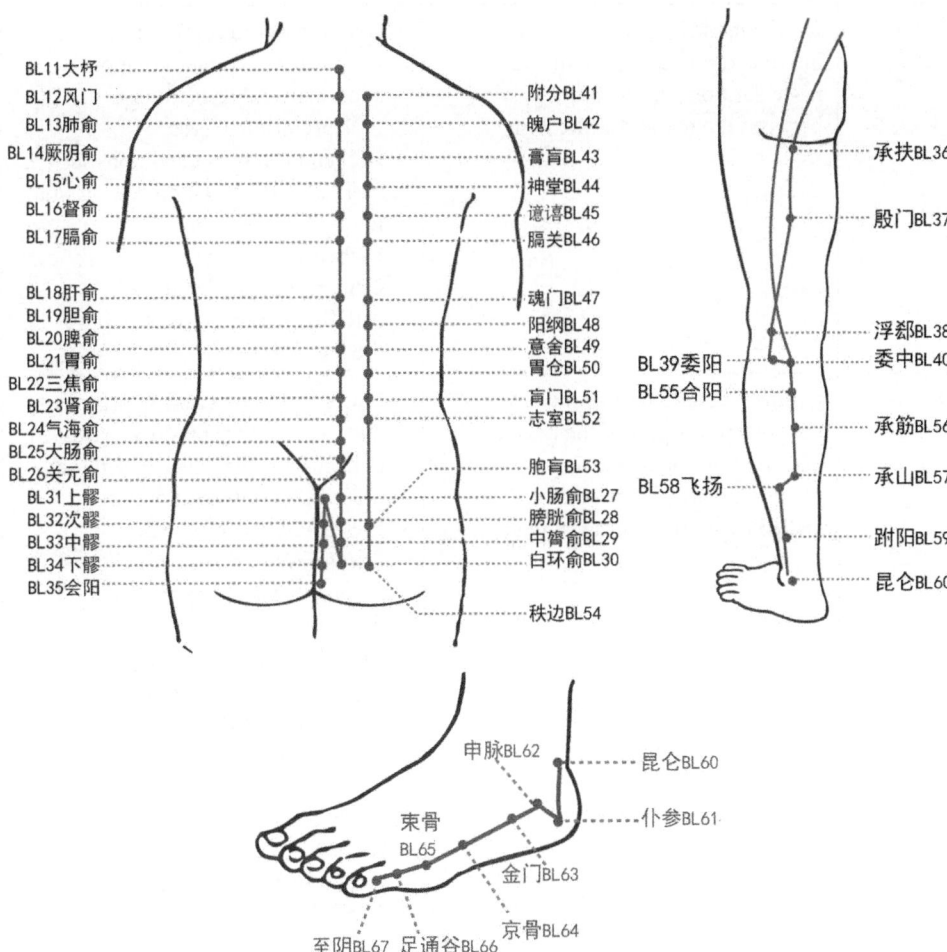

BL11大杼
BL12风门
BL13肺俞
BL14厥阴俞
BL15心俞
BL16督俞
BL17膈俞
BL18肝俞
BL19胆俞
BL20脾俞
BL21胃俞
BL22三焦俞
BL23肾俞
BL24气海俞
BL25大肠俞
BL26关元俞
BL31上髎
BL32次髎
BL33中髎
BL34下髎
BL35会阳

附分BL41
魄户BL42
膏肓BL43
神堂BL44
譩譆BL45
膈关BL46
魂门BL47
阳纲BL48
意舍BL49
胃仓BL50
肓门BL51
志室BL52
胞肓BL53
小肠俞BL27
膀胱俞BL28
中膂俞BL29
白环俞BL30
秩边BL54

BL39委阳
BL55合阳
BL58飞扬

承扶BL36
殷门BL37
浮郄BL38
委中BL40
承筋BL56
承山BL57
跗阳BL59
昆仑BL60

申脉BL62
束骨BL65
至阴BL67 足通谷BL66

昆仑BL60
仆参BL61
金门BL63
京骨BL64

Figure 2.1.7 General Chart of Points of the Bladder Channel of Foot-Taiyang

1.8 POINTS OF THE KIDNEY CHANNEL OF FOOT-SHAOYIN, KI

Name of point	Location	Indications
Yong Quan (KI-1)	On the sole of the foot, when the toes are flexed, it is located approximately in the depression at the junction of the anterior one third and the posterior two thirds of the line connecting the heel with the web margin between the bases of the second and third toes.	• Acute diseases and mental disorders such as faint, heatstroke, epilepsy, infantile convulsions • Headache, dizziness • Emptysis, sore throat • Dysuria, constipation • Heat in the soles • Running piglet

Ran Gu (KI-2)	On the medial aspect of the foot, inferior to the tuberosity of the navicular bone, at the border between the red and white flesh.	• Gynaecological conditions such as irregular menstruation, abnormal vaginal discharge, prolapse of the uterus • Urogenital system conditions such as spermatorrhoea, impotence, dysuria • Emptysis, sore throat • Diabetes • Umbilical tetanus, trismus • Atrophy and paralysis of the legs, back pain
Tai Xi (KI-3)	On the medial aspect of the foot, at the posterior aspect of the medial malleolus, in the depression between the prominence of the medial malleolus and the calcaneal tendon.	• Diseases of the five sense organs due to deficiency of kidney such as headache, dizziness, sore throat, toothache, deafness, tinnitus • Urogenital system diseases such as irregular menstruation, spermatorrhoea, impotence, frequent urination • Pain along spinal column, cold legs and swelling and pain in the medial malleolus • Lung conditions such as asthma, thoracalgia, emptysis • Diabetes • Kidney essence deficiency syndrome such as insomnia, forgetfulness
Da Zhong (KI-4)	On the medial aspect of the foot, posteroinferior to the medial malleolus, in the depression anterior to the medial attachment of the calcaneal tendon.	• Anuria, dysuria and urorrhoea • Irregular menstruation • Stiff and painful loin, heel pain • Asthma, emptysis
Shui Quan (KI-5)	On the medial aspect of the foot, posteroinferior to the medial malleolus, 1 cun inferior to Tai Xi (KI-3), in the depression medial to the calcaneal tuberosity.	• Irregular menstruation, dysmenorrhoea • Dysuria
Zhao Hai (KI-6)	On the medial aspect of the foot, in the depression inferior to the medial malleolus.	• Mental diseases such as epilepsy and insomnia • Heat type conditions of the five sense organs such as dry and sore throat, bloodshot and painful eyes • Dysuria, frequent urination • Gynaecological conditions such as irregular menstruation, dysmenorrhoea, red and white abnormal vaginal discharge • Atrophy and paralysis of the legs

Fu Liu (KI-7)	On the posteromedial aspect of the crus, 2 *cun* superior to Tai Xi (KI-3), anterior to the calcaneal tendon.	• Oedema, abdominal distension • Night sweating, fever and adiapneustia • Borborygmus, diarrhoea • Flaccid paralysis of legs, stiff and painful loins
Jiao Xin (KI-8)	On the medial aspect of the crus, 2 *cun* superior to Tai Xi (KI-3), 0.5 *cun* anterior to Fu Liu (KI-7), posterior to the medial border of the tibial bone.	• Gynaecological conditions such as irregular menstruation, dysmenorrhoea, metrorrhagia and metrostaxis • Abdominal pain, diarrhoea • Dysuria, oedema • Swelling and pain of testicles, hernia • Pain in the medial knee, thigh and popliteal fossa
Shu Fu (KI-27)	In the anterior thoracic region, just inferior to the clavicle, 2 *cun* lateral to the anterior midline.	• Cough, asthma, thoracalgia • Lack of appetite

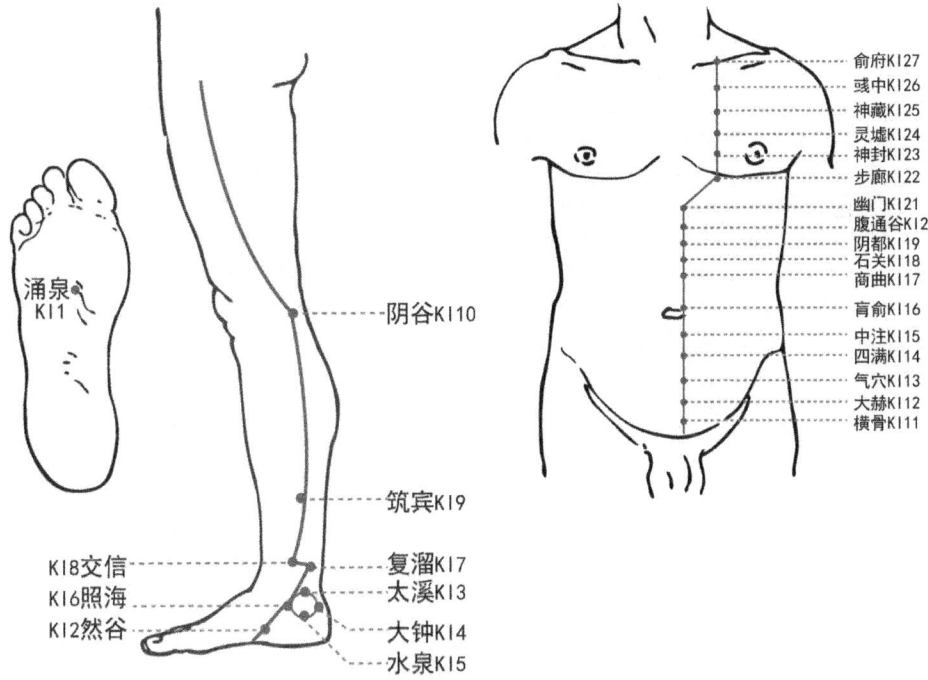

Figure 2.1.8 General Chart of Points of the Kidney Channel of Foot-Shaoyin

1.9 POINTS OF THE PERICARDIUM CHANNEL OF HAND-JUEYIN, PC

Name of point	Location	Indications
Tian Chi (PC-1)	In the anterior thoracic region, in the fourth intercostal space, 1 *cun* lateral to the nipple, 5 *cun* lateral to the anterior midline.	• Breast conditions such as acute mastitis, hypogalactia • Cough, asthma, pain in the chest and hypochondrium
Qu Ze (PC-3)	At the cubital crease, on the ulnar border of the biceps brachii tendon.	• Heart disease such as cardiodynia, palpitations • Acute gastroenteropathy such as stomach ache, vomiting, diarrhoea • Pain and restriction of the elbow and arm; fever
Jian Shi (PC-5)	On the palmar forearm, on the line connecting Qu Ze (PC-3) with Da Ling (PC-7), 3 *cun* proximal to the palmar wrist crease, between the tendons of the palmaris longus and the flexor carpi radialis.	• Cardiodynia, palpitations, mania, epilepsy • Stomach ache, vomiting • Fever, malaria • Arm pain
Nei Guan (PC-6)	On the palmar forearm, on the line connecting Qu Ze (PC-3) with Da Ling (PC-7), 2 *cun* proximal to the palmar wrist crease, between the tendons of the palmaris longus and the flexor carpi radialis.	• Heart and chest conditions such as cardiodynia, palpitations, oppression in the chest, thoracalgia • Lung diseases such as stomach ache, vomiting, hiccups • Mental diseases such as insomnia, mania • Local diseases such as arm pain, hemiplegia, numbness of the fingers
Da Ling (PC-7)	At the midpoint of the palmar wrist crease, between the tendons of palmaris longus and the flexor carpi radialis.	• Heart and chest conditions such as cardiodynia, palpitations, pain in the chest and hypochondrium • Mania • Stomach ache, vomiting • Pain in the wrist and arm
Lao Gong (PC-8)	At the centre of the palm, between the second and third metacarpal bones and near the third metacarpal bone, where the tip of the middle finger touches the palm when flexing the fingers and making a fist.	• Cardiodynia, palpitations • Mania, epilepsy • Aphtha, halitosis
Zhong Chong (PC-9)	At the centre of the tip of the middle finger.	• Acute diseases such as coma, heatstroke, fainting • Cardiodynia • Night crying in infants, stiff and swollen tongue

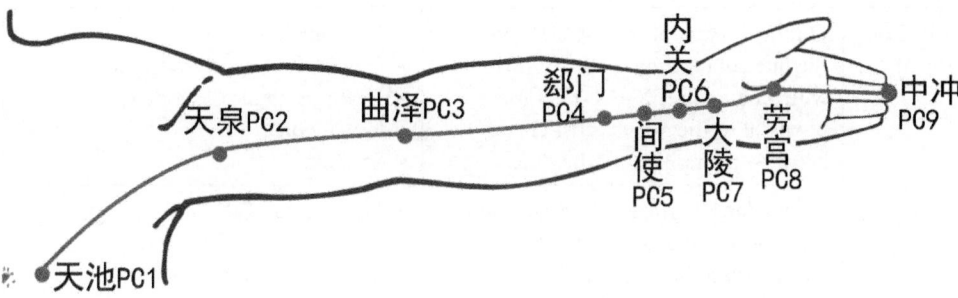

Figure 2.1.9 General Chart of Points of the Pericardium Channel of Hand-Jueyin

1.10 Points of the Sanjiao Channel of Hand-Shaoyang, SJ

Name of point	Location	Indications
Guan Chong (SJ-1)	On the ring finger, on the ulnar side of the distal phalanx, 0.1 *cun* proximal to the ulnar corner of the fingernail.	• Fever, fainting • Diseases of the five sense organs such as headache, bloodshot eyes, deafness, pharyngitis
Zhong Zhu (SJ-3)	On the dorsum of the hand, proximal to the metacarpophalangeal joint of the ring finger, in the depression between the fourth and fifth metacarpal bones.	• Diseases of head, face and the five sense organs such as headache, bloodshot eyes, tinnitus, deafness, pharyngitis • Pain and numbness of the shoulder, back, elbow and arm, and an inability to flex and extend the fingers • Fever
Yang Chi (SJ-4)	On the dorsal wrist crease, in the depression on the ulnar side of the extensor digitorum tendon.	• Conditions of the head, face and the five sense organs such as headache, bloodshot and painful eyes, deafness, pharyngitis • Wrist pain • Diabetes
Wai Guan (SJ-5)	On the dorsum of the forearm, on the line connecting Yang Chi (SJ-4) with Zhou Jian (EX-UX-1), 2 *cun* proximal to the dorsal wrist crease, between the radius and the ulna.	• Diseases of head, face and the five sense organs such as headache, cheek pain, bloodshot and painful eyes, tinnitus, deafness • Fever • Pain in the hypochondrium and upper arm • Scrofula

Zhi Gou (SJ-6)	On the dorsum of the forearm, on the line connecting Yang Chi (SJ-4) with Zhou Jian (EX-UX-1), 3 *cun* proximal to the dorsal wrist crease, between the radius and the ulna.	• Constipation • Pain in the hypochondrium • Deafness, tinnitus, sudden loss of voice • Scrofula
Tian Jing (SJ-10)	On the lateral arm, in the depression 1 *cun* proximal to Zhou Jian (EX-UX-1) when the elbow is flexed.	• Myasthenia of the arm, paralysis of the arm • Migraine, deafness • Pain in the chest and hypochondrium • Scrofula
Jian Liao (SJ-14)	On the shoulder girdle, posterior to Jian Yu (LI-15), in the depression posteroinferior to the acromion when the arm is abducted.	• Arm pain, frozen shoulder • Pain in the hypochondrium
Yi Feng (SJ-17)	Posterior to the ear lobe, in the depression between the mastoid process and the angle of the mandible.	• Diseases of head, face and the five sense organs such as deviated mouth and eyes, jaw clenching, toothache, swollen cheek, tinnitus, deafness • Scrofula
Jiao Sun (SJ-20)	On the head, with the auricle folded forward, it is located in the hairline superior to the auricular apex.	• Swollen cheeks, nebula or macule of the cornea, toothache • Stiff neck
Er Men (SJ-21)	On the face, when the mouth is slightly open, the point is located in the depression anterior to the supratragic notch, posterior to the condylar process of the mandible.	• Tinnitus, deafness, purulent ear conditions • Toothache
Si Zhu Kong (SJ-23)	On the face, in the depression at the lateral end of the eyebrow.	• Bloodshot and painful eyes, twitching of the eyelid • Headache, mania, epilepsy

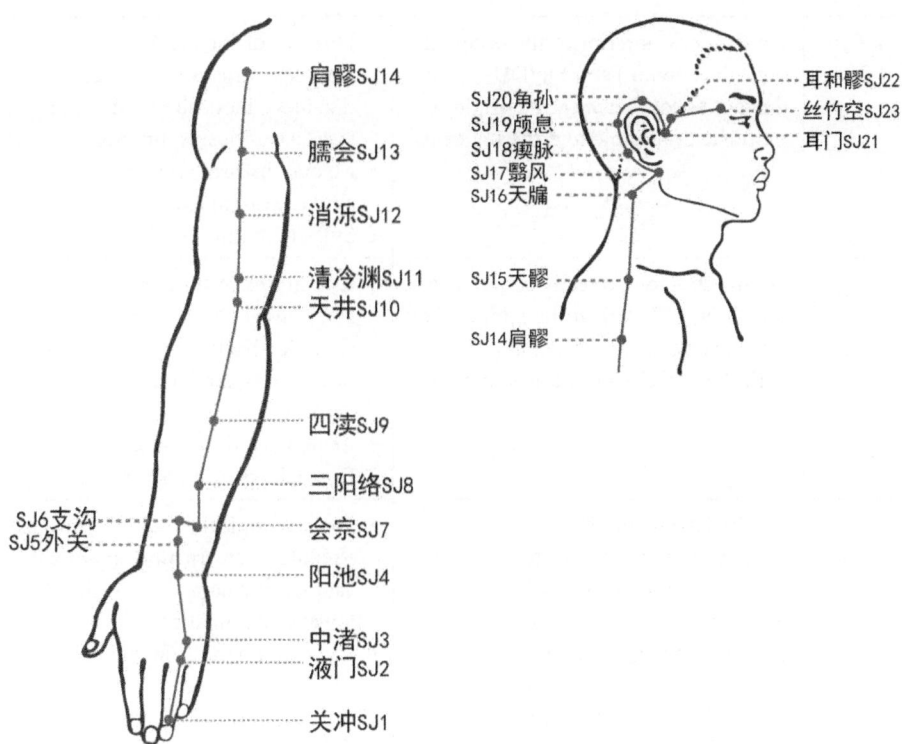

肩髎SJ14
臑会SJ13
消泺SJ12
清冷渊SJ11
天井SJ10
四渎SJ9
三阳络SJ8
SJ6支沟
SJ5外关
会宗SJ7
阳池SJ4
中渚SJ3
液门SJ2
关冲SJ1

SJ20角孙
SJ19颅息
SJ18瘈脉
SJ17翳风
SJ16天牖
SJ15天髎
SJ14肩髎

耳和髎SJ22
丝竹空SJ23
耳门SJ21

Figure 2.1.10 General Chart of Points of the Sanjiao Channel of Hand-Shaoyang

1.11 Points of the Gallbladder Channel of Foot-Shaoyang, GB

Name of point	Location	Indications
Tong Zi Liao (GB-1)	On the face, lateral to the outer canthus, on the lateral border of the orbital margin.	• Eye conditions such as bloodshot eyes, eye pain, nebula or macule of the cornea • Headache, deviated mouth and eyes
Ting Hui (GB-2)	On the face, when the mouth is open, the point is located in the depression anterior to the intertragic notch, posterior to the condylar process of the mandible.	• Ear conditions such as tinnitus, deafness, purulent ear diseases • Toothache, a deviated mouth and eyes, face pain
Yang Bai (GB-14)	On the forehead, directly superior to the centre of the pupil, 1 *cun* superior to the eyebrow.	• Head and eye diseases such as bloodshot and painful eyes, blepharoptosis, deviated mouth and eyes, headache

Feng Chi (GB-20)	On the neck, inferior to the occipital bone, level with Feng Fu (DU-16), in the depression between the origins of sternocleidomastoid and the trapezius.	• Diseases of the head, face and the five sense organs such as headache, dizziness, bloodshot and painful eyes, nasosinusitis, tinnitus • Mental diseases such as stroke, insomnia, epilepsy • Stiff and painful neck
Jian Jing (GB-21)	On the shoulder, directly superior to Ru Zhong (ST-17), at the midpoint of the line connecting Da Zhui (DU-14) with the lateral end of the acromion.	• Conditions of the shoulder, neck and arms such as pain in the shoulder, back and arm, paralysis of the arms, stiff and painful neck • Scrofula • Acute mastitis, hypogalactia • Dystocia, placenta retention
Dai Mai (GB-26)	On the lateral abdomen, 1.8 *cun* posterior to Zhang Men (LR-13), at the junction of the perpendicular line of the inferior border of the free extremity of the eleventh rib and the horizontal line of the centre of umbilicus.	• Gynaecological conditions such as irregular menstruation, abnormal vaginal discharge, amenorrhoea, lower abdominal pain • Hypochondriac pain, lumbago
Huan Tiao (GB-30)	On the lateral aspect of the hip, at the junction of the lateral one third and medial two thirds of the line connecting the prominence of the greater trochanter with the sacral hiatus.	• Waist and leg diseases such as pain in the waist and crotch, atrophy and paralysis of the legs
Feng Shi (GB-31)	On the midline of the lateral aspect of the thigh, 7 *cun* superior to the popliteal crease, in the depression where the tip of the middle finger rests, when standing up with the arms hanging alongside the thigh.	• Atrophy and paralysis of the legs • Pruritus, dermatophytosis
Xi Yang Guan (GB-33)	On the lateral aspect of the knee, 3 *cun* superior to Yang Ling Quan (GB-34), in the depression proximal to the lateral epicondyle of the femur.	• Swelling and pain of the knee and patella, popliteal tendon spasm, numbness of the crus • Dermatophytosis
Yang Ling Quan (GB-34)	On the lateral aspect of the crus, in the depression anterior and distal to the head of the fibula.	• Liver and gall bladder diseases such as jaundice, a bitter taste, hiccups, vomiting, pain in the hypochondrium • Leg and knee joint diseases such as atrophy and paralysis of the legs, swelling and pain of the knee and patella • Shoulder pain

Guang Ming (GB-37)	On the lateral aspect of the crus, 5 *cun* proximal to the prominence of the lateral malleolus, anterior to the fibula.	• Eye disease such as eye pain, night blindness, blurred eyes • Atrophy and paralysis of the legs • Swelling and pain of the breast, hypogalactia
Yang Fu (GB-38)	On the lateral aspect of the crus, 4 *cun* proximal to the prominence of the lateral malleolus, anterior to the fibula.	• Atrophy and paralysis of the legs • Migraine, pain in the outer canthus, oxter, chest and hypochondrium • Scrofula, malaria
Xuan Zhong (GB-39)	On the lateral aspect of the crus, 3 *cun* proximal to the prominence of the lateral malleolus, anterior to the fibula.	• Stiff and painful neck, distending pain in the chest and hypochondrium, atrophy and paralysis of the legs • Dementia, stroke
Zu Qiao Yin (GB-44)	On the fourth toe, lateral to the distal phalanx, 0.1 *cun* proximal to the lateral corner of the toenail.	• Diseases of the five sense organs such as headache, bloodshot and painful eyes, tinnitus, deafness, pharyngitis • Insomnia, dreaminess • Distension in the hypochondrium, swelling and pain in back of the foot

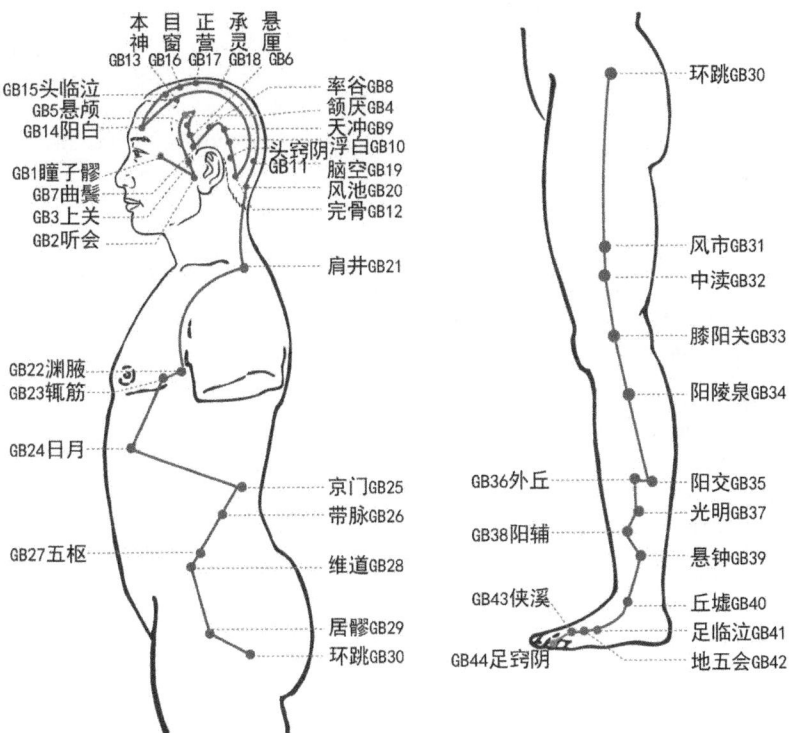

Figure 2.1.11 General Chart of Points of the Gallbladder Channel of Foot-Shaoyang

1.12 Points of the Liver Channel of Foot-Jueyin, LR

Name of point	Location	Indications
Da Dun (LR-1)	On the big toe, lateral to the distal phalanx, 0.1 *cun* proximal to the lateral corner of the toenail.	• Hernia • Amenorrhoea, metrorrhagia and metrostaxis, prolapse of the uterus, urorrhoea, dysuria • Epilepsy
Xing Jian (LR-2)	On the dorsum of the foot, between the first and second toes, proximal to the web margin, at the border between the red and white flesh.	• Stroke, epilepsy, headache, dizziness, bloodshot and painful eyes, glaucoma, deviated mouth • Irregular menstruation, dysmenorrhoea, metrorrhagia and metrostaxis, abnormal vaginal discharge • Urorrhoea, anuria and dysuria • Hernia • Distending pain in the chest and hypochondrium
Tai Chong (LR-3)	On the dorsum of the foot, in the depression proximal to the first interosseous metatarsal space.	• Headache, dizziness, bloodshot and painful eyes, deviated mouth • Stroke, epilepsy, infantile convulsions • Jaundice, hypochondriac pain, bitter taste, abdominal distension • Irregular menstruation, dysmenorrhoea, amenorrhoea, abnormal vaginal discharge • Urorrhoea, anuria and dysuria • Atrophy and paralysis of the legs, swelling and pain in back of the foot
Zhang Men (LR-13)	On the lateral abdomen, inferior to the free extremity of the eleventh rib.	• Hypochondriac pain, jaundice • Abdominal distension, diarrhoea, vomiting, masses in the abdomen
Qi Men (LR-14)	In the anterior thoracic region, directly inferior to the nipple, in the sixth intercostal space, 4 *cun* lateral to the anterior midline.	• Distending pain in the chest and hypochondrium • Abdominal distension, hiccups, vomiting • Acute mastitis

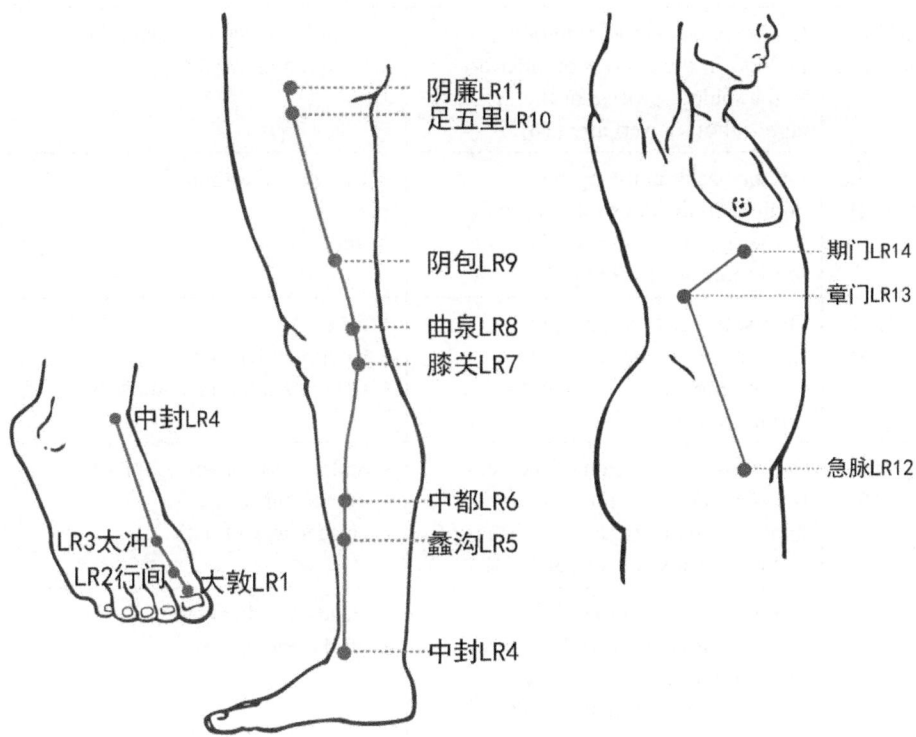

阴廉LR11
足五里LR10

阴包LR9

曲泉LR8
膝关LR7

中封LR4

中都LR6
蠡沟LR5

LR3太冲
LR2行间 大敦LR1

中封LR4

期门LR14
章门LR13

急脉LR12

Figure 2.1.12 General Chart of Points of the Liver Channel of Foot-Jueyin

1.13 Points of the Du Channel (Governor Vessel), DU

Name of point	Location	Indications
Chang Qiang (DU-1)	Inferior to the tip of the coccyx, midway between the tip of the coccyx and the anus.	• Haemorrhoids • Mania, epilepsy
Yao Shu (DU-2)	In the sacral region, on the posterior midline, at the sacral hiatus.	• Stiff and painful groin • Epilepsy
Yao Yang Guan (DU-3)	In the lumbar region, on the posterior midline, in the depression inferior to the spinous process of the fourth lumbar vertebra (L4).	• Lumbosacral pain, atrophy and paralysis of the legs • Irregular menstruation
Ming Men (DU-4)	In the lumbar region, on the posterior midline, in the depression inferior to the spinous process of the second lumbar vertebra (L2).	• Lumbago, atrophy and paralysis of the legs • Spermatorrhoea, impotence, irregular menstruation, urorrhoea, frequent urination • Diarrhoea

Zhi Yang (DU-9)	On the back, on the posterior midline, in the depression inferior to the spinous process of the eighth thoracic vertebra (T8).	• Jaundice, fever, stomach ache • Cough and asthma
Shen Zhu (DU-12)	On the back, on the posterior midline, in the depression inferior to the spinous process of the third thoracic vertebra (T3).	• Cough and asthma • Fever • Epilepsy
Da Zhui (DU-14)	On the posterior midline, in the depression inferior to the spinous process of the seventh cervical vertebra (C7).	• Fever • Cough and asthma • Epilepsy, infantile convulsions
Ya Men (DU-15)	In the posterior region of the neck, 0.5 *cun* superior to the posterior midline, inferior to the spinous process of the first cervical vertebra (C1).	• Sudden loss of voice, aphasia with a stiff tongue • Headache, stiff neck
Feng Fu (DU-16)	In the posterior region of the neck, 1 *cun* superior to the centre of posterior hairline, directly inferior to the external occipital protuberance, in the depression between the two trapezius muscles.	• Headache, dizziness • Stroke and aphasia
Bai Hui (DU-20)	On the head, 5 *cun* superior to the centre of anterior hairline, or at the midpoint of the line connecting the two auricular apexes.	• Headache, dizziness • Insomnia, forgetfulness • Rectocele, prolapse of the uterus, chronic diarrhoea
Shen Ting (DU-24)	On the head, 0.5 *cun* superior to the centre of anterior hairline.	• Headache, dizziness, insomnia • Nasosinusitis, lachrymation, eye pain
Su Liao (DU-25)	On the face, at the tip of the nose.	• Nasal congestion, nasosinusitis, hemorrhinia, acne rosacea • Apnoea
Shui Gou (DU-26)	On the face, at the junction of the upper one third and lower two thirds of the philtrum midline.	• Coma, stroke • Deviated mouth, jaw clenching • Stiff and painful groin

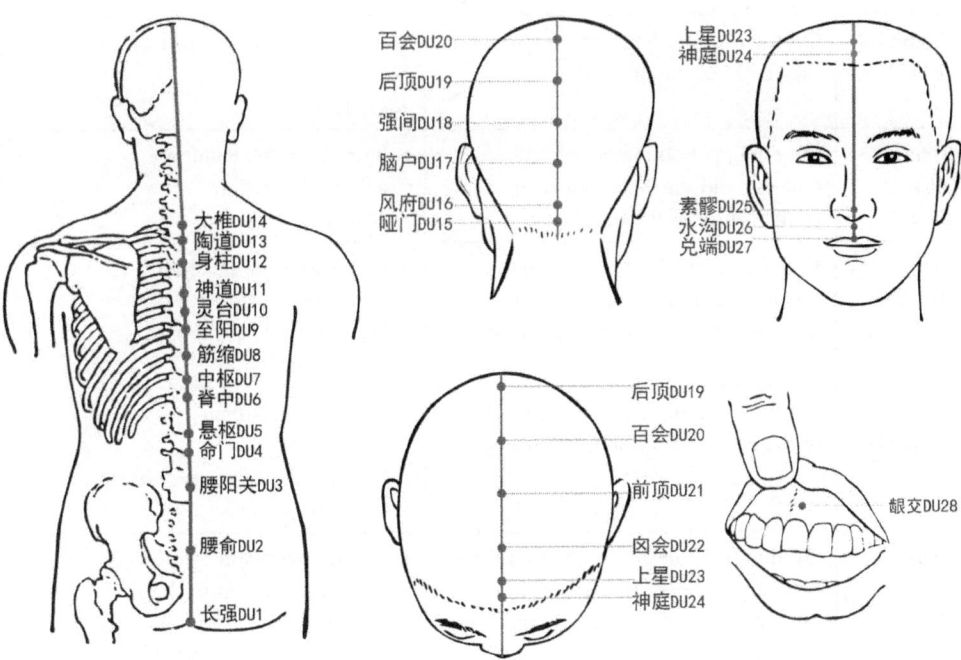

Figure 2.1.13 General Chart of Points of the Du Channel (Governor Vessel)

1.14 Points of the Ren Channel (Conception Vessel), RN

Name of point	Location	Indications
Zhong Ji (RN-3)	On the lower abdomen, on the anterior midline, 4 *cun* inferior to the centre of the umbilicus.	• Anuria and dysuria, urorrhoea, frequent urination, spermatorrhoea, impotence • Irregular menstruation, abnormal vaginal discharge, dysmenorrhoea
Guan Yuan (RN-4)	On the lower abdomen, on the anterior midline, 3 *cun* inferior to the centre of the umbilicus.	• Impotence, spermatorrhoea, urorrhoea, anuria and dysuria • Irregular menstruation, dysmenorrhoea, amenorrhoea, sterility • Abdominal pain, diarrhoea • Consumptive disease, collapse syndrome of stroke
Qi Hai (RN-6)	On the lower abdomen, on the anterior midline, 1.5 *cun* inferior to the centre of the umbilicus.	• Abdominal pain, diarrhoea • Urorrhoea, spermatorrhoea, impotence • Amenorrhoea, dysmenorrhoea, abnormal vaginal discharge, prolapse of the uterus • Consumptive disease, collapse syndrome of stroke

Shen Que (RN-8)	On the middle abdomen, in the centre of the umbilicus.	• Abdominal pain, chronic diarrhoea • Collapse • Oedema
Shang Wan (RN-13)	On the upper abdomen, on the anterior midline, 5 *cun* superior to the centre of the umbilicus.	• Stomach ache, vomiting, acid regurgitation • Mania, epilepsy
Dan Zhong (RN-17)	In the anterior thoracic region, on the anterior midline, at the same level as the fourth intercostal space, at the midpoint of the two nipples.	• Oppression in the chest, thoracalgia, asthma • Hypogalactia, acute mastitis • Vomiting
Tian Tu (RN-22)	On the neck, on the anterior midline, in the centre of the suprasternal fossa.	• Cough and asthma • Thoracalgia • Sudden loss of voice, goitre, pharynx neurosis
Lian Quan (RN-23)	On the neck, on the anterior midline, superior to the Adam's apple, in the depression superior to the hyoid bone.	• Aphasia with stiff tongue, swelling and pain in the hypoglossis; salivation with the convulsion of the tongue • Sudden loss of voice, dysphagia

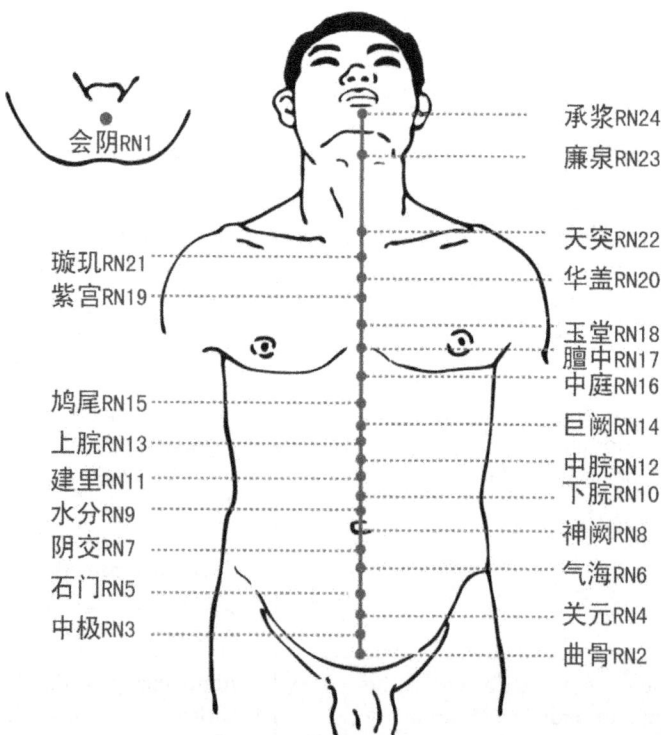

Figure 2.1.14 General Chart of Points of the Ren Channel (Conception Vessel)

2. Commonly Used Extra Points

Name of point	Location	Indications
Si Shen Cong (EX-HN-1)	Four points on the vertex, 1 *cun* anterior, posterior and lateral to Bai Hui (DU-20) respectively (Figure 2.2.1).	• Mental disorders such as headache, dizziness, insomnia, forgetfulness, epilepsy
Yin Tang (EX-HN-3)	On the forehead, midway between the medial ends of the two eyebrows (Figure 2.2.2).	• Disorders of head and face such as headache, dizziness, sinusitis, epistaxis, bloodshot and painful eyes • Febrile convulsion, insomnia
Tai Yang (EX-HN-5)	At the temporal part of the head, in the depression 1 *cun* posterior to the midpoint between the lateral end of the eyebrow and the outer canthus (Figure 2.2.3).	• Headache • Eye disease such as bloodshot and painful eyes, epidemic conjunctivitis, nebula or macule of the cornea • Deviated mouth and eyes
Qiu Hou (EX-HN-7)	On the face, at the junction of the lateral one fourth and medial three fourths of the infraorbital margin (Figure 2.2.2).	• Eye disease such as bloodshot and painful eyes, nebula or macule of the cornea, blurred eyes, glaucoma, nyctalopia
Jin Jin, Yu Ye (EX-HN-12, EX-HN-13)	In the mouth, on the left and right vein of the frenulum under the tongue (Figure 2.2.4).	• Disorders of the mouth and tongue such as stiff tongue, swelling of the tongue, aphtha, pharyngitis • Diabetes, vomiting, diarrhoea • Aphasia
Qian Zheng	0.5–1 *cun* anterior to earlobe (Figure 2.2.3).	• Deviated mouth, aphtha
Yi Ming (EX-HN-14)	On the neck, 1 *cun* posterior to Yi Feng (SJ-17) (Figure 2.2.3).	• Eye conditions such as bloodshot and painful eyes, nebula or macule of the cornea, blurred eyes, glaucoma, nyctalopia • Tinnitus, deafness
Ti Tuo	4 *cun* lateral to Guan Yuan (RN-4) (Figure 2.2.5).	• Prolapse of the uterus, hernia, abdominal pain
Zi Gong (EX-CA-1)	On the lower abdomen, 4 *cun* inferior to the centre of the umbilicus, 3 *cun* lateral to Zhong Ji (RN-3) (Figure 2.2.5).	• Gynecopathy such as prolapse of the uterus, dysmenorrhoea, uterine bleeding, sterility, irregular menstruation

San Jiao Jiu (EX-CA-2)	Draw an equilateral triangle with each side the same length as the patient's mouth. The top corner of the triangle is at the navel, and the lower side of the triangle is horizontal. The two lower corners of the triangle are the acupoints (Figure 2.2.5).	• Hernia, up-rushing gas syndrome • Umbilical pain • Sterility
Ding Chuan (EX-B-1)	On the back, inferior to the spinous process of the seventh cervical vertebra and 0.5 *cun* lateral to the posterior midline (Figure 2.2.6).	• Lung diseases such as asthma, cough • Stiff neck, pain in the shoulder and back
Jia Ji (EX-B-2)	In the back lumbar region, 0.5 *cun* lateral to the posterior midline, from the first thoracic to the fifth lumbar vertebra, 17 points on each side (Figure 2.2.6).	• Upper thoracic vertebra: disorders of the chest, heart, lung and upper limbs • Lower thoracic vertebra: disorders of the stomach and intestines • Lumbar vertebra: disorders of the lumbar region, abdomen and lower limbs
Yao Yan (EX-B-7)	In the lumbar region, in the depression inferior to the spinous process of the fourth lumbar vertebra, 3.5 *cun* lateral to the posterior midline (Figure 2.2.6).	• Lumbar pain • Irregular menstruation, abnormal vaginal discharge
Shi Xuan (EX-UE-11)	On the tips of ten fingers, 0.1 *cun* distal to the fingernails, 10 points on both sides altogether (Figure 2.2.7).	• Coma and fainting, heatstroke, fever, epilepsy • Febrile convulsions, insomnia
Si Feng (EX-UE-10)	On the palmar of the hand, midpoint of the proximal phalangeal joints, 4 points on each side (Figure 2.2.8).	• Malnutrition and indigestion syndrome in children • Whooping cough
Ba Xie (EX-UE-9)	On the dorsum of the hand; with a loose fist, it is proximal to the web margins between 5 fingers, at the border between the red and white flesh, 8 points on both hands altogether (Figure 2.2.9).	• Venomous snake bite, swelling and pain on the dorsum of the hand, numbness of the fingers • Eye pain, restless fever
Luo Zhen Xue, Wai Lao Gong (EX-UE-8)	On the dorsum of the hand, between the second and third metacarpal bones, 0.5 *cun* proximal to the metacarpophalangeal joint (Figure 2.2.10).	• Stiff neck • Swelling and pain on the dorsum of hand, numbness of the fingers

Yao Tong Dian (EX-UE-7)	On the dorsum of the hand, between the second and third, fourth and fifth metacarpal bones respectively, at the midpoint of the metacarpophalangeal joints and the dorsal wrist crease, 2 points on each side (Figure 2.2.10).	• Acute lumbar sprain
Bi Zhong	At the midpoint of the wrist crease and elbow crease, between the radius and ulna (Figure 2.2.11).	• Paralysis and spasm of the arms, neuralgia in the forearm, hysteria
Jian Qian	Sitting straight with the shoulder hanging, at the midpoint of the line connecting the anterior axillary fold with Jian Yu (LI-15) (Figure 2.2.11).	• Pain in the shoulder and arm, frozen shoulder
Bai Chong Wo (EX-LE-3)	With the knee flexed, it is on the medial aspect of the thigh, 3 *cun* superior to the medial border of the patella, 1 *cun* superior to Xue Hai (SP-10) (Figure 2.2.12).	• Parasitic accumulation • Rheumatism, prurigo, eczema, skin ulcer on the lower portion of the body
He Ding (EX-LE-2)	Superior to the knee, in the depression at the midpoint of the superior patellar border. (Figure 2.2.12)	• Knee pain, weakness of legs and feet, tuberculous arthritis, dermatophytosis
Xi Yan (EX-LE-5)	With the knee flexed, in the depressions medial and lateral to the patellar ligament, known as Nei Xi Yan on the medial and Wai Xi Yan on the lateral side (Figure 2.2.12).	• Knee pain, tuberculous arthritis, leg pain, dermatophytosis
Dan Nang (EX-LE-6)	On the superior lateral aspect of the crus, 2 *cun* directly inferior to the depression anteroinferior to the small head of the fibula Yang Ling Quan (GB-34) (Figure 2.2.12).	• Disorders of the gallbladder such as cholecystitis, cholelithiasis, biliary ascariasis, gallbladder colic • Atrophy and paralysis of the legs, hypochondriac pain
Lan Wei (EX-LE-7)	On the superior lateral aspect of the crus, 5 *cun* inferior to Du Bi (ST-35), one finger's breadth lateral to the anterior border of the tibia (Figure 2.2.12).	• Appendicitis, dyspepsia • Atrophy and paralysis of the legs
Ba Feng (EX-LE-10)	On the dorsum of the foot, proximal to the web margins between the 5 toes, at the border between the red and white flesh, 4 points on each side, 8 points in total (Figure 2.2.12).	• Venomous snakebite, swelling and pain on the dorsum of the foot • Myasthenia of the foot • Dermatophytosis

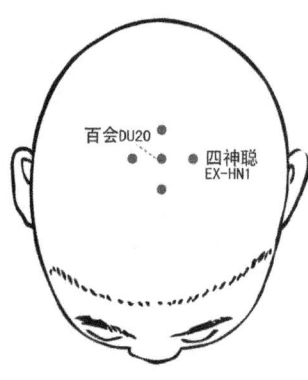

Figure 2.2.1

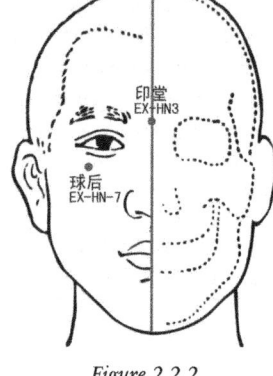

Figure 2.2.2

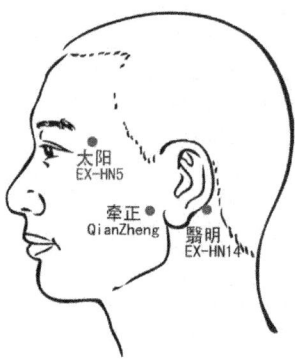

Figure 2.2.3

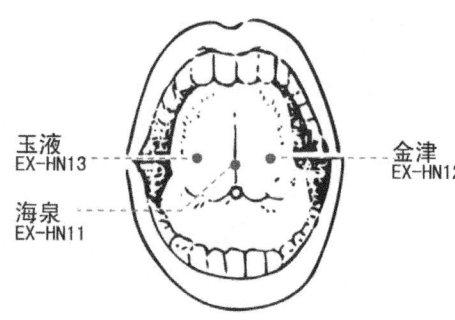

Figure 2.2.4

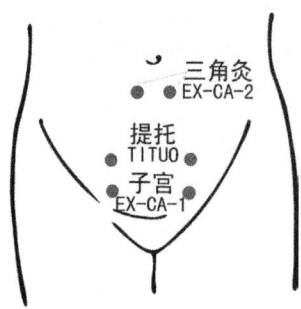

Figure 2.2.5

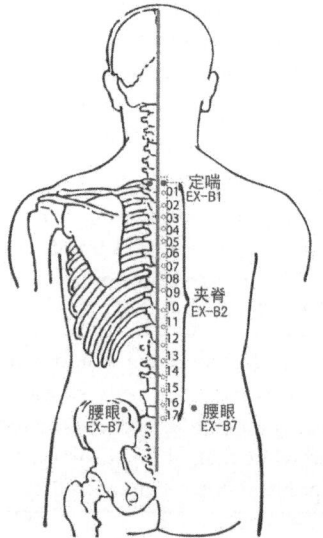

Figure 2.2.6

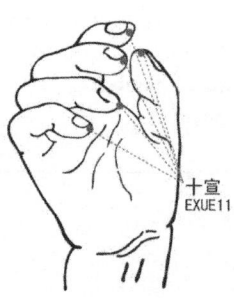

Figure 2.2.7

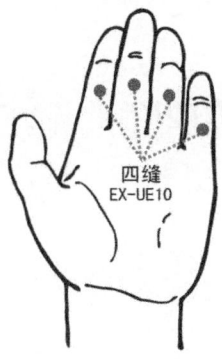

四缝
EX-UE10

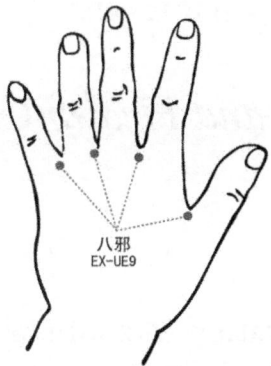

八邪
EX-UE9

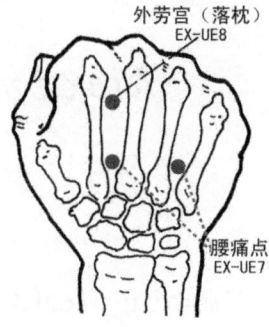

外劳宫（落枕）
EX-UE8

腰痛点
EX-UE7

Figure 2.2.8   Figure 2.2.9   Figure 2.2.10

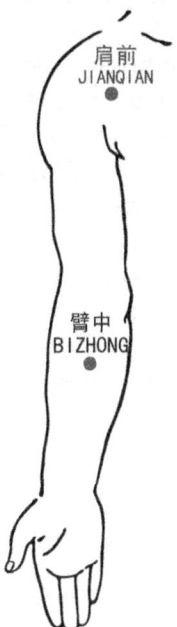

肩前
JIANQIAN

臂中
BIZHONG

Figure 2.2.11

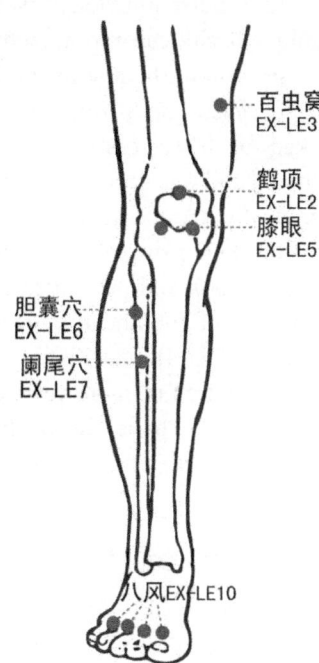

百虫窝
EX-LE3

鹤顶
EX-LE2

膝眼
EX-LE5

胆囊穴
EX-LE6

阑尾穴
EX-LE7

八风 EX-LE10

Figure 2.2.12

CHAPTER 3

Moxibustion and Health Cultivation

1. Defining Health Cultivation Moxatherapy

Moxatherapy for health cultivation refers to the method of applying moxa to certain acupoints to regulate qi and blood, warm and open the channels and collaterals, warm and nourish the organs, and prolong life. In ancient times it was referred to as 'counter moxa'. Moxatherapy for health cultivation is not only used for improving one's health, but can also be used to nurse individuals weakened by prolonged illness back to health. It is one of the unique health cultivation methods from China.

The use of moxatherapy for health cultivation has a long history. The famous Tang Dynasty physician Sun Si-Miao was active and healthy well into his eighth decade, and when asked for the secret of his longevity he replied, 'I used to have many illnesses, and often suffered and was short of breath. A physician taught me to moxa Qi Hai (RN-6), and my qi gradually became abundant. Perform moxa one or two times each year to protect one's qi from being dispelled. Additionally, it is appropriate for any case of qi vacuity, extreme exhaustion and prolonged unresolved illness.' In *Bian Que Xin Shu* he also stated, 'During periods of good health, frequent moxibustion of Guan Yuan (RN-4), Qi Hai (RN-6), Ming Men (DU-4), and Zhong Wan (RN-12) may not result in immortality, but will guarantee a hundred or more years of life.' These quotations show that in ancient times health cultivation experts already had plentiful experience in the use of moxatherapy. Today it is still an effective and popular method to maintain good health.

2. The Effects of Health Cultivation Moxatherapy

2.1 WARM AND OPEN THE CHANNELS, MOVE QI AND INVIGORATE BLOOD

In the chapter *Ci Jie Zhen Xie* in *Ling Shu* it states, 'If the blood in the vessels is congealed and stagnated, regulate it with fire.' The flow of qi and blood demonstrates the characteristics of moving when warmed and congealing when cold. Moxibustion is warming; therefore it can warm and open the channels and collaterals to stimulate the movement of qi and blood.

2.2 FOSTER AND SUPPLEMENT ORIGINAL QI, PROTECT AGAINST DISEASE

In the book *Bian Que Xin Shu* it says 'Real origin [qi] is the ruler of the body. When real qi is strong the individual is strong; when real qi is weak the individual sickens; when real qi deserts, the individual dies. The best method for cultivating life is moxibustion.' As a warm, acrid, yang medicinal, it promotes the body's internal fire. The two yangs work together, making real origin (qi) abundant, with the end result of strength and health.

'When right qi is internally preserved, pathogens cannot invade.' Moxibustion has the function of fostering and supplementing original qi and protecting against disease.

2.3 FORTIFY THE SPLEEN AND BOOST THE STOMACH TO FOSTER AND SUPPLEMENT THE LATER HEAVEN, ACQUIRED CONSTITUTION

Moxibustion has a definite strengthening effect on the spleen and stomach systems. As stated in *Zhen Jiu Zi Sheng Jing*, 'Cases of disinterest in eating, swelling and distension in the epigastric region and stomach, sallow-yellow facial complexion are commonly known as spleen-stomach disease, and Zhong Wan (RN-12) should be heated with moxa.' Applying moxa to Zhong Wan (RN-12) can warm and move spleen yang, supplement the centre and boost qi. Frequent moxa on Zu San Li (ST-36) will not only cause the functioning of the digestive system to be exuberant, increasing the absorption of nutrition and nourishing the whole body, but can also achieve the effects of preventing and curing disease, resisting debilitation and protecting against the effects of ageing.

2.4 UPLIFT YANG QI, CONSTRAIN AND PROTECT THE SKIN AND EXTERIOR

The chapter *Jing Mai* in the *Ling Shu* asserts 'downward movement should be treated with moxa'. In the case of sinking qi vacuity, clear yang will not be uplifted and dispersed, causing the skin and [body] hairs to lose control of wind and cold. Defensive qi and yang, then, don't combine and the interstices are insecure. Frequent application of moxibustion can uplift yang qi, secure the skin, improve resistance to external pathogens, regulate nourishment and defence, and achieve the effects of strengthening the body, preventing disease and treating disease.

3. Key Points for the Application of Health Cultivation Moxatherapy

Acupoints should be selected on the basis of the patient's constitution and necessary health preservation requirements. Lit moxa cones should be placed at the acupoints, bringing a tolerable level of warmth to the local area.

The points can be treated for 3–5 minutes, or 10–15 minutes at the most. Generally speaking, health cultivation moxibustion is carried out for a slightly shorter time, while moxa for rehabilitation is applied for slightly longer. During spring and summer the treatment time is shortened, and it is lengthened during autumn and winter. Moxibustion on the limbs and chest is conducted for a shorter time, while it is done for longer on the abdomen and back. The elderly, women and children should receive moxa for a shorter time, while healthy youths can receive longer treatments.

The traditional method of measuring the length of a moxibustion treatment is to count the number and size of the moxa cones. A moxa cone is a unit that is formed by squeezing loose moxa into a cone shape. They can be formed in large, medium and small sizes: large cones are the size of a broad bean; medium cones are the size of a soybean, and small cones are the size of a grain of wheat. As a unit of measure, 'one cone' means one cone that is entirely burnt through. In actual practice the choice of number and size is based on the strength of the individual's constitution: stronger patients are given large cones, while the weaker individuals receive small cones.

4. Matters Requiring Attention in Health Cultivation Moxatherapy

4.1 APPLY MOXA REGULARLY

Living within a natural environment, humans are constantly affected by environmental changes, especially those relating to the climate and weather. For this reason, regular yearly, seasonal, monthly, and daily moxibustion can help the body to adapt to weather changes and strengthen resistance against disease in a timely fashion.

4.2 PERSEVERANCE IS GOLDEN

People usually seek emergency help from doctors when they encounter illness, and relax their vigilance once their sickness has passed. Health cultivation requires patience and perseverance; longevity results from long-term use of moxibustion, and vice-versa.

4.3 COMBINE MOXATHERAPY WITH OTHER METHODS

The five viscera and six bowels are interconnected and form a whole. If one organ is diseased it will affect other organs, therefore application of various types of moxa can be used concurrently or combined with other health cultivation techniques to both prevent and cure disease.

4.4 TAKE CARE TO PREVENT BURNING

Moxa burns easily, so when applying moxa take care to prevent the ember from falling and burning the patient. This is especially true in the case of the elderly and children. Be careful to completely extinguish the ember after moxa to prevent accidental fire.

5. Common Acupoints for Health Cultivation Moxatherapy

Generally speaking, the majority of the acupoints that are used during acupuncture health cultivation can also be used for moxatherapy health cultivation. However, moxatherapy health cultivation also includes a certain number of points contraindicated for acupuncture.

5.1 ZU SAN LI (ST-36)

This point can fortify the spleen and boost the stomach, promote digestion, strengthen the body and lengthen lifespan. Moxa of Zu San Li in the middle-aged and elderly can also prevent stroke. It both prevents ageing and strengthens the body.

Moxibustion Method:

- Pole Moxa or Cone Moxa: 15–20 minutes each treatment, or until the acupoint reddens. Conduct one treatment either every other day, 10 times a month, or every day from Chu Yi to Chu Ba (the first and eighth day of a month on the traditional lunar calendar) for even better effects.

Health preservation experts in ancient times advocated the use of scarring moxibustion on this point. Prolonging the recovery period of the moxa sore strengthens the body and lengthens the lifespan. The quotation 'If a body at ease is desired, Zu San Li (ST-36) should often be wet' refers to this type of moxibustion. Modern research has proved that moxa of Zu San Li (ST-36) improves the immune function and has a definite effect on the enterogastric and cardiovascular systems. (Figure 3.5.1, Figure 3.5.2)

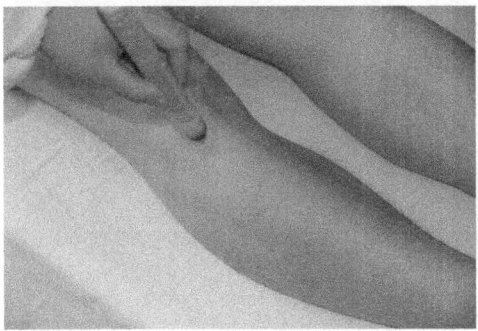 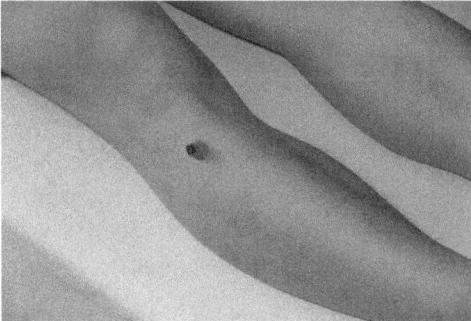

Figure 3.5.1 Pole Moxa   *Figure 3.5.2 Cone Moxa*

5.2 Shen Que (RN-8)

This point can restore consciousness and stem qi desertion, warm and supplement original yang, fortify movement of spleen and stomach, and prolong the lifespan.

Moxibustion Method:

- Gentle Pole Moxa: 10–20 minutes each time, one treatment per day. After 10 days stop treatment for 10–20 days, and then repeat (Figure 3.5.3). Moxa can also be performed on an insulating medium, for example by filling the umbilicus cavity with salt and placing a moxa cone on the top. It has the effect of lengthening the lifespan. (Figure 3.5.4)

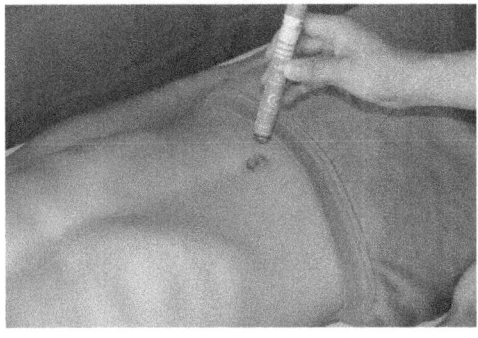 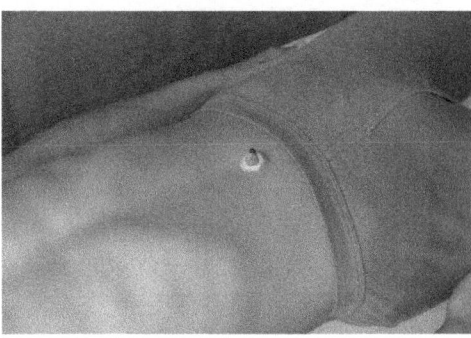

Figure 3.5.3 Gentle Pole Moxa   *Figure 3.5.4 Cone Moxa on Salt*

5.3 Guan Yuan (RN-4)

Moxa of this point can warm the kidneys and secure the root, supplement qi and return yang, free and regulate the thoroughfare and controlling vessels, rectify qi and harmonize blood. It is an important point for cultivating qi, caring for health and strengthening the constitution. It is also a common health cultivation acupoint for the elderly. Long-term moxa of this point can strengthen the qi of the whole body, causing original qi to be abundant and rehabilitating vacuity injury; for this reason it can be the primary point for treatment of all vacuity-taxation injuries. It can prevent and treat an insufficiency of yang qi, debilitated health, aversion to cold and weakness, as well as seminal emissions, premature ejaculation, impotence and diarrhoea. This method is contraindicated for pregnant women.

Moxibustion Method:

- Gentle Pole Moxa: Moxa each point for 10–20 minutes until each point reddens and feels hot; repeat the treatment 1–2 times per week. In the autumn and winter the treatment can be done daily for 10 or more consecutive days, stopped for 10–20 days, then continued. (Figure 3.5.5)

- Moxa on Ginger: Perform moxibustion for 10–20 minutes each time using medium size moxa cones. Perform treatments either daily, every other day or once every 3 days. One course of treatment consists of 10–15 treatments. (Figure 3.5.6)

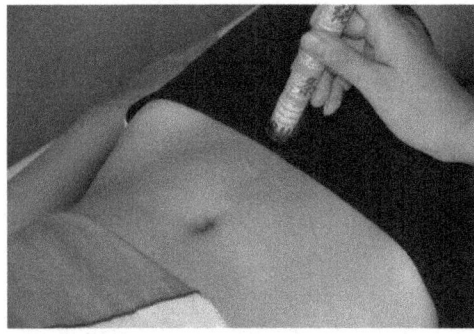
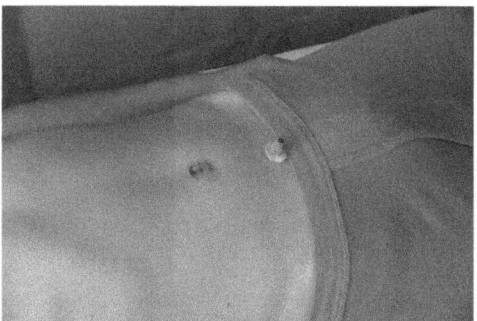

Figure 3.5.5 Gentle Pole Moxa   *Figure 3.5.6 Moxa on Ginger*

5.4 Qi Hai (RN-6)

Qi Hai is an important point for cultivating qi and maintaining health. Frequent moxa of this point can cultivate and supplement original qi, and regulate and rectify the qi dynamics. Moxibustion of this point is indicated for diarrhoea, impotence, seminal emissions, irregular menstruation, or other conditions attributed to an insufficiency of original qi and irregular lower burner qi dynamics. When treating these conditions, moxa regulates and rectifies the root cause.

Moxibustion Method:

- Gentle Pole Moxa: Moxa each point for 10–20 minutes every other day, for approximately 4–5 treatments per month. The point should become warm and redden. (Figure 3.5.7)

- Cone Moxa: Apply 3 cones to each point. Only one treatment is necessary. Blistering moxa may also be used: 5–7 cones are used each time, and 10 times constitutes one treatment course, which is repeated after several days of rest. (Figure 3.5.8)

- Moxa on Fu Zi: Grind Fu Zi (Aconiti Radix Lateralis) into powder, then mix it with a small amount of wheat flour into a paste cake 0.3–0.5cm thick. When it has dried pierce it several times with a needle. Place the Fu Zi cake on the umbilicus and place the moxa cone on top to perform moxibustion. Each time use 3–5 cones. Repeat 1–2 times per week for a total of 10 times, and then repeat after a rest of 5–10 days. (Figure 3.5.9)

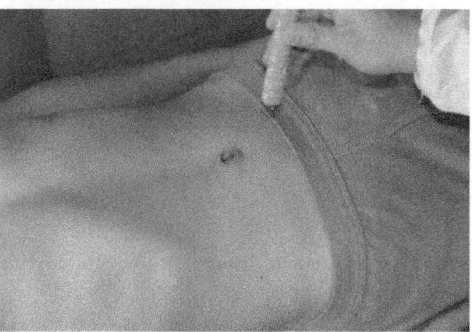

Figure 3.5.7 Gentle Pole Moxa

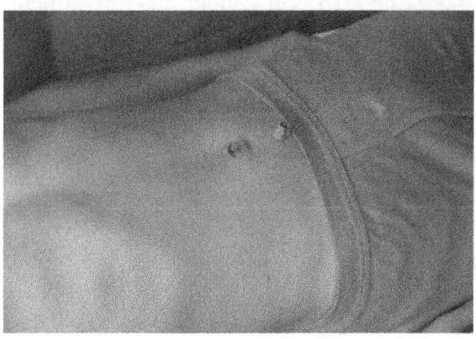
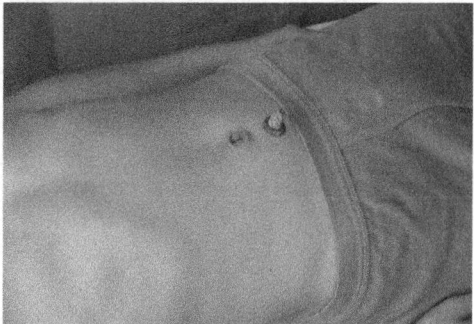

Figure 3.5.8 Cone Moxa   *Figure 3.5.9 Moxa on Fu Zi*

5.5 GAO HUANG (BL-43)

Moxa of this point can perfuse and free yang qi, kill worms and calm panting. In the text *Qian Jin Yao Fang* (*Important Formulas Worth a Thousand Gold*) it states, 'This moxibustion method will make yang qi healthy and exuberant.' A common folk custom is for children to moxa this point when they reach 17 or 18 years of age. The goal is to raise their ability to resist disease to prevent tuberculosis and common cold.

Moxibustion Method:

- Gentle Pole Moxa: 5–10 minutes each time. (Figure 3.5.10)

- Cone Moxa: 7–15 cones; every other day for a total of 5–6 times per month. (Figure 3.5.11)

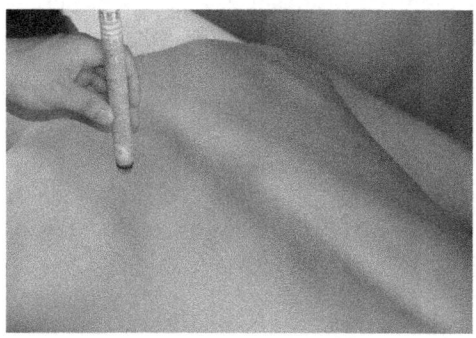 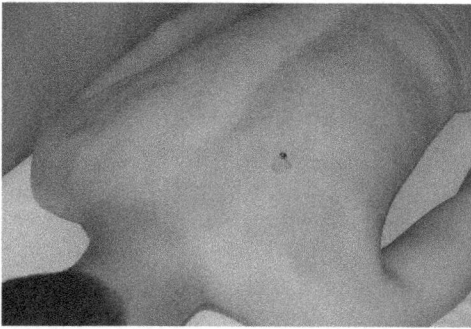

Figure 3.5.10 Gentle Pole Moxa   *Figure 3.5.11 Cone Moxa*

5.6 ZHONG WAN (RN-12)

This is an important strengthening point, as it fortifies spleen and boosts stomach qi, thereby cultivating and supplementing acquired constitutional essence. It can regulate the gastrointestinal functions and promote digestive absorption, causing the body to have abundant nutrition and effulgent qi and blood.

Moxibustion Method:

- Gentle Pole Moxa, Direct Cone Moxa, and Cone Moxa on Ginger: Each treatment consists of moxa for 10–20 minutes using 5–7 cones, which should be repeated every other day. Ten treatments make up one course of treatment. (Figure 3.5.12, Figure 3.5.13, Figure 3.5.14)

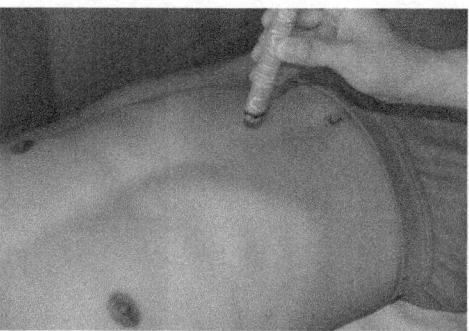

Figure 3.5.12 Gentle Pole Moxa

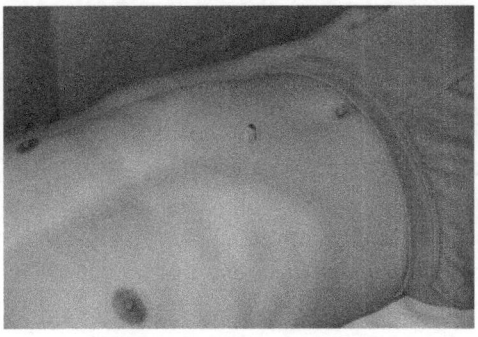

Figure 3.5.13 Direct Cone Moxa

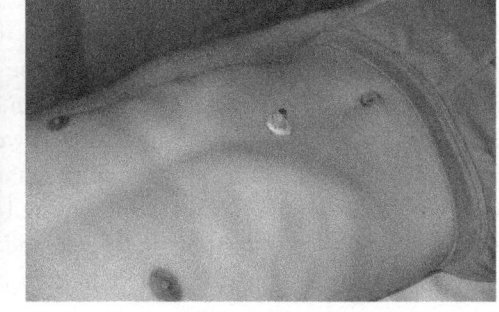

Figure 3.5.14 Cone Moxa

5.7 Shen Zhu (DU-12)

This is a health cultivation point for children. It can free yang and rectify qi, expel wind, reduce heat, clear the heart, quiet the emotions, lower counterflow, and stop coughing. It is indicated in *Yang Sheng Yi Yan Cao* that 'For children, moxa of Shen Zhu (DU-12) and Tian Shu (ST-25) once per month can guarantee health. Children with worm qi can be given moxa continuously; this is more effective than herbal medicine.' Gentle moxa of Shen Zhu is common. Shen Zhu can also fortify the brain and quiet the spirit, promote brain development, fortify the entire nervous system, increase intelligence, diffuse lung qi and improve the body's ability to resist disease and prevent the occurrence of respiratory system disease.

Moxibustion Method:

- Gentle Pole Moxa: Moxa for 5–10 minutes every other day for a total of 10 treatments per month. Cone Moxa: 1–3 cones per treatment every 2 or 3 days, or once per week. (Figure 3.5.15)

- Moxa on Ginger: Moxa for 10–20 minutes every day or every other day, for a total of 4–5 times each month. (Figure 3.5.16)

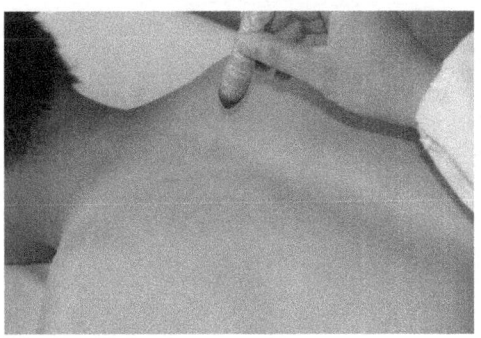
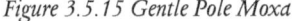

Figure 3.5.15 Gentle Pole Moxa

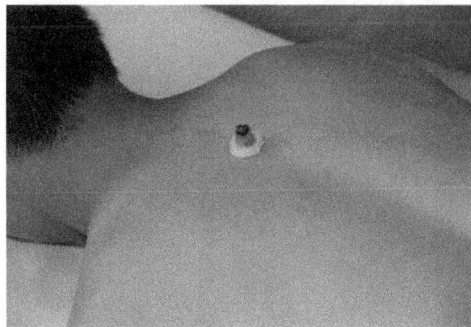

Figure 3.5.16 Moxa on Ginger

5.8 Da Zhui (DU-14)

Da Zhui is the confluence point of the governing vessel and the three yang channels of the hands and feet. It governs yang qi of the whole body, and is an important point for vitalizing yang qi, strengthening the body and maintaining health. Its usage can protect against and cure various vacuity-taxation as well as common cold diseases and symptoms. It can also clear the brain, quiet the spirit, enhance intelligence and regulate the functions of the brain. Modern research has discovered that moxibustion of Da Zhui has excellent effects of reducing inflammation, fever and spasms, as well as eliminating jaundice, protecting against meningitis and flu, and increasing white blood cells.

Moxibustion Method:

- Gentle Pole Moxa and Pecking Sparrow Moxa: Moxa for 5–10 minutes each time every 2 or 3 days for a total of 10 days per month. (Figure 3.5.17, Figure 3.5.18)

- Cone Moxa: Use 3 cones in each treatment. (Figure 3.5.19)

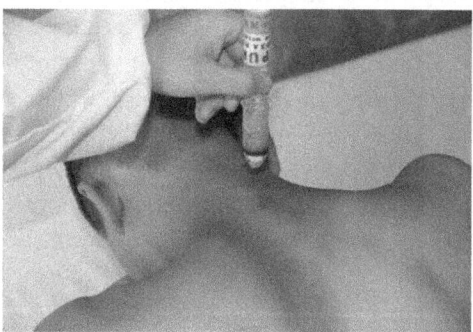

Figure 3.5.17 Gentle Pole Moxa

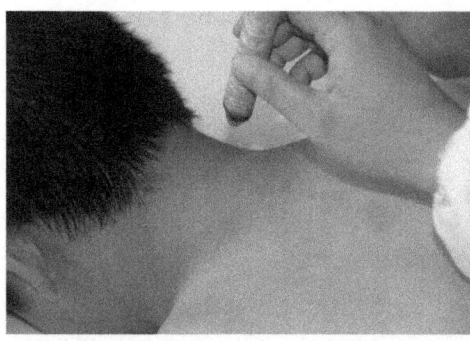

Figure 3.5.18 Pecking Sparrow Moxa

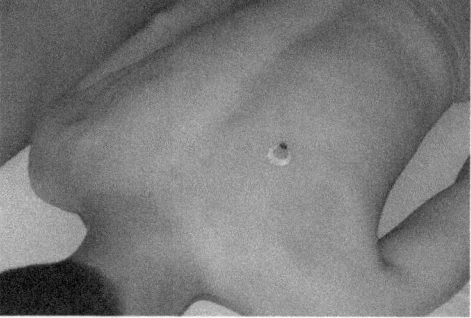

Figure 3.5.19 Cone Moxa

5.9 Feng Men (BL-12)

This point has the function of coursing wind and resolving the exterior, and diffusing lung qi. It can, therefore, prevent and treat common cold and respiratory system diseases. Individuals with vacuity constitutions who easily contract common colds will achieve even better results. Moxa of this point has efficacy in preventing and treating sores and boils, abscesses and rhinitis.

Moxibustion Method:

- Gentle Pole Moxa and Pecking Sparrow Moxa: Moxa for 5–10 minutes every 2–3 days for a total of 10 treatments per month. This method is often used to prevent and cure stroke and high blood pressure. (Figure 3.5.20, Figure 3.5.21)

- Cone Moxa on Ginger: Use 10–15 cones once every day or every other day for a total of 4–5 times per month. This method is appropriate for preventing and treating flu. (Figure 3.5.22)

- Cone Moxa on Garlic: Use 5–7 cones once per day or every other day. This is usually used to prevent and cure sores, boils, abscesses and rhinitis. (Figure 3.5.23)

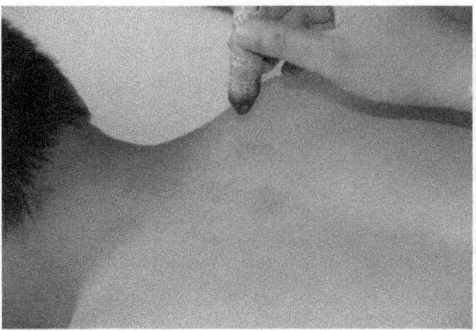
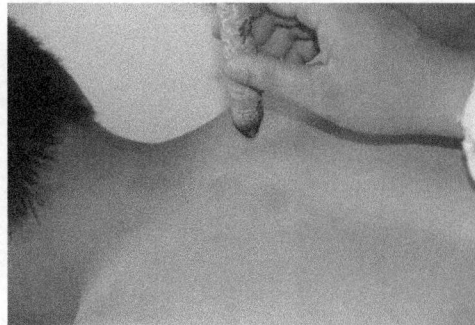

Figure 3.5.20 Gentle Pole Moxa　　　　　*Figure 3.5.21 Pecking Sparrow Moxa*

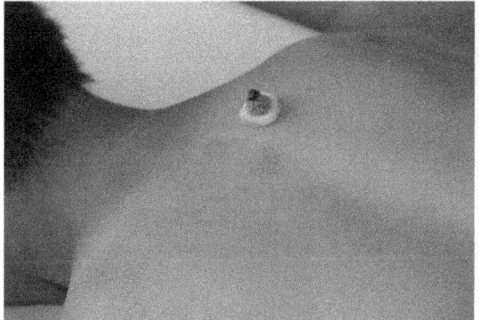
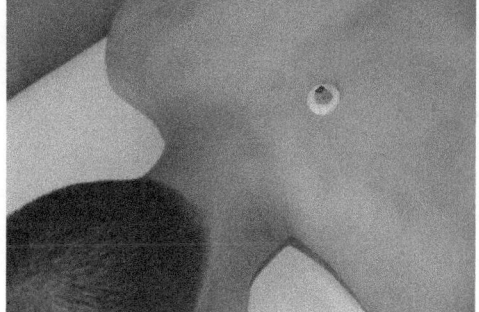

Figure 3.5.22 Cone Moxa on Ginger　　　　*Figure 3.5.23 Cone Moxa on Garlic*

5.10 MING MEN (DU-4)

The Chinese name for this point, *ming men*, means 'the gate of life'. This point is an important point for enriching kidney qi, invigorating yang, cultivating qi and maintaining health. It is often used in the case of deficient kidney qi and individuals with vacuous and cold bodies. It is especially effective in the case of seminal emissions, impotence, premature ejaculation, gynaecological disease, diarrhoea, and cold limbs and abdomen.

Moxibustion Method:

- Gentle Pole Moxa: 10–20 minutes every day or every other day. Continue for 3–6 months. (Figure 3.5.24)

- Direct Cone Moxa: 10–15 cones each time, once every other day or every 3–5 days. A treatment course consists of one month; continue for 1–3 courses. (Figure 3.5.25)

- Cone Moxa on Fu Zi: Grind Fu Zi (Aconiti Radix Lateralis) into a powder, mix with a small amount of wheat flour, and form into a paste cake 0.3–0.5cm thick. When it has dried pierce it several times with a needle. Place the Fu Zi cake on the umbilicus and place the moxa cone on top and ignite to perform moxibustion. When the cake is dry it can be replaced with another. Use 3–5 cones each time every day or every other day; continue for 1 month. (Figure 3.5.26)

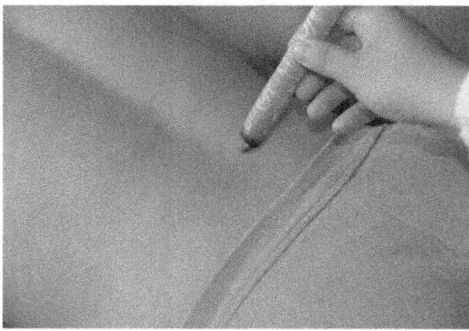

Figure 3.5.24 Gentle Pole Moxa

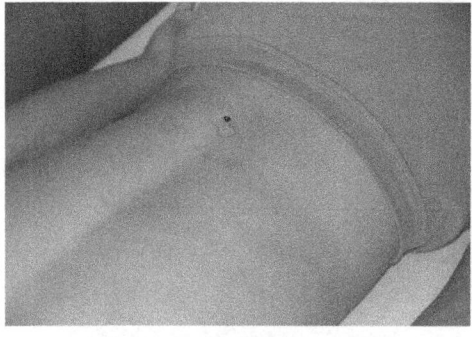
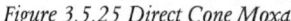

Figure 3.5.25 Direct Cone Moxa

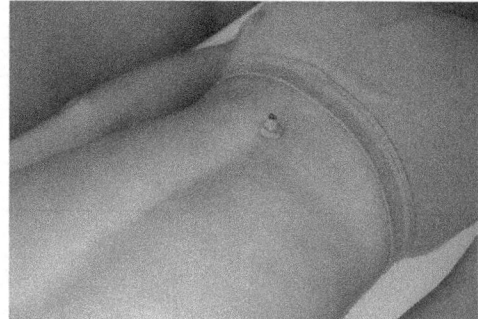

Figure 3.5.26 Cone Moxa on Fu Zi

5.11 SHEN SHU (BL-23)

BL-23 is the back transport point of the kidney, which is the root of ore-heavenly energy and the spring source for the entry and exit of essential qi. If kidney qi is abundant, essential qi will be abundant, movements nimble, brain intelligent, eyes clear, reproductive force strong, and digestive absorption and metabolism will both be vigorous. Moxa of Shen Shu can supplement and boost kidney essence, warm and open original yang, strengthen the body and the lower back, and delay the effects of ageing; so it is a common method for health cultivation. It also has special efficacy in the case of urinary and reproductive system diseases such as nephritis and seminal emission.

Moxibustion Method:

- Gentle Pole Moxa: 10–20 minutes every day or every other day. Continue for 3–6 months; one treatment course consists of 7–10 treatments. (Figure 3.5.27)

- Direct Cone Moxa: Use 3–7 cones each treatment, once every other day or every 3–5 days. One treatment course consists of one month. Continue for 2–3 months. (Figure 3.5.28)

- Warm Needle Moxa: 1–3 cones each time or for 10–20 minutes; repeat once per day or once every other day. One treatment course consists of one month. (Figure 3.5.29)

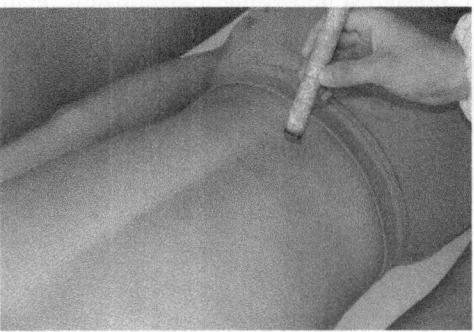

Figure 3.5.27 Gentle Pole Moxa

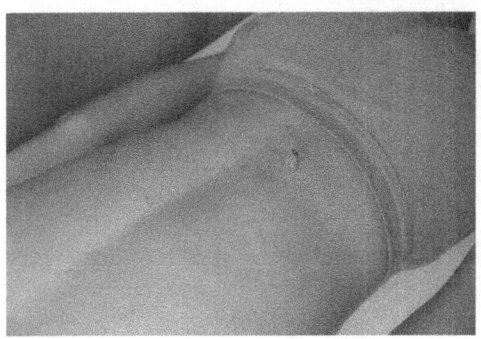
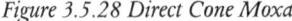

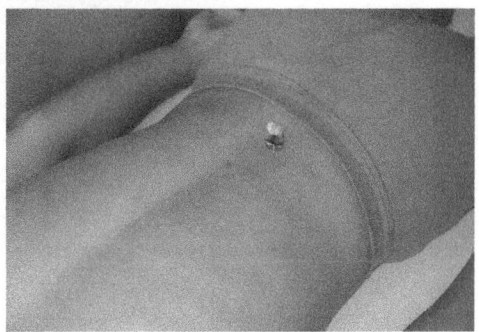

Figure 3.5.28 Direct Cone Moxa   *Figure 3.5.29 Warm Needle Moxa*

5.12 Qu Chi (LI-11)

Qu Chi is the uniting point for the large intestine channel. It can regulate the gastrointestinal functions, and protect against and treat diarrhoea, constipation and other gastrointestinal diseases. Qu Chi is located at the elbow, and moxa of this point warms the channel, dissipates cold, soothes the channels, and quickens the collaterals, making the functions of the upper limb more agile. It has a relatively good efficacy in preventing and treating common conditions such as shoulder inflammation, elbow inflammation and tennis elbow.

Qu Chi also has strong heat clearing and wind dispelling functions. It is an important point for reducing heat effusion in the case of different types of inflammatory heat effusion and diseases such as common cold and wind papules.

Moxibustion Method:

- Gentle Pole Moxa: 10–15 minutes every 1–2 days for a total of 4–5 times per month. Continue until a healthy constitution is achieved. (Figure 3.5.30)

- Cone Moxa: 3 cones each time; only one treatment is necessary. Blistering moxa can also be used: 3–5 cones each time, every other day or once per week. (Figure 3.5.31)

- Moxa on Ginger: 5–7 cones each treatment, once every day or every other day. Ten times constitutes one course of treatment. This method is most appropriate for health-protection directed at upper-limb functionality. (Figure 3.5.32)

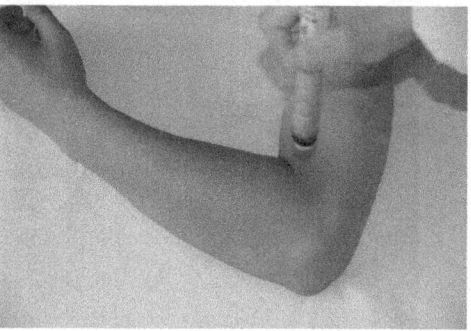

Figure 3.5.30 Gentle Pole Moxa

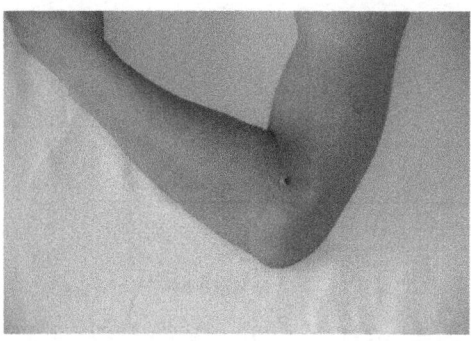

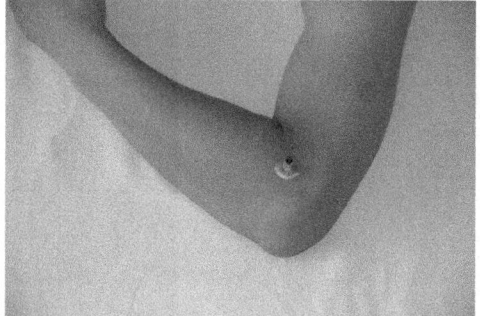

Figure 3.5.31 Cone Moxa   *Figure 3.5.32 Moxa on Ginger*

5.13 He Gu (LI-4)

He Gu is an important point for preventing and treating disease of the head, face and sensory organs. In ancient times it was said that 'He Gu is responsible for the face and mouth', and indeed it shows good efficacy in treating diseases of the five sensory organs. He Gu can be used to relieve pain and is the first point of choice when treating various types of pain syndromes. It can also dispel wind, disperse cold, resolve the exterior and regulate gastrointestinal functions. It is one of the most common life enriching health-cultivation points used extensively in self-healing.

Moxibustion Method:

- Gentle Pole Moxa: 10–20 minutes every day or every other day. Continue for 3–6 months. (Figure 3.5.33)

- Direct Cone Moxa: 3–5 cones per treatment, every other day or every 3–5 days. One month is one course of treatment; continue for 1–3 courses. (Figure 3.5.34)

- Moxa on Garlic: 3–5 cones per time, every day or every other day. This method is usually used in treatment of diseases of the head, face and sensory organs. (Figure 3.5.35)

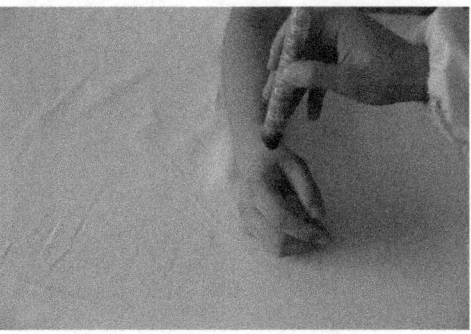

Figure 3.5.33 Gentle Pole Moxa

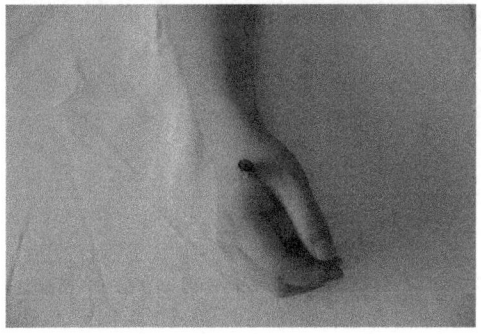
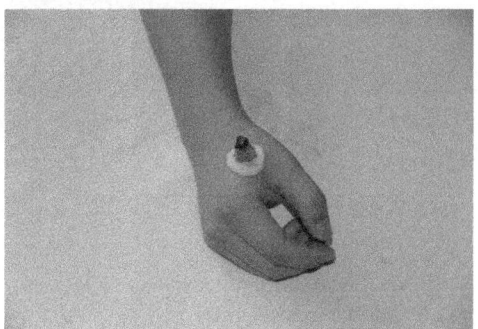

Figure 3.5.34 Direct Cone Moxa   *Figure 3.5.35 Moxa on Garlic*

5.14 SAN YIN JIAO (SP-6)

San Yin Jiao is the intersection point of the three yin foot channels, and treats disease of the liver, spleen and kidney. It has the functions of fortifying spleen, harmonizing stomach, supplementing and boosting liver and kidney, regulating menstruation and governing reproduction. Young people can moxa San Yin Jiao to prevent diseases of the reproductive system. Modern research has shown that this point has a regulatory function on the urinary, reproductive, digestive, endocrine and cardiovascular systems.

Moxibustion Method:

- Gentle Pole Moxa and Pecking Sparrow Moxa: 20–30 minutes each time, every day or every other day. Continue for at least one month. (Figure 3.5.36, Figure 3.5.37)

- Cone Moxa: 5–10 cones each time, every other day or once per week. Continue for 1–3 months. (Figure 3.5.38)

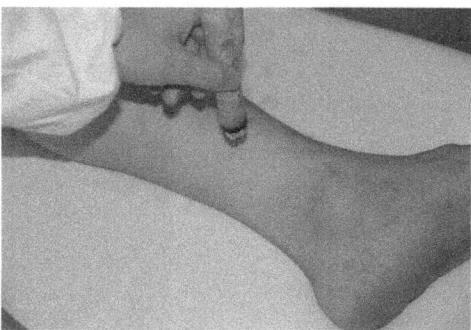

Figure 3.5.36 Gentle Pole Moxa

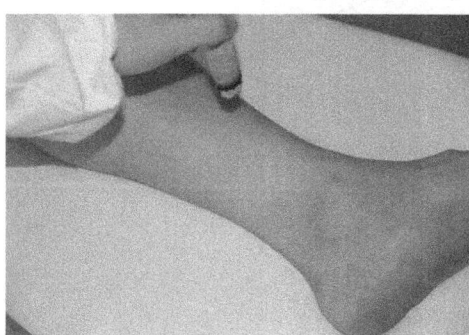
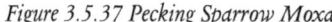

Figure 3.5.37 Pecking Sparrow Moxa

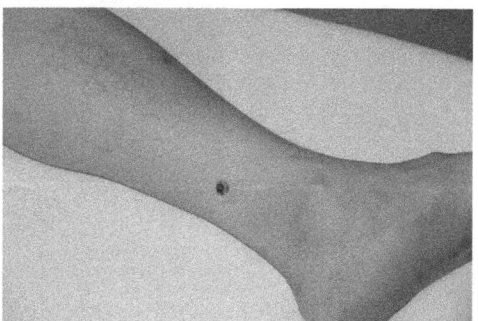

Figure 3.5.38 Cone Moxa

5.15 Yong Quan (KI-1)

Yong Quan is a point of the Foot-Shaoyin Kidney channel. This point can enrich and supplement kidney's essential qi, enhance the functional activity of the viscera and bowels, strengthen the body and resist the effects of ageing. It is a commonly used health-protection point for the elderly. Regular moxa of this point has the effects of making the body healthy, strengthening the heart and lengthening the lifespan.

Moxibustion Method:

- Moxa on Ginger: 5–10 medium-sized cones per time; stop when the local area is reddened and warm. Repeat every day or every other day. One course of treatment consists of 10 treatments; pause for 5–7 days then repeat. (Figure 3.5.39)

- Direct Moxa: 3–5 medium-sized cones per treatment; when the skin has a scorching feeling quickly replace the cone to prevent blistering. (Figure 3.5.40)

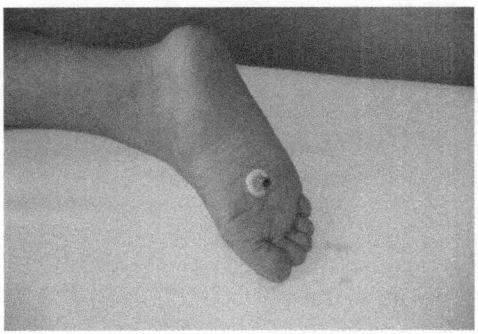

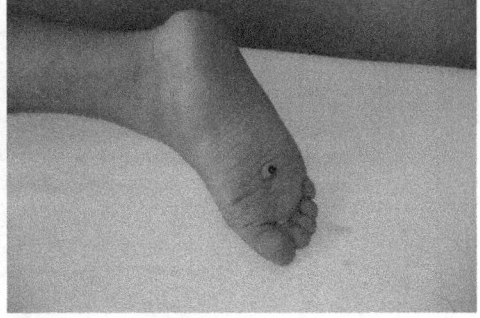

Figure 3.5.39 Moxa on Ginger   *Figure 3.5.40 Direct Moxa*

6. Common Methods of Health Cultivation Moxibustion

6.1 SPLEEN-STOMACH REGULATION

In Chinese medicine the spleen and stomach are considered to be the 'root of later, acquired heaven' and the 'source of qi and blood formation'; meaning that they are responsible for digestion, absorption, and transformation of qi and blood essence, which the body requires. When spleen and stomach are functioning normally qi and blood will be abundant and the body will be healthy. If there is dysfunction the opposite will occur: qi and blood will be insufficient and the constitution will be vacuous and weak. This moxibustion method can enhance movement and transformation of spleen and stomach, regulate gastrointestinal function, and promote digestion and absorption of nutritional material and metabolism. In this way it achieves the goal of life-enhancement and health-protection. This method is appropriate for any age group, and is a common method for preventing disease and protecting health.

Acupoints: Zu San Li (ST-36), Pi Shu (BL-20), Wei Shu (BL-21), Zhong Wan (RN-12), Tian Shu (ST-25).

Moxibustion Method:

- Gentle Pole Moxa: 10–20 minutes each time, every day or every other day. Continue for 3–6 months; one course of treatment consists of 7–10 treatments. In the case of symptoms of poor digestion, poor appetite, epigastric region distension and diarrhoea it is necessary to moxa every day, and to continue until the gastrointestinal function returns to normal. (Figure 3.6.1)

- Moxa on Ginger: Place ginger on the points listed above and use 5–10 cones per treatment. Repeat every other day or once per week, and continue for 20–30 days. This method is appropriate for individuals who are particularly averse to cold and have poor gastrointestinal function. (Figure 3.6.2)

- Moxa on Fuzi Cake: Grind Fu Zi (Aconiti Radix Lateralis) into powder, mix with a small amount of wheat flour, and form into a paste cake 0.3–0.5cm thick. When it has dried pierce it several times with a needle. Place the cake on the umbilicus, place the moxa cone on top, and ignite to perform moxibustion. When one cake is dry it can be replaced to continue the treatment. Each time use 5–7 cones, and repeat treatment every day or every other day; continue for 1–3 months. This is appropriate in the case of severe vacuity and cold. (Figure 3.6.3)

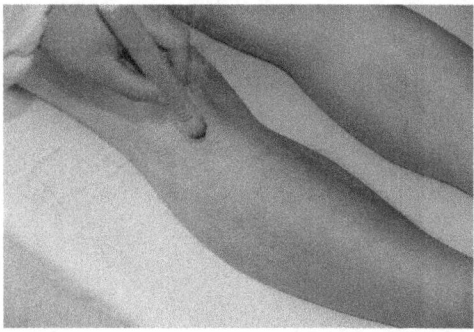

Figure 3.6.1 Gentle Pole Moxa at Zu San Li (ST-36)

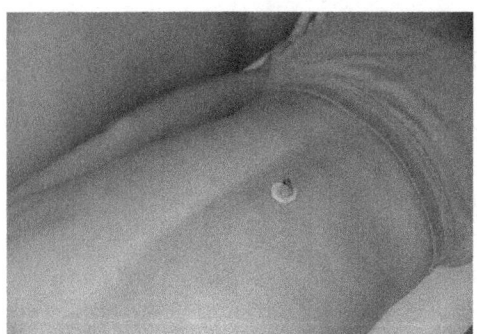 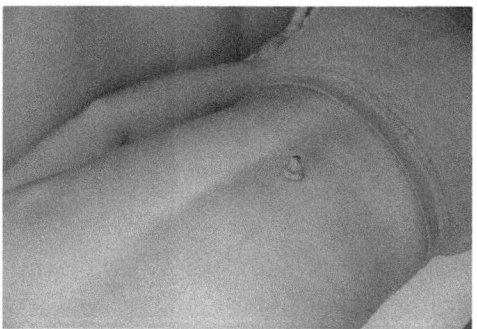

Figure 3.6.2 Moxa on Ginger at Pi Shu (BL-20)   *Figure 3.6.3 Moxa on Fu Zi at Wei Shu (BL-21)*

6.2 COMMON COLD PREVENTION

In Chinese medicine it is thought that a tendency to catch colds and suffer from flu, cough, asthma, and other respiratory system diseases is due to insufficiency of lung qi. This results in a weakened resistance to external pathogen function, making it easier to be injured by external pathogens. The warming and medicinal effects of moxibustion stimulate the related points to enhance lung function and improve the body's ability to resist external pathogens, preventing occurrence of the above diseases.

Acupoints: Fei Shu (BL-13), Da Zhui (DU-14), He Gu (LI-4), Zu San Li (ST-36), Dan Zhong (RN-17).

Moxibustion Method:

- Gentle Pole Moxa or Pecking Sparrow Moxa: 10–20 minutes every day or once every other day. Continue for at least one month. During the flu season this method can be applied to prevent flu. When an individual first catches a cold, perform the treatment 1–2 times per day, and moxa each point for 20 minutes; this can remove or reduce cold symptoms. (Figure 3.6.4)

- Direct Moxa: For individuals with constitutional vacuity who easily catch colds, use an extra small (half a grain of rice) moxa cone on the acupoint; when it has finished burning replace it with another. Use 3–7 cones each time and repeat every day or every 3 days. Continue for 1–6 months. (Figure 3.6.5)

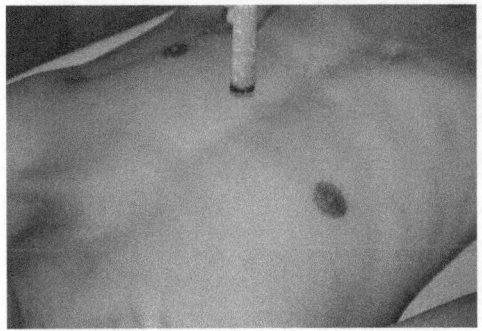
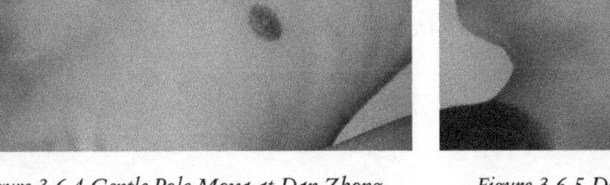

<table>
<tr><td>Figure 3.6.4 Gentle Pole Moxa at Dan Zhong (RN-17)</td><td>Figure 3.6.5 Direct Moxa at Fei Shu (BL-13)</td></tr>
</table>

6.3 HEALTH-NOURISHING SPIRIT-QUIETENING

This method can supplement and boost essential qi, quicken blood, open vessels, supplement and nourish heart-blood, improve the heart function, tranquilize and quiet the spirit, and promote sleep. It causes blood vessels to be full, the heart, spirit, qi, and blood to be regulated. Patients will be full of vigour and will be agile in thinking. It is a common method for preventing cardiovascular disease, nourishing life, protecting health, and extending one's lifespan. It can prevent and cure heart palpitations, insomnia, forgetfulness, and other symptoms related to cardiovascular disease.

Acupoints: Nei Guan (PC-6), Xin Shu (BL-15), Shen Men (HT-7), Zu San Li (ST-36), Dan Zhong (RN-17), Ju Que (RN-15).

Moxibustion Method:

- Gentle Pole Moxa: 5–10 minutes every day or every other day. Continue for 20–30 days, pause 7–10 days, and then continue. (Figure 3.6.6)

- Direct Cone Moxa: 3–5 cones each time. Moxa until the local area becomes red and moist, with a slightly yellow centre. After moxibustion the area should not be painful or blistered. Repeat once per week or every 10 days. (Figure 3.6.7)

- Moxa on Ginger: 3–7 cones each time, once every other day or once per week; continue for 20–30 days. (Figure 3.6.8)

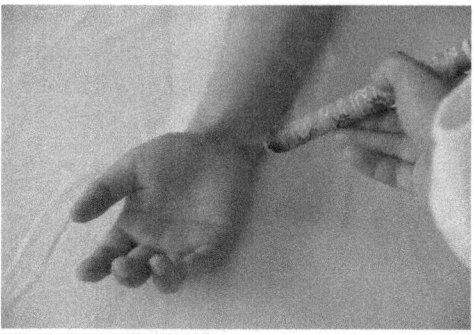

Figure 3.6.6 Gentle Pole Moxa at Shen Men (HT-7)

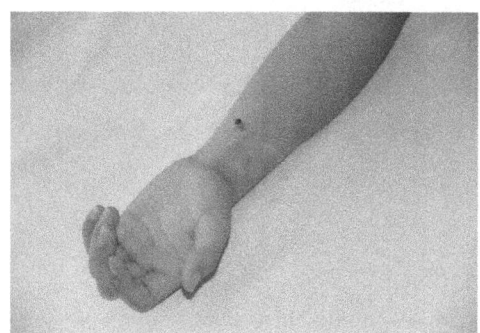

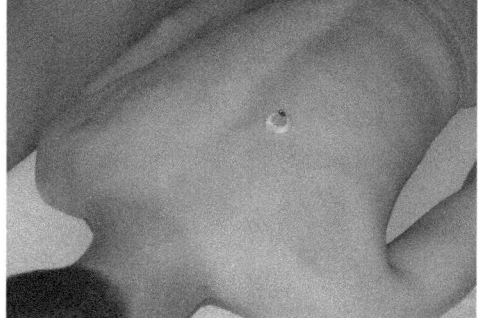

Figure 3.6.7 Direct Cone Moxa at Nei Guan (PC-6)   *Figure 3.6.8 Moxa on Ginger at Xin Shu (BL-15)*

6.4 Fortify-Brain Boost-Intelligence

This method can free the channels and collaterals, increase blood flow to the brain, regulate cerebral nerve function, vitalize energy levels, eliminate exhaustion, and improve thinking and memory ability. It is used as a self-health care method, and is especially recommended during periods of tense study and work to keep the mind alert and energy levels high.

Acupoints: Bai Hui (DU-20), Tai Yang (M-HN-9), Feng Chi (GB-20), Feng Fu (DU-16), Da Zhui (DU-14), He Gu (LI-4), Zu San Li (ST-36).

Moxibustion Method:

- Gentle Pole Moxa: 10–15 minutes every day or once every other day; continue for 1–3 months; pause for 7–10 days then continue. (Figure 3.6.9)

- Direct Moxa: 2–3 cones per point, once every 3 days or once per week. (Figure 3.6.10)

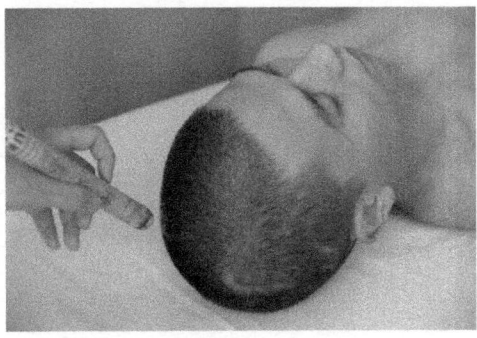

Figure 3.6.9 Gentle Pole Moxa at Bai Hui (DU-20)

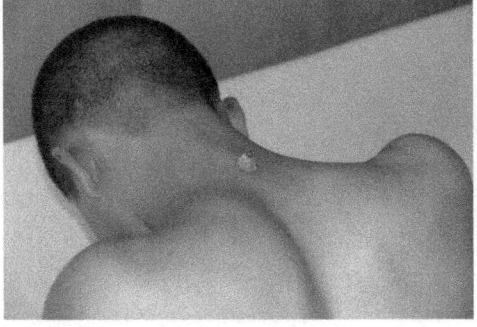

Figure 3.6.10 Direct Moxa at Da Zhui (DU-14)

6.5 SUPPLEMENT-KIDNEY STRENGTHEN-BODY

This method focuses on enriching and supplementing kidney essence and qi. It has the functions of cultivating and supplementing original qi, supplementing and nourishing qi and blood, balancing yin and yang, and regulating the endocrine system. It is an important life-enhancement and health protection method, and when used on children, it can promote their physical development; when used on middle-aged adults, abundant kidney essence results in abundant energy and physical health; when used on the elderly it can strengthen the sinews and bones, and prevent ageing. It has a regulatory effect on many organs involved in respiratory, digestive, cardiovascular, reproductive, nervous, and endocrine systems.

Acupoints: Shen Shu (BL-23), Tai Xi (KI-3), Guan Yuan (RN-4), Yong Quan (KI-1), San Yin Jiao (SP-6), Guan Yuan Shu (BL-26).

Moxibustion Method:

- Gentle Pole Moxa: 10–20 minutes, every other day or every 3 days; continue for 1–3 months with a 7–10 day rest before repeating. (Figure 3.6.11)

- Direct Cone Moxa: 5–7 cones per point, or until the local area reddens without blistering; repeat every other day or every 3 days and continue for 1–3 months. (Figure 3.6.12)

- Moxa on Ginger: Use 5–10 cones every 1–3 days or once per week; continue for 20–30 days. This method is appropriate for individuals with kidney vacuity who are averse to cold. (Figure 3.6.13)

- Moxa on Fu Zi: Grind Fu Zi (Aconiti Radix Lateralis) into a powder, mix with a small amount of wheat flour, and form into a paste cake 0.3–0.5cm thick. When it has dried pierce it several times with a needle. Place the cake on the umbilicus and place the moxa cone on top to commence moxibustion. When the cake is dry it can be replaced with another. Use 5–10 cones each time every other day or once per month; continue for 1–3 months. This is appropriate for individuals with vacuity and cold who are averse to cold and have loose bowel movements. (Figure 3.6.14)

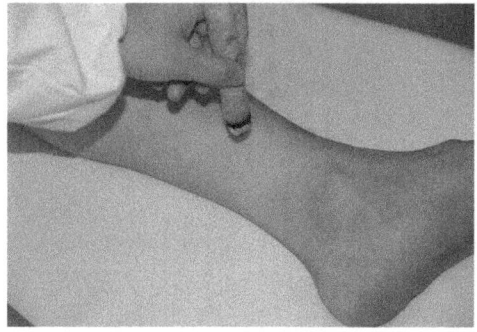

Figure 3.6.11 Gentle Pole Moxa at San Yin Jiao (SP-6)

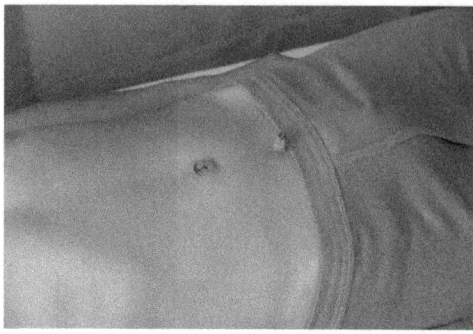

Figure 3.6.12 Direct Cone Moxa at Guan Yuan (RN-4)

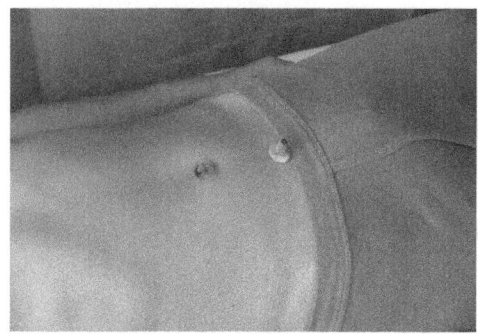

Figure 3.6.13 Moxa on Ginger at Guan Yuan (RN-4)

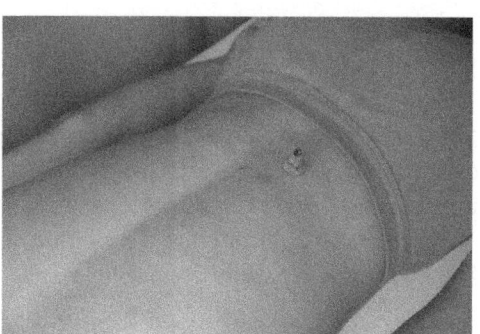

Figure 3.6.14 Moxa on Fu Zi at Shen Shu (BL-23)

6.6 Eye Health Protection

This method focuses on freeing the channel vessels, qi and blood of the eye area. It protects the eyes, helps vision to recover, nourishes blood, clears the eyes, and can also prevent and treat many different eye diseases. It is appropriate for any age group.

Acupoints: Guang Ming (GB-37), Qu Chi (LI-11), Gan Shu (BL-18), He Gu (LI-4), Tai Yang (M-HN-9), Yang Bai (GB-14), Si Bai (ST-2).

Moxibustion Method:

- Hanging Pole Moxa: Moxa each point for around 10 minutes; repeat 1–2 times per week. (Figure 3.6.15)

- Direct Moxa: 2–3 cones per point; repeat once every 2–3 days and do not cause scarring. (Figure 3.6.16)

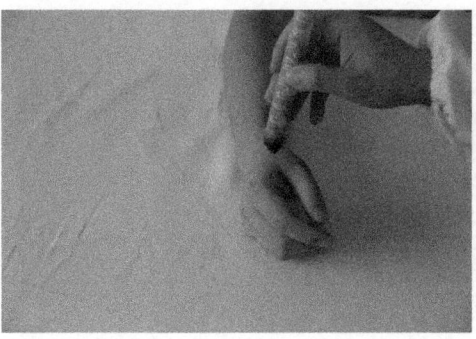

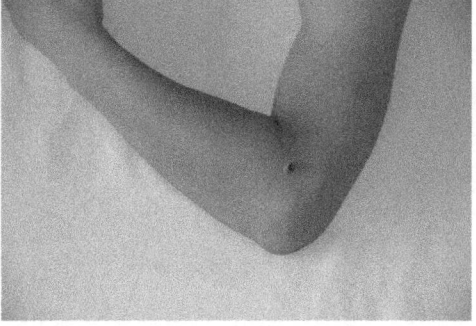

Figure 3.6.15 Hanging Pole Moxa at He Gu (LI-4)   *Figure 3.6.16 Direct Moxa at Qu Chi (LI-11)*

6.7 CHILDREN'S HEALTH CULTIVATION

During the process of children's development the full functionality of many organs is still incomplete. In Chinese medicine this is called a 'tender yin and tender yang' constitution: the viscera and bowels are tender and fragile, and physical qi has not yet become filled. On the basis of this physiological characteristic, physicians in various dynasties created many health cultivation methods, which are listed below.

Acupoints:

- To strengthen the body and protect health, choose Shen Zhu (DU-12) and Tian Shu (ST-25).

- To fortify spleen and harmonize stomach, choose Zhong Wan (RN-12), Pi Shu (BL-20), Shen Que (RN-8) and Tian Shu (ST-25).

- To supplement lung and boost qi, choose Feng Men (BL-12), Fei Shu (BL-13), Shen Zhu (DU-12), Da Zhui (DU-14) and Gao Huang (BL-43).

- To fortify the brain and boost intelligence choose Shen Zhu (DU-12), Da Zhui (DU-14), Gao Huang (BL-43) and Shen Shu (BL-23).

Moxibustion Method:

- Gentle Pole Moxa: 5–10 minutes every other day or once every 3 days; continue for 1–3 months, pause for 7–10 days and then continue. In the case of new-born infants whose body is relatively weak, one may begin to moxa Shen Zhu (DU-12) 3–6 months after birth: perform once per week or month and continue for 3–6 months. (Figure 3.6.17)

- Direct Moxa: 1–2 cones per point; repeat once every 7–10 days. (Figure 3.6.18)

- Moxa on Ginger: 3–5 cones per point; repeat once every 1–3 days or once per week; continue for 1–3 months. (Figure 3.6.19)

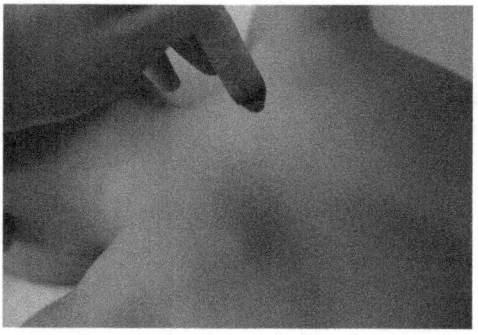

Figure 3.6.17 Gentle Pole Moxa at Shen Zhu (DU-12)

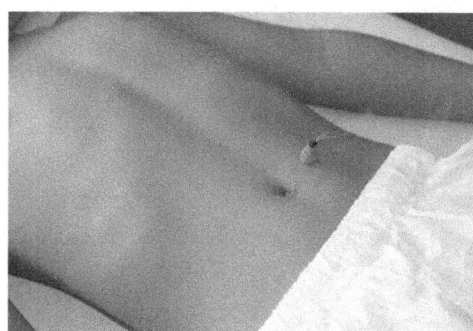

Figure 3.6.18 Direct Moxa at Tian Shu (ST-25)

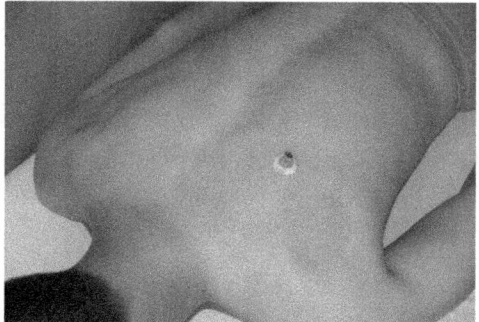

Figure 3.6.19 Moxa on Ginger at Gao Huang (BL-43)

- Moxa on Garlic: 3–5 cones each time; once every 1–3 days or once per week; continue for 1–3 months. (Figure 3.6.20)

- Moxa on Salt: Choose Shen Que (RN-8); 3–10 cones each time; once every other day or once per week; moxa for 10–30 minutes each time. (Figure 3.6.21)

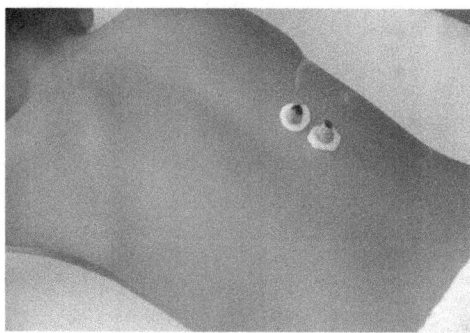

Figure 3.6.20 Moxa on Garlic at Pi Shu (BL-13) and Wei Shu (BL-21)

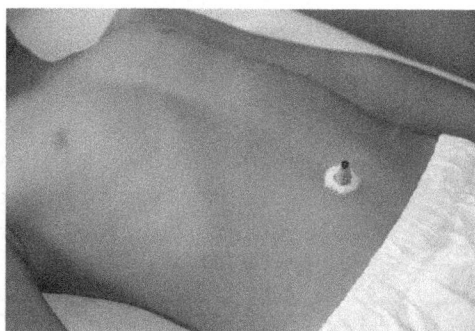

Figure 3.6.21 Moxa on Salt at Shen Que (RN-8)

6.8 MIDDLE-AGED AND ELDERLY HEALTH CULTIVATION

Moxa has the functions of enriching the kidney and liver, boosting and invigorating yang qi, quickening and moving qi and blood, and opening the channels and collaterals. It has the ability to regulate blood pressure, lower blood lipids, and strengthen the organs. As it can prevent disease, protect health and postpone ageing, it is an important health cultivation method for the middle-aged and elderly.

Acupoints:

- The combination of Zu San Li (ST-36) and Qu Chi (LI-11) can regulate blood pressure and prevent and treat stroke.

- Qi Hai (RN-6) can boost qi and secure essence, supplement kidney and assist yang.

- The combination of the three points Fei Shu (BL-13), Feng Men (BL-12) and Da Zhui (DU-14) can be used on individuals with weak constitutions who easily catch colds, or patients with respiratory system disease.

- The combination of San Yin Jiao (SP-6), Shen Shu (BL-23) and Guan Yuan (RN-4) will strongly fortify spleen and supplement kidney.

Moxibustion Method:

- Gentle Pole Moxa: Perform for 10–20 minutes per point each session. Best results are obtained by performing the treatment at 11 o'clock in the morning. Perform once every other day or every 3 days. If the individual does not have any obvious complaints, then performing the treatment once per week or 1–2 times per month will suffice. Alternatively, treatment can take place for 4–8 days in a row at the beginning of each month. Individuals who diligently continue for several months or for many years will definitely see results. (Figure 3.6.22)

- Moxa on Ginger: 5–7 cones per point per session. One treatment every 1–3 days or once per week; continue for 1–3 months. For individuals with spleen and kidney vacuity and cold, a larger number of large cones should be used. (Figure 3.6.23)

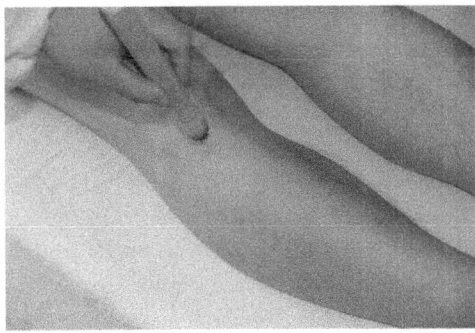
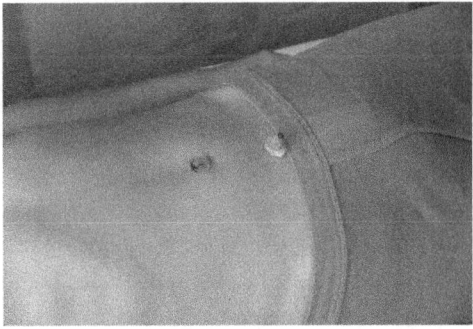

Figure 3.6.22 Gentle Pole Moxa at Zu San Li (ST-36)

Figure 3.6.23 Moxa on Ginger at Guan Yuan (RN-4)

7. Health Cultivation Moxibustion Customized for the Individual and Time

7.1 DIFFERENT TIMES AND SEASONS

As we live in a natural environment, weather and climate changes can affect our physiological functioning and pathological changes.

- Health Cultivation Moxibustion for Spring and Summer: In the spring and summer seasons dampness begins to change to heat; yang qi opens, and the interstices open and discharge. Especially after the beginning of summer and the weather becomes burning hot, it is easy to sweat and people tend to eat raw and cold foods and fruits. This makes it easy for wind, cold, summer-heat, damp, and fire pathogens to enter the skin and interstices or be carried into the intestines and stomach along with food. For these reasons, health cultivation moxibustion during this time focuses on lung, spleen, and stomach, and securing and protecting lung-defence. To resist invasion by external pathogens, regulation of the intestines and stomach and fortification of movement of spleen-earth can reduce the occurrence of disease. Moxibustion health cultivation can focus on the respiratory and digestive systems by choosing channel points on the lung, spleen, and stomach channels.

- Health Cultivation Moxibustion for Autumn and Winter: During autumn and winter the climate changes from cool to cold; yin becomes exuberant and yang vacuous. The interstices become dense and yang qi internally constrained. In order to increase the ability to resist cold, fortifying and securing the waist and knees by nourishing the kidney will strengthen the constitution. Health cultivation moxibustion may be carried out on the points of the kidney channel.

At the same time, it is also obvious that disease caused by summer-heat pathogens is also seasonal. Summer-heat is usually combined with damp, so during summer-heat days, moxibustion health-protection can be carried out on the spleen channel to fortify spleen and disinhibit damp. During autumn the weather is dry, so one should enrich yin and moisten dryness. Performing moxibustion on Tai Xi (KI-3) and Shui Quan (KI-5) on the kidney channel, Qu Chi (LI-11) on the large intestine channel, and Chi Ze (LU-5) on the lung channel will help to lessen autumn dryness.

7.2 DIFFERENT GEOGRAPHICAL ENVIRONMENTS

Due to differences in altitude and climatic conditions, as well as different living habits, people living in different areas will not have the same physiological activity or pathological characteristics. For these reasons, health cultivation moxibustion should also adjust to the local environment and the individual's living habits. For example, in the high plains of the Chinese Northwest, the weather is cold and dry with little rain. Inhabitants of rural areas spend much of their time in a windy and cold environment, and eat a lot of beef, mutton, and dairy products. Their constitutions are relatively strong, making it difficult for external pathogens to invade; for this reason, they mostly suffer from internal injury diseases. In their case, health cultivation moxibustion should be performed primarily on the back-transport points and points of Foot-Taiyang Bladder channel, as well as the point Zu San

Li (ST-36) on the Foot-Yangming Stomach channel. In the Southeast lies the ocean and beaches; low altitude areas where flatlands and marshes abound, and the climate is hot and rainy. Inhabitants of these areas eat seafood and love salt; their skin tends to be dark and their interstices open. For these reasons they often suffer from abscesses and sores and easily contract external pathogens. Moxibustion should focus on the points Xue Hai (SP-10), He Gu (LI-4) and Ge Shu (BL-17) to invigorate blood, resolve toxins, move qi and transform stasis to promote the expulsion of toxins.

The cold weather of the Northwest tends to cause combined external cold and internal heat patterns that call for the dispersion of external cold and cooling internally. In contrast, the outward draining of yang qi and resultant creation of internal cold in the heat of the Southeast calls for contraction of the outward draining yang qi and warming of the internal cold. In the case of externally contracted wind-cold pattern, in the cold Northwest large amounts of moxa should be used, while in the hot Southeast the amount of moxa used should be less: these are examples of how to adjust moxatherapy for different climates.

PART II

Techniques and Methods

CHAPTER 4

Materials and Manufacture

1. Materials

From ancient times until today, Ai Ye has been the material of choice for performing moxibustion. However, other moxibustion mediums are also used depending on the disease being treated.

1.1 Ai Ye and Ai Rong

Ai Ye is also known as mugwort or Artemisiae Argyi Folium.

- Functions: Ai Ye is aromatic, bitter, slightly warm, and non-toxic. In *Ben Cao Cong Xin* it is recorded that 'The affect of Ai Ye is pure yang; it can return yang that is verging on expiration, open the twelve channels, mobilize the three yin, rectify blood and qi, expel cold-damp, warm the uterus, stop all bleeding, warm the centre and relieve depression, regulate menstruation and quiet the foetus [...] by performing moxibustion, all channels can be penetrated and a hundred diseases can be eliminated.' Here the properties of Ai Ye as a moxibustion medium are described: it can open the channels and activate collaterals, eliminate yin cold, return yang and stem counterflow.

- Ai Rong: Ai Ye is processed into fine and soft Ai Rong (mugwort floss; Artemisiae Argyi Folium Tritum). The advantages of this form are that it can be easily shaped into different sized moxa cones, it burns easily, and is aromatic; the heat produced while burning is gentle and can penetrate the skin deeply. Additionally, Ai Ye is produced in many different regions, it is easy to harvest, requires simple processing and is economical. For these reasons, it has been used in the clinical application of acupuncture and moxibustion for thousands of years.

- Gathering and Processing: Between March and May of each year thick fresh mugwort leaves are gathered (Figure 4.1.1) and dried in the sun. When dry they are pulverized in stone mortars, sieved to remove debris, and then sun-dried again. This sequence is repeated several times until the final result is pale yellow, clean and soft mugwort floss (Figure 4.1.2). Generally speaking, direct moxibustion is performed using fine floss, while indirect moxibustion is done using coarse floss. Poor quality mugwort floss is hard and does not clump together easily; care should be taken because it does not burn evenly and the bursts of flame and heat may scatter floss and cause unintentional burns.

- Storage: Mugwort floss is superior when aged, so it should be stored for a certain length of time after processing. Because of its absorbent nature, it is easily affected by humidity. If the storage conditions are not ideal, it can become mildewed, rotten, and moth-eaten, affecting how it burns. For these reasons, it should be stored in a dry area or sealed in a dry container. In dry, sunny weather it should be taken out and sun-dried to prevent mildew and rot.

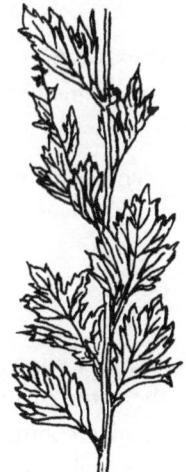

Figure 4.1.1 Ai Ye (mugwort)

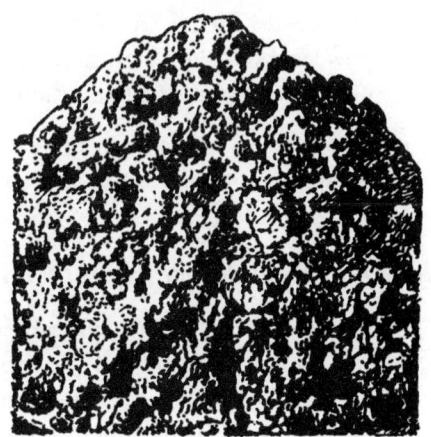

Figure 4.1.2 Ai Rong (mugwort floss)

1.2 OTHER MATERIALS

While Ai Ye is the most common moxibustion medium, there are other materials that can be used in its place. There are two classes, burning and non-burning.

*Burning**

- Deng Xin Cao: Also known as Deng Xin and Deng Cao, the marrow of the stalk of Deng Xin Cao (Junci Medulla) is sweet, bland, slightly cold, and enters the heart and small intestine channels. It has the functions of clearing the heart and disinhibiting urine. It is named Deng Xin Cao ('lamp wick grass') because it can be used in oil lanterns. It is the combustive material used in juncibustion/lantern-fire moxa.

- Beeswax: Beeswax, called Huang La or Huang Zhan in Chinese, refers to the processed wax excreted by oriental bees. It is sweet, bland and balanced. It functions to astringe, engender flesh, stop pain and resolve toxins. It is the material used in Beeswax moxa.

- Mulberry Twig: Mulberry twig (Mori Ramulus) is bitter, balanced and enters the liver channel. It dispels wind-damp, opens the channels and collaterals, disinhibits urine and lowers blood pressure. It is used in Sang Zhi (mulberry twig) moxa.

- Sulphur: This product refers to natural sulphur or refined products containing sulphur. Sulphur is warm in nature and sour in flavour. When it is placed on top of a sore and burned to treat scabs, stubborn lichen, and swelling and toxin of flat abscesses, the treatment method is called Sulphur Moxa.

- Peach Twig: The tender twigs of the peach tree are used. They are bitter in flavour, and when used in moxibustion can treat cold heart and abdomen pain, wind-cold-damp impediment, and flat abscess of the tarsal bone.

- Medicinal Lozenge: A variety of herbs and other medicinals can be ground into powder and melted with sulphur to form a medicinal lozenge (medicinal tablet) to use as a medium for moxibustion.

- Medicinal Twist: A variety of medicinals in powder form can be twisted together in cotton paper to use as a moxibustion medium.

Non-burning (Medicinal Applications)

- Mao Gen: Mao Gen (Ranunculi Japonici Herba et Radix), also known as Ye Qin Cai, Qi Pao Cao, and Lao Hu Jiao Zhua Cao, refers to the entire plant. It is acrid, warming and toxic. It abates jaundice, brings malaria under control and calms panting. After the fresh herb is pounded into pulp it can be applied to an acupoint to perform Mao Gen Moxa.

- Ban Mao: Dried Ban Mao (Mylabris) is acrid, cold, highly toxic and enters the large intestine, small intestine, liver and kidney channels. It is used to attack with toxins and expel stasis. This product contains Ban Mao shell, and as it has the effects of reddening and blistering skin and membrane, it can be used to perform Ban Mao Moxa.

- Han Lian Cao: Han Lian Cao (Ecliptae Herba), also known as Mo Han Cao, is sweet, sour, cool and enters the liver and kidney channels. Its functions are to cool blood and stop bleeding, and supplement and boost liver and kidney. The fresh herb is pound into a pulp or sun-dried and used in Hao Lian Moxa.

- Bai Jie Zi: Bai Jie Zi (Sinapis Albae Semen), is acrid, warm, and enters the lung and stomach channels. It functions to disinhibit qi and eliminate phlegm, warm the stomach and disperse cold, free the channels and stop pain, dissipate knots and disperse swelling. After the mustard glucoside undergoes hydrolysis, it has a strong stimulating effect on the skin. When ground into powder it is used in moxibustion.

- Gan Sui: Gan Sui (Kansui Radix) is bitter, cold and toxic. It enters the spleen, lung and kidney channels. Its functions are to drain accumulation of fluid in the body, break accumulations and knots, and free urine and stools. When ground into powder it can be used in moxibustion.

- Bi Ma Zi: Bi Ma Zi (Ricini Semen) is cultivated throughout China. It is sweet, acrid, balanced and toxic, and it enters the large intestine and lung channels. Its functions are to disperse swelling, expel pus, draw out toxins, lubricate the intestines and free stools. It can also be used as a medium for performing moxibustion.

2. The Manufacture of Moxa Cones and Poles

2.1 CONE MOXA

When performing moxa cone moxibustion, the burning cone-shaped clump of moxa is called a 'moxa cone'. When a moxa cone is burnt completely, this is called 'one cone' (the unit of measurement for burning moxa cones).

Method of Manufacture

Moxa cones are usually made by twisting the moxa floss into shape by hand (Figure 4.1.3). Pure aged moxa floss is placed on a flat board, and the thumb, first and middle fingers are used to pinch and twist the floss into a small round cone shape with a pointed top and flat bottom. This shape is steady and level, and when burning the temperature starts low and increases from there, making it easier for patients to tolerate. A moxa cone device (Figure 4.1.4) can also be used to manufacture the cones. The device has cone shaped depressions, each with a small hole in the tip. Moxa floss is placed in the holes, and a round metal stick is used to force the floss tightly into the hole, which forms small moxa cones when they are removed. The size of the cone depends on what condition it will be used to treat, and there are three standard sizes: small cones, the size of a grain of wheat, can be placed directly on acupoints to perform direct moxibustion; medium cones are the size of a halved jujube pit; and large cones, the size of a halved olive, are usually used for indirect moxibustion (insulated moxibustion). The medium cones are used most often in the clinic: they are 1cm in height, 0.8cm in diameter, 0.1g in weight, and burn for approximately 3–5 minutes. (Figure 4.1.5)

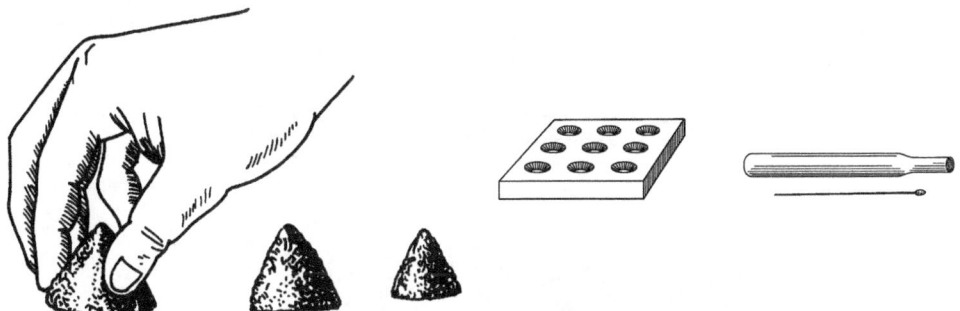

Figure 4.1.3 Manufacture of Moxa Cones by Hand   *Figure 4.1.4 Moxa Cone Devices*

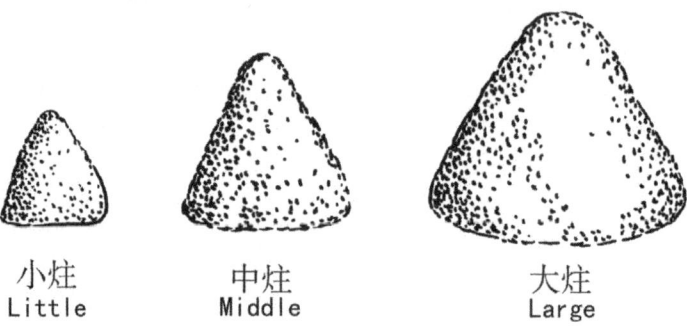

小炷
Little

中炷
Middle

大炷
Large

Figure 4.1.5 Moxa Cones

2.2 POLE MOXA

Also called rolled or stick moxa, this refers to a long round pole composed of rolled moxa floss. Depending on whether or not other herbs are included, it is divided into two types: pure pole moxa and medicinal pole moxa. Generally the pole is 20cm long and 1.2cm in diameter.

Method of Manufacture

- Pure Pole Moxa: 24g of processed aged moxa floss is spread on a 26 x 26cm (8 x 8 *cun*) piece of soft and durable mulberry paper, then rolled up tightly into a pole measuring 1.5cm (0.35 *cun*) in diameter, and glued or pasted shut. (Figure 4.1.6)

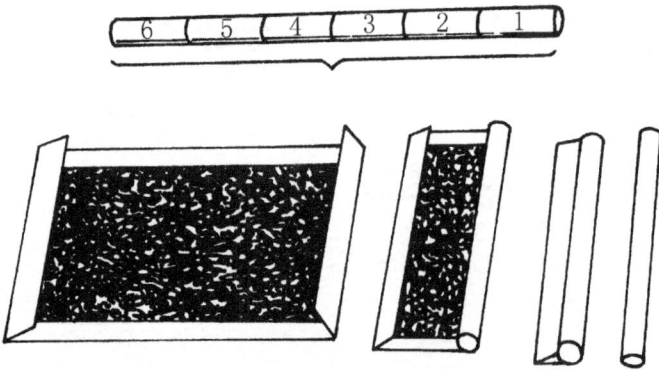

Figure 4.1.6 Pole Moxa

- Medicinal Pole Moxa: There are a variety of different types, but the most common are: Regular Medicinal Pole Moxa, Tai Yi Needle, Lightning-Fire Needle, Hundred-Effusions Amazing Needle, Disperse-Impediment Amazing Fire Needle, Yin-Pattern Poison-Dispersing Needle, etc.

- ○ Regular Medicinal Pole Moxa: Grind equal amounts of Rou Gui (Cinnamomi Cortex), Gan Jiang (Zingiberis Rhizoma), Mu Xiang (Aucklandiae Radix), Du Huo (Angelicae Pubescentis Radix), Xi Xin (Asari Herba), Bai Zhi (Angelicae Dahuricae Radix), Xiong Huang (Realgar), Cang Zhu (Atractylodes), Mo Yao (Myrrha), Ru Xiang (Olibanum), and Chuan Jiao (Zanthoxyli Pericarpium) into powder. Combine 6g of the powder with moxa floss to make one moxa pole.

- ○ Tai Yi Needle (also called Tai Yi Amazing Needle): Grind 125g of Ren Shen (Ginseng Radix), 250g of Shen San Qi (Notoginseng Radix), 62.5g of Shan Yang Xue (Naemorhedi Goral Sanguis), 500g of Qian Nian Jian (Homalomenae Rhizoma), 500g of Zuan Di Feng (Schizophragmatis Radicis Cortex), 500g of Rou Gui (Cinnamomi Cortex), 500g of Chuan Jiao (Zanthoxyli Pericarpium), 500g of Ru Xiang (Olibanum), 500g of Mo Yao (Myrrha), 250g of Chuan Shan Jia (Manis Squama), 500g of Xiao Hui Xiang (Foeniculi Fructus), 2000g of Qi Ai (Crossostephii Folium), 1000g of Gan Cao (Glycyrrhizae Radix), 2000g of Fang Feng (Saposhnikoviae Radix), and a small amount of She Xiang (Moschus) into powder. Using one layer of cotton paper and two layers of gaofang paper (41x40cm), mix 25g of powder into the mugwort floss and wrap tightly. On the outside wrap it thickly with 6–7 layers of mulberry paper and store in a dry place.

- ○ Lightning-Fire Needle (also called Lightning-Fire Amazing Needle): 94g of Moxa Floss, and 9g each of Chen Xiang (Aquilariae Lignum Resinatum), Mu Xiang (Aucklandiae Radix), Ru Xiang (Olibanum), Yin Chen (Artemisiae Scopariae Herba), Qiang Huo (Notopterygii Rhizoma et Radix), Gan Jiang (Zingiberis Rhizoma), and Chuan Shan Jia (Manis Squama) into powder. Place one piece of cotton paper on the table and fold another piece in half and place on top. Spread the moxa floss on top, and tap it lightly with a wooden ruler to make it spread evenly out in a square. Use a spoon to spread the medicinal powder over the floss. Wrap tightly, paint with egg white, then wrap thickly with 6–7 layers of mulberry paper and store in a dry place.

- ○ Hundred-Effusions Amazing Needle: 9g each of Ru Xiang (Olibanum), Mo Yao (Myrrha), Sheng Chuan (Aconiti Radix Cruda), Fu Zi (Aconiti Radix Lateralis Praeparata), Xue Jie (Daemonoropis Resina), Chuan Wu (Aconiti Radix), Cao Wu (Aconiti Kusnezoffii Radix), Tan Xiang Mo (Santali Albi Lignum), Jiang Xiang Mo (Dalbergiae Lignum Pulveratum), Da Bei Mu (Fritillariae Thunbergii Bulbus), and She Xiang (Moschus), 49 pieces of Mu Ding Xiang (Caryophylli Fructus), and 100g of Qi Ai (Crossostephii Folium). The method of manufacture is the same as that of Tai Yi Needle.

- ○ Disperse-Impediment Amazing Fire Needle: 1 Wu Gong (Scolopendra), 3g each of Wu Ling Zhi (Trogopteri Faeces), Xiong Huang (Realgar), Ru Xiang (Olibanum), Mo Yao (Myrrha), A Wei (Ferulae Resina), San Leng (Sparganii Rhizoma), Mu Bie (Momordicae Semen), E Zhu (Curcumae Rhizoma), Gan Cao (Glycyrrhizae Radix), Pi Xiao (Natrii Sulfas Non-Purus), 6g each of Nao Yang Hua (Rhododendri Mollis Flos), Liu Huang (Sulphur), Chuan Shan Jia (Manis

Squama), Ya Zao (Gleditsiae Fructus Abnormalis), 9g of She Xiang (Moschus), 1.5g of Gan Sui (Kansui Radix), and 60g of Moxa Floss. The method of manufacture is the same as that of Tai Yi Needle.

∘ Yin-Pattern Poison-Dispersing Needle: 3g each of Ru Xiang (Olibanum), Mo Yao (Myrrha), Qiang Huo (Notopterygii Rhizoma et Radix), Du Huo (Angelicae Pubescentis Radix), Chuan Wu (Aconiti Radix), Cao Wu (Aconiti Kusnezoffii Radix), Bai Zhi (Angelicae Dahuricae Radix), Xi Xin (Asari Herba), Ya Zao (Gleditsiae Fructus Abnormalis), Liu Huang (Sulphur), Chuan Shan Jia (Manis Squama), Da Bei Mu (Fritillariae Thunbergii Bulbus), Wu Ling Zhi (Trogopteri Faeces), Rou Gui (Cinnamomi Cortex), Xiong Huang (Realgar), 1g each of Chan Su (Bufonis Venenum) and She Xiang (Moschus), and 30g of Moxa Floss. The method of manufacture is the same as that of Tai Yi Needle.

CHAPTER 5

Classes of Moxibustion and Their Operation

1. Classes of Moxatherapy

Moxatherapy has been used to treat disease since ancient times. In the beginning there was only moxibustion, but later many different methods developed from the original form. They are generally classified into moxa combustion methods using the herb Ai Ye (moxa; mugwort; Artemisiae Argyi Folium) and non-moxa combustion methods. 'Moxa' moxibustion includes, for example, cone moxa, pole moxa, warm-needle moxa. Of these, cone and pole moxa are applied the most often in clinical practice and compose the majority of moxatherapy theory. Cone moxa can be further divided into direct and indirect moxibustion depending on whether the moxa is in direct contact with the skin or if it is separated from the skin using another layer of material. Common non-moxa combustion methods include lantern-fire combustion, medicinal combustion and electronic heat moxibustion. The classification of combustion methods is shown in Figure 5.1.1.

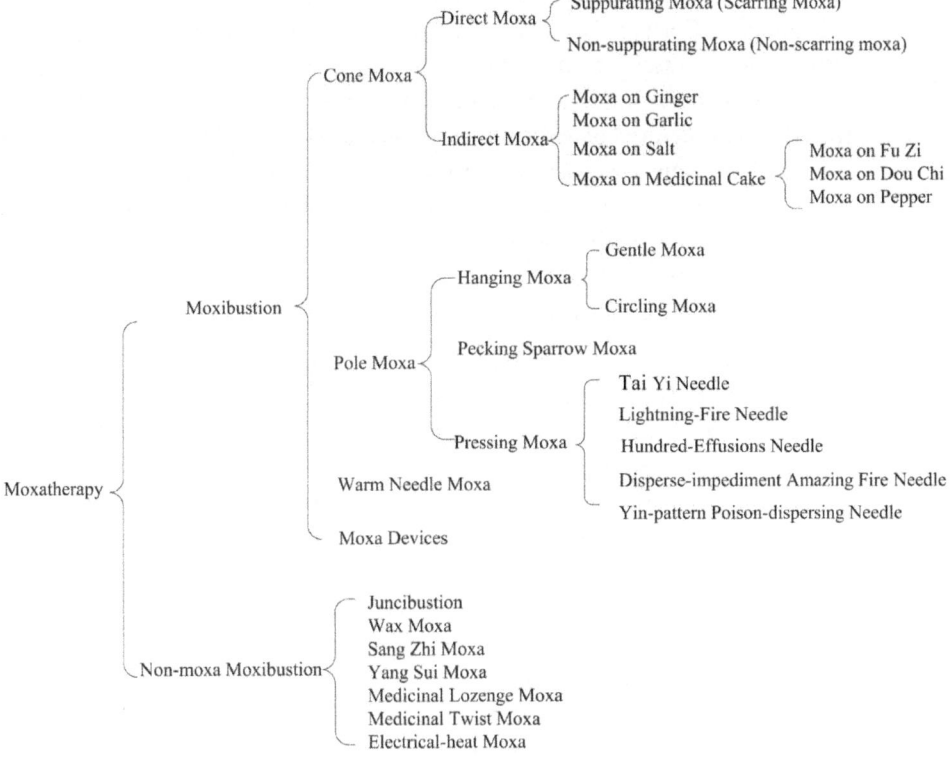

Figure 5.1.1 Classification of Moxibustion Methods

2. Operation of Moxatherapy

2.1 MOXIBUSTION

Cone Moxa

Placing cones of moxa on acupoints to perform moxibustion is called cone moxibustion. It can be divided into direct and indirect moxibustion.

DIRECT MOXIBUSTION

Placing moxa cones directly on the skin to perform moxibustion is called direct moxibustion. Depending on whether the moxibustion is intended to result in burning and suppuration or not, direct moxibustion is further divided into scarring and non-scarring moxibustion.

- Scarring Moxa:* Also known as suppurative moxibustion or burning moxibustion. The moxa cone is in direct contact with the skin during moxibustion and results in burning; the local tissue festers and suppurates, leaving a permanent scar (Figure 5.2.1). The method is as follows:

  - Locate the Point: As this method takes a relatively long time and is extremely painful, it is necessary for the patient to assume a comfortable and level position. After the position is assumed, a stick or brush dipped in gentian violet is used to mark the position of the point to be treated.

  - Perform Moxibustion: First make a moxa cone as required; other than pure moxa, aromatic medicinals such as Ding Xiang (Caryophylli Flos) and Rou Gui (Cinammomi Cortex) (i.e. Ding Gui San (Clove and Cinnamon Powder)) can also be added to assist the heat in penetrating deeply. Next, daub a small amount of scallion juice or Vaseline on the area to assist with sticking and strengthen the stimulation. After placing the cone on the point, light it with a stick of incense. Each time a cone burns through, swab the area with a piece of gauze dipped in cool water, then repeat the above procedure. Between 7–9 cones can be used each time. As this method is rather painful, the practitioner can lightly tap on the surrounding area to reduce the sensation of burning. Besides this, anaesthesia can also be used to prevent pain.

  - Apply Medicinal Paste: After finishing moxibustion, wipe the local area clean, then apply Yu Hong Gao or a bandage; the covering should be replaced every 1–2 days. Several days later, the treated area should gradually develop a non-bacterial suppurative reaction. If there is excessive pus, the medicinal paste should be changed frequently. After approximately 30–40 days the scab on the moxibustion sore will fall off, leaving a scar. During the period of suppuration, care should be taken to keep the local area clean to prevent infection and other inflammatory complications. At the same time, the overall efficacy of this treatment can be improved by consuming more nutritious foods to promote the normal granulation of the moxibustion sore. This method was common in ancient China and, besides being used as part of regular health-care maintenance, was used primarily to treat stubborn and difficult to treat diseases such as asthma, sloughing flat abscess, pulmonary consumption and wind-damp-cold impediment.

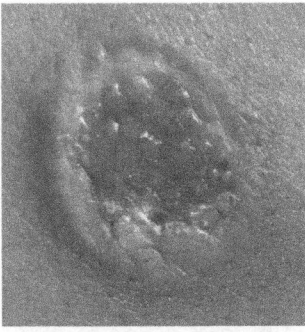

Figure 5.2.1 Scarring Moxa

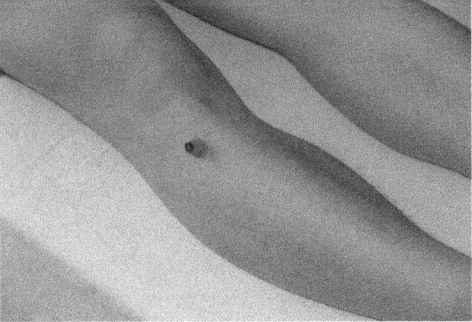

Figure 5.2.2 Non-scarring Moxa

- Non-scarring Moxa: Also referred to as non-suppurative moxa. In this method application of moxibustion is limited by how much heat the patient can tolerate, and does not create a moxibustion sore or scarring (Figure 5.2.2). The method is as follows: first wipe a small amount of Vaseline on the area to be treated, then place a small moxa cone on the moxa point and light it. Do not wait for the moxa to burn down to the level of the skin; once the patient has a sensation of burning, use tweezers to remove or extinguish the moxa cone, then replace it with a new cone. Use between 3 and 7 cones, and stop when the skin reddens slightly. Patients can more easily tolerate this method, as it does not leave a scar. It is indicated for vacuity-cold diseases and syndromes, and various types of paediatric vacuity syndromes, including abdominal pain, diarrhoea, lower back pain, menstrual pain and impotence.

INDIRECT MOXIBUSTION

Also known as insulated moxibustion. In this method a layer of material is first placed on the point, then the moxa cone is placed on top (see Figure 5.2.3). Many different types of material can be used. The heat felt by the patient is relatively mild, and it combines moxibustion with a medicinal function. It is easy for patients to tolerate and is used more often than direct moxibustion. It is indicated, for example, in the treatment of chronic diseases and sores.

- Moxa on Ginger: Cut fresh ginger into slices 0.3cm thick and pierce the centre several times to make holes. Place a moxa cone on top then place the ginger on the skin. When the patient has a sensation of burning the ginger slice can be raised off the skin for a moment, turned around, and replaced on the same area to continue moxibustion. This can be repeated several times. Alternatively, when the patient feels burning, a piece of paper or thin cardboard can be placed under the ginger. Continue until local reddening occurs (Figure 5.2.4). Raw ginger is acrid in flavour and slightly warm in nature. It has the effect of resolving the exterior, dissipating cold, warming the centre and controlling vomiting. For these reasons, this method is often used in cases of externally contracted exterior patterns and vacuity-cold diseases like common cold, cough, wind-damp impediment pain, vomiting, abdominal pain and diarrhoea.

- Moxa on Garlic: Cut a single clove of garlic into slices 0.3cm thick, and pierce the centre of the slice several times to make holes. Place the garlic on an acupoint or affected area and perform moxibustion. After burning 4 moxa cones replace the garlic slice (Figure 5.2.5). Between 5–7 cones can be applied to each acupoint. Extra attention is necessary as stimulation of garlic juice on the skin leads to easy formation of blisters. Garlic is acrid in flavour and warm in nature. It has the effect of resolving toxins, fortifying the stomach and killing worms. This method is most often used in the treatment of pulmonary consumption, accumulation lumps in the centre of the abdomen, and pre-ruptured sores and boils.

- Long-Snake Moxa (Attachment): Also known as spread moxa, in this method 500g of garlic is mashed into paste and spread along the patient's spine, from Da Zhui (DU-14) to Yao Shu (DU-2) in a long ribbon approximately 2.5cm thick and 6cm wide. Both sides are lined with tissue paper, and then medium sized moxa cones are placed at Da Zhui and Yao Shu. Moxibustion continues until the patient can taste garlic in their mouth (Figure 5.2.6). After moxibustion, warm water is used to soak the tissue paper and the garlic paste is wiped away. Due to the stimulation from the garlic and heat, blisters will form along the skin over the spine, which require care and attention. This method is a popular folk remedy and is used for treating stubborn vacuity-taxation impediment.

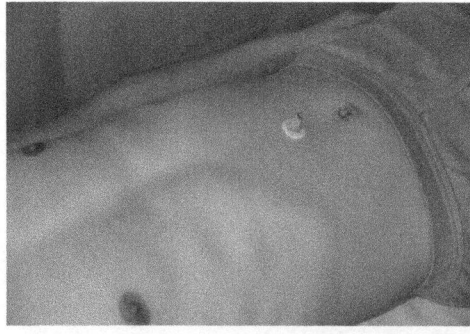
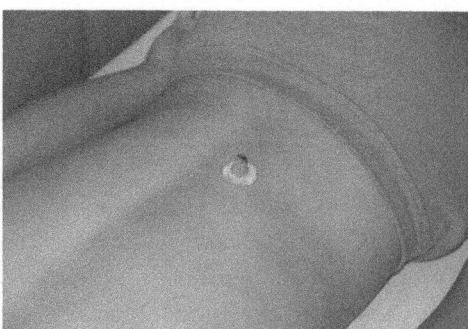

Figure 5.2.3 Indirect Moxa   Figure 5.2.4 Moxa on Ginger

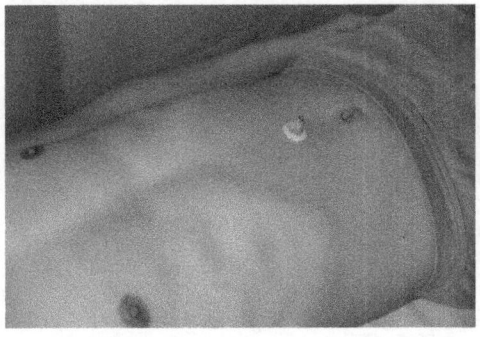
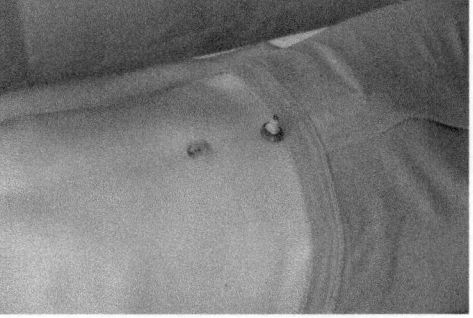

Figure 5.2.5 Moxa on Garlic   *Figure 5.2.6 Long-Snake Moxa*

- Moxa on Salt: Also known as Shen Que (RN-8) moxa, this method is only used on the umbilical region (Figure 5.2.7). With the patient lying supine with knees bent, fill the umbilicus with pure dry edible salt, place a slice of ginger on top, and place the moxa cone on top of the ginger to perform moxibustion. If the patient's umbilicus protrudes, wet strands of noodle can be used to encircle the area, like the mouth of a well. This is filled with salt and moxibustion is performed as above. This method has the effect of renewing yang and stemming counterflow in cases of qi desertion syndromes such as copious sweating and yang collapse presenting with cold limbs and hidden pulse. In the case of acute abdominal pain, vomiting and diarrhoea, dysentery, reversal cold of the limbs and vacuity qi desertion patterns, large moxa cones can be used to continuously perform moxibustion. Moxibustion should continue until the sweating ceases, the pulse is no longer hidden, the body's warmth returns and other symptoms show improvement.

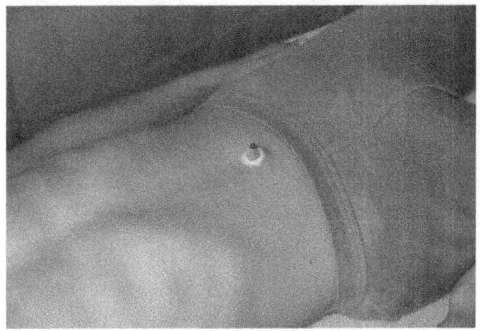
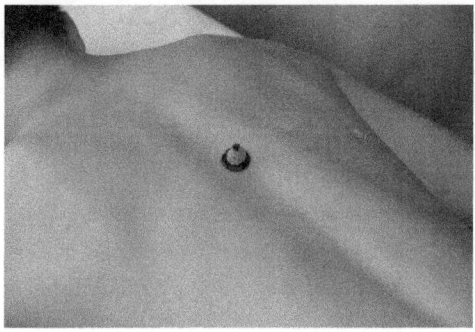

Figure 5.2.7 Moxa on Salt   *Figure 5.2.8 Moxa on Fu Zi (cake)*

- Moxa on Fu Zi (Cake): This method is performed by placing the moxa cones on top of slices of Fu Zi (Aconiti Radix Lateralis Praeparata) or on a Fu Zi cake, which is made by grinding the Fu Zi into a powder and mixing with yellow wine to form cakes measuring 0.3cm thick and 2cm in diameter (Figure 5.2.8). As Fu Zi is acrid and warming, it has the effect of warming the kidneys and supplementing yang. It is therefore used in the treatment of various types of yang vacuity patterns such as impotence and premature ejaculation. It is also used in external medicine to treat sores that fail to close, or yin-vacuity sores that do not suppurate or disperse. The choice of location for moxibustion can be based on the condition of the illness. When the cake is dry replace it with a fresh one and continue until the skin is reddened. In recent times Fu Zi or other warming aromatic medicinals have been used to make pre-made medicinal cakes for performing indirect moxibustion. During moxibustion a layer of gauze can be placed under the cake to prevent burning. Medicinal cakes can be re-used.

- Moxa on Fermented Soybeans: Mild fermented soybeans (Dou Chi) are ground into powder and passed through a filter. According to the size of the sore, mix an appropriate amount of powder with yellow wine to make a cake. The cake should be neither too hard nor too soft, and should be approximately 0.3cm thick. Place it around the sore and light moxa cones on top. Do not injure the skin and repeat once per day until the sore is completely resolved (Figure 5.2.9). Fermented soybeans are bitter in flavour and cold in nature, and have the effect of resolving the exterior, promoting sweating and eliminating vexation. This method is indicated for sores and flat abscesses of the back, and swollen hard malignant sores that do not rupture or heal. It is most effective in the case of dark coloured sores, and can promote healing of sores.

- Moxa on Pepper: Mix the desired amount of white pepper powder with flour and water to form cakes 0.3cm thick and 2cm in diameter with a slight depression in the middle. Fill the depression with medicinal powder Ding Xiang (Caryophylli Flos), She Xiang (Moschus), Rou Gui (Cinnamomi Cortex), and place a moxa cone on top (Figure 5.2.10). Between 5–7 cones may be used or until the patient feels a comfortable level of warmth. Pepper is acrid in flavour and hot in nature, so it has the effect of warming the middle and dispersing cold. It is usually used for treating stomach cold with vomiting, abdominal pain with diarrhoea, wind-cold-damp impediment and facial numbness.

- Moxa on Ba Dou: Grind 10 Ba Dou (crononis fructus) seeds into a powder and mix with 3g of white flour to form a paste, and then squeeze it into a small flat cake. Place the cake on Shen Que (RN-8) and place a moxa cone on top to perform moxibustion. This can be combined with moxa on scallion for even better results. An alternative method is to mix the Ba Dou seed powder with Huang Lian (Coptidis Rhizoma) powder instead of flour (Figure 5.2.11). Moxibustion can be performed daily or every other day, and 5–8 cones can be used each time. This type of indirect moxibustion has the effect of freeing bowel movements, disinhibiting urine, rectifying qi and relieving pain, dispersing accumulation and dissipating binds. It can be used in the case of food accumulation, abdominal pain, diarrhoea, constipation, urinary stoppage, tightness of the chest and scrofula.

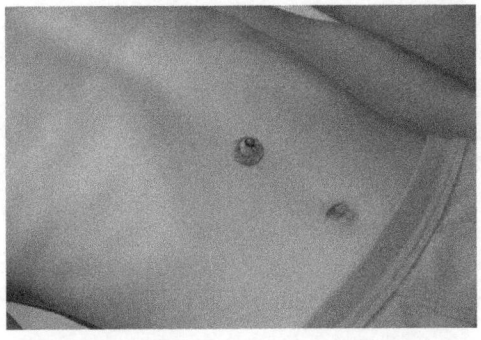

Figure 5.2.9 Moxa on Fermented Soybeans

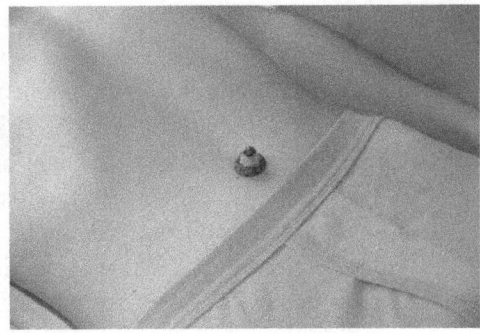

Figure 5.2.10 Moxa on Pepper

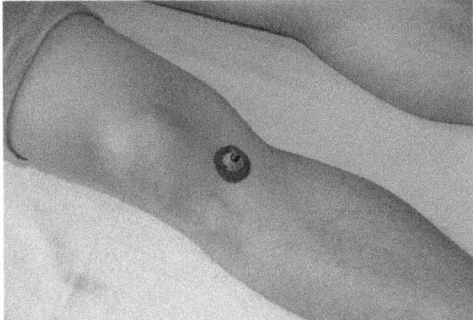

Figure 5.2.11 Moxa on Ba Dou

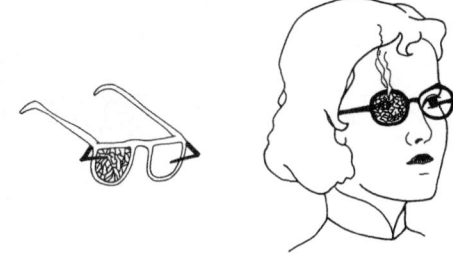

Figure 5.2.12 Moxa on Walnut Shell

- Moxa on Yellow Earth: Mix clean yellow soil with water to form a mud cake approximately 0.6cm thick and 5cm wide. Make several holes through it with a needle and place it on the affected area. Between 7–21 moxa cones are used per session, with a new cake used each time the cone is replaced. This method has the effects of quickening blood and dissipating stasis, and can be used in the treatment of swelling and toxins resulting from welling and flat abscesses, as well as in the case of injury due to knocks and falls.

- Moxa on Walnut Shell: This method is also referred to as 'Eye Moxa on Walnut Shell'. Split a walnut open along the centreline and remove the nut. Bend thin metal wire to resemble the frame from a pair of glasses, with two curved extensions from the outside of the frame to in front of the eyes. Before moxibustion, soak the walnut shells in chrysanthemum water for 3–5 minutes, and then place them over the eyes (or eye). Place 1.5cm long segments of moxa pole on the frame extensions, light the moxa, and then place the glasses frame on the patient's face (Figure 5.2.12). This method has the effect of dispelling wind and brightening the eyes, quickening blood and freeing the collaterals, and reducing inflammation and pain. It is indicated for conjunctivitis, near-sightedness, central retinitis and optical nerve atrophy.

- Moxa on Wheat Flour: Mix wheat flour with water to form a small cake approximately 0.5cm thick. Pierce it many times with a needle, place it on the affected area, and place a moxa cone on top to commence moxibustion (Figure 5.2.13). Wheat flour is made by grinding the wheat and sieving out the bran. According to Ben Cao Gang Mu, its nature and flavour is as follows: 'The nature of new wheat is hot, old wheat is balanced. Wheat flour is sweet and warm.' It enters the heart, spleen and kidney channels, and has the functions of nourishing the heart, boosting the kidney, eliminating heat, allaying thirst and dispersing swelling. This method is appropriate for use in the case of malign sores, welling abscess swelling and external injury with blood stasis.

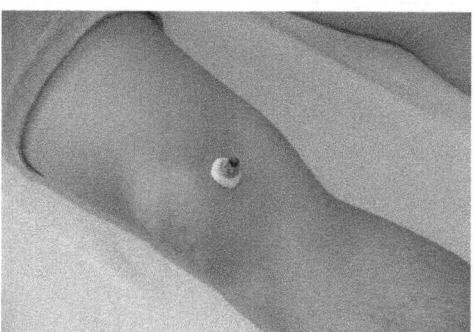

Figure 5.2.13 Moxa on Wheat Flour

Pole Moxa

Pole Moxa is a type of moxibustion that makes use of specially manufactured rolls of moxa to warm, smoke or burn acupoints. If medicinals of an acrid, warming and aromatic nature are combined with the moxa floss, it is called medicinal pole moxibustion. There are two types of pole-moxibustion: hanging moxibustion and pressing moxibustion.

Hanging Moxa

In this method the lit end of the moxa pole is suspended above the area receiving moxibustion treatment. The burning end is kept approximately 3cm away from the surface of the skin, and moxibustion is performed for 6–20 minutes; the skin should be warm and reddened but not burned. There are three methods of performing hanging moxibustion: gentle moxibustion, circling moxibustion and pecking sparrow moxibustion.

- Gentle Moxa: One end of the moxa pole is lit and is pointed at the acupoint from a distance of 2–3cm. Moxibustion is performed for 6–15 minutes; the skin should be warm and reddened but not burnt (Figure 5.2.14). When treating patients that are unconscious or have lessened sensitivity at the acupoint, or when treating children, the practitioner may place the index and middle fingers on the skin at either side of the acupoint in order to judge the level of heat and adjust the distance and duration accordingly. Gentle moxibustion is appropriate for a variety of conditions and syndromes.

- Pecking Sparrow Moxa: While performing moxibustion using this method, the burning end of the moxa pole does not maintain a fixed distance from the surface of the skin, but rather moves up and down like a sparrow pecking seeds off the ground (Figure 5.2.15). It is used in the treatment of children's diseases or when reviving an unconscious patient.

- Circling Moxa: When using this method, the distance between the burning tip of the moxa pole and the surface of the skin does not change, but the position is not fixed, and the tip of the pole moves from left to right or in a circle (Figure 5.2.16). It is used in the treatment of pain due to wind damp impediment, neuroparalysis, and conditions featuring a relatively large area of pathology.

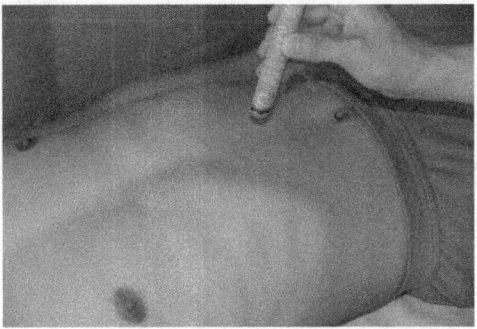

Figure 5.2.14 Gentle Moxa

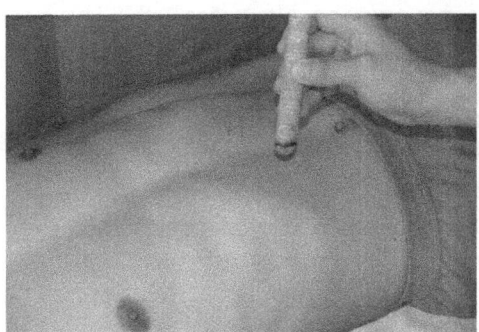
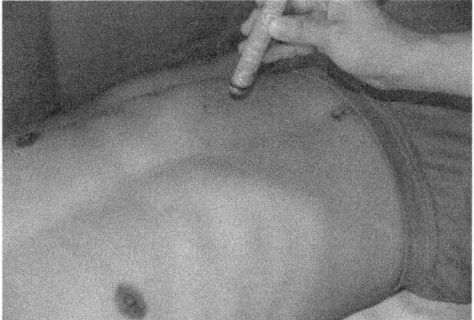

Figure 5.2.15 Pecking Sparrow Moxa

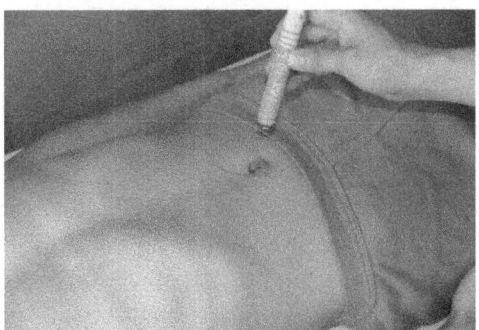

Figure 5.2.16 Circling Moxa

PRESSING MOXA

During moxibustion, a layer of cloth or several layers of tissue are placed over the area to be treated. The burning end of a medicinal moxa pole is then pressed on the cloth or paper, causing heat to penetrate deeply (Figure 5.2.17). As there are various uses of this method and different medicinal formulas, it can be divided into categories such as Tai Yi Amazing Needle, Lightning-Fire Amazing Needle, Hundred-Issuances Amazing Needle.

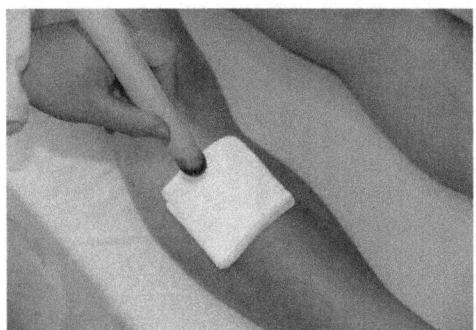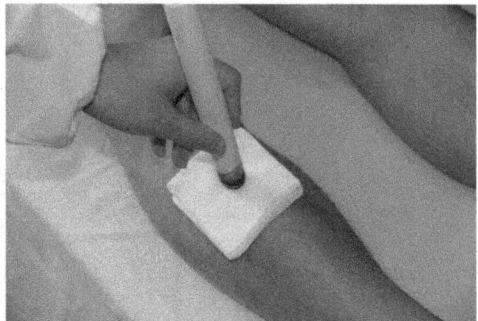

Figure 5.2.17 Pressing Moxa

- Tai Yi Needle (also called Tai Yi Amazing Needle): Use an ethanol lamp to light one end of the medicine pole and wrap it in several layers of coarse cloth. Press the burning end on an acupoint or diseased area until it is no longer hot. Light it again and repeat the procedure 5–7 times per acupoint. Alternatively, 6–7 layers of cotton paper or cloth can be placed on the acupoint first, and then the burning end of the moxa pole is pressed directly upon the cloth for 1–2 seconds. If the ember is extinguished it can be lit again. This procedure should be repeated 5–7 times. This method has the following objectives: to open the channels and invigorate the collaterals, disperse stasis and move blood, warm the centre and disperse cold, expel wind and damp, repel turbidity and resolve toxins, diffuse impediment and stop pain. It can be used in the case of wind-cold-damp impediment, atrophy pattern and vacuity-cold pattern.

- Lighting-Fire Needle (also called Lightning-Fire Amazing Needle): This method was first mentioned in the 6th chapter of *Ben Cao Gang Mu* and is the predecessor of Tai Yi Needle. The method of operation is similar to that of Tai Yi Needle. It has the functions of warming the centre and transforming damp, rectifying qi to stopping pain, dispelling wind and opening the collaterals, soothing the sinews and invigorating blood. It can be used in such cases as wind-cold-damp impediment, joint tetany pain, atrophy pattern, abdominal pain and diarrhoea.

- Hundred-Effusions Amazing Needle: This is a type of pressing-moxibustion and is, in fact, very similar to Tai Yi Needle. It first appeared in the work *Zhong Fu Tang Gong Xuan Liang Fang* by the Qing Dynasty physician Ye Gui. It has the function of quickening blood and dispelling stasis, transforming phlegm and dissipating knots, tracking down wind and diffusing impediment, moving qi and stopping pain. It can be used in cases of unilateral wind in the head, frozen shoulder, crane's-knee wind, hemiplegia, lump glomus, lower back pain, small intestine mounting qi, welling and flat abscess.

- Disperse-Impediment Amazing Fire Needle: This method was recorded in the 2nd chapter of *Chuan Ya Wai Bian*. The method of operation is very similar to that of Tai Yi Needle. It has the functions of opening the channels and invigorating the collaterals, dispersing stasis and quickening blood, dispersing impediment and breaking apart accumulations, transforming phlegm and softening hardness, dispelling impediment and settling pain. It is primarily for treating patterns such as emaciation due to partiality to certain foods, as well as abdominal masses and lump glomus.

- Yin-Pattern Poison-Dispersing Needle: This method was also recorded in *Chuan Ya Wai Bian*, and the method of operation is the same as Tai Yi Needle. It has the functions of warming the channels and opening the collaterals, dispersing stasis and quickening blood, transforming phlegm and dispersing knots, dispersing yin and resolving toxins. It is primarily used to treat yin-pattern, welling and flat, abscesses.

- Fire-Needle Pad Moxibustion (also known as Pad Moxibustion): Decoct 15g of dry ginger slices to obtain 300ml of liquid, and mix with wheat flour to form a thin paste. Apply the paste to 5–6 layers of clean white cotton cloth (non-synthetic cloth) to make a hard pad. After the pad has dried cut it into squares approximately 10x10cm in preparation for use. When performing moxibustion, place the square pads on the area to be treated, then press the lit end of the moxa pole on the pad and hold it there for approximately 5 seconds or until a burning sensation is felt. Repeat 5 times then change to another acupoint. The local skin should be reddened. This method has the functions of soothing sinews and quickening collaterals, dispelling impediment and stopping pain, boosting kidney and strengthening yang, stopping cough and stabilizing panting. Clinically it is used in the treatment of joint pain, orthopaedic pain patterns, enuresis, yang-fistula, asthma, and chronic stomach and intestine conditions.

WARM NEEDLE MOXA

This method combines acupuncture needling and moxibustion, and is applicable to all diseases that require both retained needles and moxibustion. The method of operation is as follows: after needling and obtaining the arrival of qi, retain the needle at an appropriate depth. Place a 1.5cm long segment of moxa pole on the handle of the needle or squeeze a small amount of moxa floss onto the end of the handle and commence moxibustion. When burning is complete, knock off the ash and remove the needle (Figure 5.2.18). This method, combining acupuncture and moxibustion, is simple and easy to perform. The heat from the burning moxa floss is conveyed through the needle into the body, achieving the treatment goal by maximizing the effects of both needle and moxa. When using this method it is important to prevent the burning ember from falling onto the skin or cloth. The patient should be instructed not to move during treatment, and a thick piece of paper or cardboard can be placed under the burning moxa to protect against burns in the event of falling moxa. This method has the functions of warming the centre and expelling cold, resolving wind and alleviating damp, dispelling impediment and opening the collaterals, dispersing stasis and quickening blood, strengthening the body and maintaining health. It can be used to treat patterns such as wind-cold-damp impediment, and can also be used to support health and improve immune function.

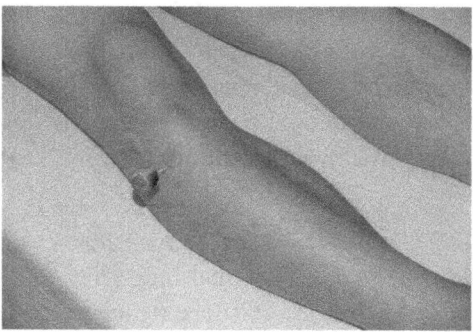

Figure 5.2.18 Warm Needle Moxa

Moxa Devices

This refers to devices that are used specifically for performing moxibustion. Commonly used examples include the Moxa Tube, Moxa Box and Moxa Frame. First mugwort floss or pole moxa is placed in the device and ignited, and then the device is used to apply heat to acupoints or the area of disease until the local area is reddened. This method has the effect of warming the centre and dispersing cold, dispelling wind and eliminating damp, soothing the sinews and quickening the collaterals, diffusing impediment and reducing pain. It is indicated for the following patterns: wind-cold-damp impediment, abdominal pain, diarrhoea, abdominal distension, and atrophy pattern. As it is also appropriate for women, children and nervous patients, its usage is quite common.

2.2 Other Moxibustion Methods

In this section other methods of moxibustion are introduced. These methods do not make use of the herb Ai Ye (moxa; mugwort; Artemisiae Argyi Folium), as seen in conventional moxibustion, but rather use other herbs or materials to achieve a similar effect. In some methods the herbs are spread or applied to the treatment area and no combustion is involved. They include such practices as 'heavenly moxibustion', 'juncibustion' or 'lantern-fire moxibustion', 'medicinal application' and 'joss stick moxibustion'.

Non-combustion Medicinal Moxibustion

Heavenly Moxa (Medicinal Blistering Method)

Heavenly moxibustion is also known as 'self moxibustion', 'medicinal moxibustion' and 'blistering moxibustion'. In this method medicinal herbs that have a stimulating or irritating effect on the skin are spread or otherwise applied to acupoints or diseased areas. The treatment effect results from hyperaemia and blistering of the local area. As the outcomes of reddening and blistering are similar to those resulting from moxibustion, this method is known as 'heavenly' or 'natural' moxibustion. In most cases a single type of medicinal herb is used, although in some cases compound formulas are used.

- Mao Gen Leaf Moxa: Mao Gen (Ranunculi Japonici Herba et Radix), also known as 'tiger paw grass', refers to the entire herb, including the root. Mao Gen is acrid, warm and toxic. Method: pound an appropriate amount of fresh Mao Gen leaf to a pulp and apply to acupoints or the diseased area. At first a feeling of itchiness or heat will be apparent, which is followed by reddening and hyperaemia, then blistering. After the blisters recede a darker, skin pigmentation will remain, which will fade naturally. The herb is usually applied for 1–2 hours. Application on Jing Qu (LU-8), Nei Guan (PC-6), and Da Zhui (DU-14) can treat malaria; application to Xi Yan (MN-LE-16) (with special care taken to avoid infection of blisters) can treat crane's-knee wind; when combined with table salt to form pellets and applied to Shao Shang (LU-11) and He Gu (LI-4) it can treat acute conjunctivitis.

- Garlic Paste Moxa: Pound garlic (purple-skinned garlic is best) into a pulp and apply 3–5g to each acupoint. Retain for 1–3 hours or until a burning sensation or blistering occurs. This method is used primarily in the treatment of various bleeding disorders, swelling and pain of the throat, dysentery, vomiting and neurodermitis. It can also be used for menstrual pain (dysmenorrhoea). If applied to Yong Quan (KI-1) it can treat expectoration of blood (haemoptysis) and nosebleed; if applied to He Gu (LI-4) it can treat tonsillitis; if applied to Yu Ji (LU-10) it can treat painful swelling of the throat.

- Bai Jie Zi Moxa: Bai Jie Zi (Sinapis Albae Semen) is acrid in taste, warm in nature, and associates with the lung channel. Its function is to warm the lung and dispel phlegm, disinhibit qi and disperse knots, disperse swelling and stop pain. Bai Jie Zi moxibustion is most effective in treating cold-phlegm panting and cough. Grind Bai Jie Zi into a powder and mix with vinegar into a paste. Apply 5–10g of the paste to each acupoint, cover with a thin layer of plastic sheet, and fix with adhesive tape. Alternatively, grind 1g of the herb into a powder; place it in the middle of a round bandage 3cm in diameter, and stick the bandage directly onto an acupoint. The herb is usually retained for 2–4 hours, or until hyperaemia and reddening or blistering occurs. This method is applicable in cases of patterns such as wind-cold-damp impediment pain, pulmonary tuberculosis, wheezing and panting, and deviated mouth and eyes. In the clinic it is common to use compound formulas based on Bai Jie Zi during the three days representing the periods of greatest heat (san fu tian) to treat bronchial asthma and bronchitis. A common compound formula and its usage are as follows: 21g mix-fried Bai Jie Zi (Sinapis Albae Semen), 21g Yuan Hu (Corydalis Rhizoma), 12g Gan Sui (Kansui Radix), 12g Xi Xin (Asari Herba). Grind the above herbs into a powder and place them in a receptacle in preparation for use. On each of the three days attributed to greatest heat mix 1/3 of the powder with fresh ginger juice and a small amount of She Xiang (Moschus) to make a paste, then spread the paste on 6 pieces of oilpaper each 3cm in diameter. Apply these to Fei Shu (BL-13), Xin Shu (BL-15), Ge Shu (BL-17), Gao Huang (BL-43), Bai Lao (DU-14) and Dan Zhong (RN-17), and fix with adhesive tape. Retain the herbs for 4–6 hours each time. Perform once every

10 days; namely once on the first, middle and last days of greatest heat. A course of treatment consists of three treatments per year for three years in a row, for a total of 9 treatments. As this treatment can cause blistering, it should be used with care when treating patients with a tendency for allergic hypersensitivity.

- Han Lian Cao Moxa: Pound fresh Han Lian Cao (Ecliptae Herba) into a pulpy paste, apply to acupoints, and fix in place with a sticking plaster. Retain the herbs for 1–4 hours or until reddening and hyperaemia or blistering occur. This method is appropriate for treating malaria.

- Ban Mao Moxa: Ban Mao (Mylabris) is acrid, warm and toxic. It enters the liver and stomach channels and can break concretions and dissipate knots, attack toxins and erode sores, as well as fight tumours. Grind an appropriate amount of Ban Mao in advance. To use, first cut a small hole (approximately the size of a soybean) in the middle of an adhesive plaster and stick the plaster on the acupoint so the treatment area is exposed and the surrounding skin is protected. Apply a small amount of Ban Mao powder into the hole and fix in place with another piece of adhesive plaster. Retain until blistering occurs. Other options include: mix the Ban Mao powder with Vaseline and spread it on the acupoint or diseased area; soak the Ban Mao powder in vinegar or 95% alcohol for 10 days, and then spread it on the diseased area. The herb is usually retained for 2–3 hours. This method is usually used to treat asthma, psoriasis, neurodermatitis, neuralgia, and arthritis. As Ban Mao is highly toxic and stimulating to the skin, take care not to allow non-treatment areas (especially the mouth) to be exposed to the powder.

- Wei Ling Xian Moxa: Pound Wei Ling Xian (Clematidis Radix) leaves (tender ones are best) into a paste and mix in a small amount of cane sugar. Apply the paste to an acupoint and cover with disinfectant gauze. When a sensation of crawling ants occurs immediately remove the herbs. Blistering is desirable but the stimulation should not be too strong. Apply to Zu San Li (ST-36) to treat haemorrhoids with descent of blood; apply to Tai Yang (M-HN-9) to treat acute conjunctivitis; apply to Shen Zhu (DU-12) to treat hundred-day cough (whooping cough); apply to Tian Rong (SI-17) to treat tonsillitis.

- Cong Bai (Scallion White) Moxa: Clean an appropriate amount of Cong Bai (Allii Fistulosi Bulbus), mash into a pulp and apply to an acupoint or diseased area. In the case of mastitis it can be applied directly to the diseased area. In the treatment of infantile malnutrition, mash scallion white, fresh ginger and fresh Gan Ji Cao (Rungiae Herba) into a pulp and apply to Yong Quan (KI-1) before bed; remove in the morning upon arising from bed.

- Ban Xia Moxa: Mash equal amounts of mix-fried Ban Xia (Pinelliae Rhizoma) and scallion whites into a pulp and apply to acupoints or the diseased area. This method is used in the treatment of acute mastitis. Another optional method is to roll the medicinal paste into a stick shape and insert it into the nostril. Retain for 30 minutes and repeat twice per day.

- Ba Dou Shuang Moxa: Grind equal amounts of Ba Dou Shuang (Crotonis Fructus Pulveratus) and Xiong Huang (Realgar) into a powder and mix evenly. Place a meng-bean sized amount of powder in the centre of a 1.5 x 1.5cm piece of adhesive plaster and place one behind each of the patient's ears on the mastoid process (equivalent to GB-12) and retain for 7–8 hours. This can successfully treat malaria if applied 5–6 hours before it occurs.

MEDICINAL APPLICATION MOXIBUSTION

This type of moxibustion is also known as medicinal effect moxibustion. Although this method, like heavenly moxibustion, involves the application of medicinals on acupoints, it differs in that blistering usually does not occur. It makes use of the therapeutic effect of the medicinal to achieve the treatment goal. The medicinals used are primarily acrid, fragrant, mobile and penetrating, and provide a certain degree of stimulation to the acupoints or skin. For these reasons, this method is considered a form of moxibustion. As there are a various medicinals used, all with different therapeutic effects, the range of application of this technique is broad.

- Ma Qian Zi Moxa: Grind an appropriate amount of Ma Qian Zi (Strychni Semen) into a powder, apply to an acupoint and fix with adhesive plaster. An example of its common application is on Xia Che (ST-6) and Di Cang (ST-4) in the treatment of facial paralysis (Bell's palsy).

- Tian Nan Xing Moxa: Grind an appropriate amount of Tian Nan Xing (Arisaematis Rhizoma) into a powder and mix with raw ginger juice to make a paste. Apply to an acupoint, cover with a layer of plastic and gauze, and tape in place. It can be used to treat facial paralysis by applying the paste to Xia Che (ST-6) and Quan Liao (SI-18).

- Gan Sui Moxa: Grind an appropriate amount of Gan Sui (Kansui Radix) into a powder, apply it to an acupoint, and fix in place with adhesive plaster. Alternatively, combine the Gan Sui powder with an appropriate amount of wheat flour and add warm water to make a doughy paste. It can be applied directly to an acupoint, covered with oilpaper, and fixed in place with adhesive tape. Examples of its use include application to Da Zhui (DU-14) to treat malaria; application to Fei Shu (BL-13) to treat asthma; and application to Zhong Ji (RN-3) to treat retention of urine.

- Wu Zhu Yu Moxa: Grind an appropriate amount of Wu Zhu Yu (Evodiae Fructus) into a powder and mix with vinegar into a thick paste. Apply the paste to an acupoint, cover with a sheet of plastic, and fix in place with an adhesive plaster. It can be replaced every 1–2 days, with a course of treatment consisting of 7 applications. Some treatment examples include bilateral application to Yong Quan (KI-1) for treating high blood pressure, mouth ulcers and oedema in children; application to the umbilicus to treat malnutrition, cold pain in the epigastric region, stomach-cold vomiting, and vacuity-cold chronic diarrhoea. It can also be combined with Huang Lian (Coptidis Rhizoma): grind both into a powder and mix with vinegar to form a thick paste, and apply to Yong Quan (KI-1) to treat acute tonsillitis.

- Sheng Fu Zi Moxa: Grind an appropriate amount of Sheng Fu Zi (Aconiti Radix Lateralis Cruda) into a powder and add water to make a thick paste. Apply to an acupoint, cover with a thin layer of plastic wrap, and fix in place with adhesive tape. This can be used to treat toothache when applied to Yong Quan (KI-1).

- Wu Bei Zi Moxa: Grind equal amounts of Wu Bei Zi (Galla Chinensis Galla) and He Shou Wu (Polygoni Multiflori Radix) into a powder and mix with vinegar into a thick paste. Apply to an acupoint, cover with oilpaper and fix with adhesive tape. An example of its use is in the treatment of enuresis: apply to the umbilicus Shen Que (RN-8) before sleeping and remove in the morning.

- Bi Ma Ren Moxa: Take an appropriate amount of Bi Ma Ren (Ricini Semen), remove the hulls and pound into a pulp. Apply it to an acupoint and fix in place with an adhesive plaster. Some examples of its application include: Yong Quan (KI-1) in treating difficult delivery; Bai Hui (DU-20) in treating uterine prolapse, rectal prolapse and gastroptosia.

- Xi Xin Moxa: Grind an appropriate amount of Xi Xin (Asari Herba) into a powder and add a small amount of vinegar to make a thick paste. Apply to the acupoint, cover with oilpaper and fix with adhesive plaster. Apply to Yong Quan (KI-1) or Shen Que (RN-8) to treat infantile stomatitis.

- Fresh Ginger Moxa: Pound an appropriate amount of fresh ginger into a pulp and apply to an acupoint or diseased area. Cover with oilpaper or gauze and fix with adhesive tape. It can be used to treat frost damage when applied to the injured area.

- Jing Jie Sui Moxa: Smash an appropriate amount of Jing Jie Sui (Schizonepetae Flos) then heat it in a pan. Quickly insert into a cloth bag and apply to the area of disease. It is applicable in the treatment of urticaria.

- Wu Mei Moxa: Take an appropriate amount of the flesh of Wu Mei (Mume Fructus), add vinegar, and pound into a pulp. Apply it to the diseased area. When treating corns and calluses, first soak the patient's feet in warm water, scrape off the surface layer of the cuticle, then paste the medicinal pulp onto the area. Retain for 12 hours.

- Fennel Moxa: Take 100g of fennel, 50g of dried ginger, and 500g of vinegar residue (Aceti Residuum). Heat them in a pan, place them in a cloth bag and apply to the acupoint of the diseased area for 5–10 minutes. This method can be used to treat patterns such as cold pain of the abdomen and cold impediment.

- Ya Dan Zi Moxa: Pound an appropriate amount of Ya Dan Zi (Bruceae Fructus) into a pulp, apply to the diseased area and fix in place with adhesive plaster. Take care not to apply to healthy skin. It is primarily applicable to verruca vulgaris.

- White Pepper Moxa: Grind an appropriate amount of white pepper into a powder, apply to the acupoint, and fix in place with adhesive plaster. Application to Da Zhui (DU-14) can treat malaria.

- Wu Jing Hua Moxa: Take 100g of Wu Jing Hua (Brassicae Rapae Flos) and soak in vinegar for 1 day. Add 12g of Xiong Huang (Realgar), 20g of Dan Nan

Xing (Arisaema cum Bile), and 10g of white pepper and grind into a powder in preparation for use. Insert an appropriate amount of the powder into the umbilicus level with the surface of the abdomen and fix in place with adhesive tape. This method can be used to treat epilepsy.

Medicinal Moxibustion

- Sulphur Moxa:* In this form of moxibustion sulphur is used as the combustive material. In the early Song Dynasty Wang Huai-Yin recorded the following in the 61st chapter of *Tai Ping Shen Hui Fang*: 'Sulphur moxibustion should be used in the case of chronic channel atrophy. Take a small amount of sulphur, depending on the size of the sore, place it on the fire, then take out a burning piece with silver tweezers and apply it to the sore 3–5 times until the pus appears and the sore is dry.' This method is used in the treatment of stubborn sores and their associated fistulas.

- Wax Moxa: In this method wax is melted to perform moxibustion. The first step is to use wheat flour to make dough, form it into a wet snake, and circle it around the swollen root of the sore. It should be approximately 3cm in height. Surround the dough ring with several layers of cloth to prevent the skin from being burnt. Place several pieces of wax (approximately 1cm high) inside the ring. Heat up a bronze (or steel) spoon and use it to melt the wax until there is a mild burning sensation. If the fistula is relatively deep, more wax can be added until the dough ring is full. If the heat causes the wax to bubble and the treatment area feels itchy, followed by unbearable pain, immediately cease the treatment. When finished sprinkle a small amount of cold water on the wax, and when it is cool remove the cloth, dough ring and wax. This method is similar to the modern style of wax therapy. In Zhou Hou Fang this method is recorded as a treatment for bites by rabid dogs, and today it is used in cases such as wind-cold-damp impediment, innominate toxic swelling, sores and shank sores.

- Tobacco Moxa: When no moxa is available, tobacco (in the form of a cigarette) may be used instead. This method warms the channels, disperses cold and activates blood.

- Juncibustion:* This method is also known as Deng Cao moxibustion, oil-twist moxibustion, Thirteen Yuan Xiao fire, or, in Jiangsu Province, light-the-lantern fire. In this method Deng Xin Cao (Junci Medulla) is dipped in either sesame or Su Zi (Perillae Fructus) oil, lit and then quickly applied to an acupoint to burn the skin. Deng Xin Cao is a perennial herb, the medicinal component is obtained by removing the skin, retaining the marrow of the stalk and drying it in the sun. The method of use is as follows: first dip the Deng Xin Cao in sesame oil and light it, then quickly apply the lit end to the chosen acupoint and remove immediately. When this is done, there will be a slight 'pop-pop' sound. Juncibustion has the effects of coursing wind and dissipating the exterior, moving qi and disinhibiting phlegm, resolving depression and opening the chest, arousing the clouded spirit and settling convulsions. It is primarily used to treat disease patterns such as infantile wind due to fright, stupor, convulsions, hordeolum, acute tonsillitis, cervical tuberculosis lymphadenitis and parotitis.

- Tao Zhi Moxa: In this method Tao Zhi (a peach twig; Persicae Ramulus) is used as the moxibustion medium. A tender twig, 16–20cm in length and approximately as thick as a thumb, from a rosaceae or mountain peach is dried. When performing moxibustion, place 3–5 layers of cotton paper on the treatment area. Dip the peach twig in sesame oil and light. Extinguish the flame and press the end on the paper over the acupoint or diseased area. It can be performed once every day or every other day. Each area should receive moxibustion until it reddens. This method is primarily for treating cold pain in the upper abdomen, wind-cold-damp impediment and bone flat abscess (suppurative osteomyelitis).

- Sang Zhi Moxa: In this method Sang Zhi (a mulberry twig; Mori Ramulus) is used as the moxibustion medium. A twig or piece of wood from the mulberry tree is cut to a length of 23cm and the thickness of a finger. The end is first lit, then extinguished, and applied to the area of disease. It can be performed 3–5 times per day, each time for 5–10 minutes. Tender twigs can be collected at the end of spring or beginning of summer; the leaves are removed and the twig is sun-dried. It is bitter and balanced, and when taken internally it can dispel wind-damp, disinhibit the joints, and move water-qi. Mulberry twig moxibustion is primarily used in the treatment of swelling and toxins or sores: in the case of sores that have not yet ulcerated, it has the effect of drawing out toxins and stopping pain; in the case of ulcerated sores it can supplement and boost yang qi, eliminate putridity and engender flesh. It also has the effect of warming yang and dispelling cold, freeing stasis and dispersing binds. It is often used in the treatment of scrofula and streaming sores.

- Zhu Ru Moxa: In this method, Zhu Ru (Bumbusae Caulis in Taenia) is used instead of moxa. Zhu Ru is the shavings of the inner layer of bamboo stalks. It is sweet and cool, and when taken internally can clear heat, cool blood, transform phlegm and halt vomiting. When used to perform moxibustion, Zhu Ru has the effect of resolving toxins, dispersing swelling, and stopping pain. It is primarily used to treat welling abscess swelling, insect bites and snakebites.

- Ma Ye Moxa: The leaves and flowers of Da Ma (Cannabis) are used to perform moxibustion. Ma Ye (Cannabis Folium) is acrid and toxic: when taken internally it can treat malaria, asthma and kill roundworms. When used to perform moxibustion, it has the effect of dispersing swelling and dispelling binds, engendering flesh and closing sores. It can be performed once every day and 5–10 cones can be used. It primarily treats sores and haemorrhoids.

- Matchstick Moxa:* In this method a matchstick is used as the moxibustion medium. After the matchstick is lit, it is quickly applied to an acupoint and a 'pa' or 'pop' noise can be heard and the skin will turn slightly red. For repletion pattern, draining method is used whereby the match is quickly applied to the acupoint but not pressed, then blown to quickly disperse the heat. For vacuity pattern the supplementation method is used whereby the match is applied to the acupoint for a moment then the point is pressed; causing the fire qi to slowly penetrate the skin. To treat mumps apply to Jiao Sun (SJ-20); to treat nosebleeds apply to Shao Shang (LU-11); to treat swollen tonsils apply to Yi Feng (SJ-17) and Jiao Sun (SJ-20).

- Aluminum Moxa: 20g of mercuric chloride, 20g of Hua Jiao (Zanthoxyli Pericarpium) flour, 10g of sodium chloride, and water and glycerine (in a 1:5 ratio) are combined with 100g of another disease-specific medicinal powder to make a thick paste. Apply the paste to a piece of aluminum foil, and then apply it to the treatment area. Once a replacement reaction occurs between the aluminium and mercury, the aluminium will oxidize rapidly, forming oxide on the surface of the aluminium and creating heat. Usually a sensation of heat or burning will be felt on the acupoint or the treatment area; this is called aluminium moxibustion. It is applicable in the case of patterns such as wind-cold-damp impediment, wind-cold cough, lung vacuity asthma, spleen and stomach vacuity weakness and menstrual disorders.

- Medicinal Lozenge Moxa: Combine many different types of herbs, grind and melt together with sulphur to create lozenges. These are placed on the skin and lit to perform moxibustion. By changing the herbs and acupoints, this can be used to treat a variety of patterns. For example, Xiang Liu Bing is used to treat cold-damp qi; Yang Sui Bing is used to treat streaming sores that are chronic, internally ulcerated and painless; Jiu Ku Dan is used to treat patterns such as wind impediment, external injuries, infantile convulsions, deviated eyes and mouth, and, for women, upper abdominal lump glomus with intermittent acute pain.

- Medicinal Twist Moxa: Use an equal amount of Xi Niu Huang (Bovis Bezoar Occidentale), Xiong Huang (Realgar), Ru Xiang (Olibanum), Mo Yao (Myrrha), Ding Xiang (Caryophylli Flos), She Xiang (Moschus) and Huo Xiao (Nitrum) (Xi Niu Huang can be replaced by Pen Sha (Borax) and Cao Wu (Aconiti Kusnezoffii Radix)). Wrap the medicinal powder in purple cotton paper and twist tightly into a string-like shape the diameter of a cigarette. When performing moxibustion, cut off a piece, approximately 0.2–0.3 *cun* long, place it on the treatment area and light. When treating wind impediment and scrofula place it on the area of disease; when treating water distension, diaphragm qi and stomach qi conditions, place it on relevant acupoints.

- Joss Stick Moxa:* In this method a joss stick is applied directly to an acupoint or diseased area to treat the disease. First the treatment area is disinfected with 75% alcohol, then a technique similar to 'pecking sparrow moxibustion' is used to bring the burning tip of the joss stick close to the acupoint or diseased area; when the patient has a sensation of burning the joss stick is immediately lifted away. This is repeated for 3–5 minutes, during which the ember touches the acupoint 2–3 times. This can be used to treat asthma, dribbling urinary block, acute folliculitis, warts and corns. Cautions: this method should be used with care on the weak, elderly and those with chronic organic diseases. The joss stick should be narrow, as if it is too wide it can create too much heat and burn the skin. If small blisters result from moxibustion, they can be allowed to naturally recede; if large blisters appear, they should be drained using a sterilized needle, daubed with gentian violet, then covered with sterilized gauze.

• Magic Lantern Therapy: An effective method for treating welling and flat abscess sores, it is also known as fumigation therapy. The method of operation is as follows: grind 6g each of Zhu Sha (Cinnabaris), Xiong Huang (Realgar), Xue Jie (Daemonoropis Resina), and Mo Yao (Myrrha), and 1.2g of She Xiang (Moschus) into powder. Wrap ⅓ of the powder in cotton paper and twist into a piece 1.7 *cun* long. Dip it in sesame oil then light on fire. Hold the smoking tip approximately half a *cun* from the sore, and circle around it starting from the outside and working inwards. When performing the fumigation, point the tip upward and let the smoke slowly penetrate into the body, dispersing pathogenic toxins with fire qi. Generally speaking, at the beginning 3 twists can be used, and later 4–5 twists can be used. As the sore gradually disappears the above fumigation method can still be used, but after fumigation external medicinals should immediately be applied around the root of the sore. The medicinals should be applied in an area 2 to 3 *fen* larger than the area of the sore, and Wan Ying Gao (Myriad Applications Paste) should be applied to the sore itself. This method should be discontinued when the sore has ulcerated and is discharging pus.

2.3 SPECIALIZED MOXIBUSTION METHODS

Medicinal Fumigation and Steaming Moxibustion

Steam from medicinal liquid and fumigation moxibustion is applied to channels and acupoints to achieve the treatment objective. In Wu Shi Er Bing Fang, the oldest Chinese medical document, the use of the steam from boiling Qiu Zhu to treat 'fire rot' is recorded. In the Qing Dynasty, the physician Wu Shi-Ji recorded in his book *Li Yu Pian Fang* the usage of steam from *Bu Zhong Yi Qi Tang* to treat enduring dysentery in vacuous individuals as well as flooding and prolapse of the rectum. This method can be used to treat different patterns by varying the medicinal formula used and area to receive the steam treatment. In modern times medicinal steam devices have been used in the treatment of rheumatoid arthritis.

• Cong Bai Steam Treatment: Grind 500g of chopped Cong Bai (Allii Fistulosi Bulbus), 60g of Pu Gong Ying (Taraxaci Herba), and 15g of Ya Zao (Gleditsiae Fructus Abnormalis) into powder, decoct in water, then pour into a large mug and allow the steam to flow over the treatment area. This method is appropriate for acute mastitis in the early stages before suppuration has occurred.

• Gou Ji Gen Steam Treatment: Pound an appropriate amount of Gou Ji Gen (Lycii Cortex) into a pulp, decoct in water and pour into a basin or cup to allow the steam to flow over the treatment area. Appropriate for the treatment of haemorrhoids.

• Cottonseed Steam Treatment: Decoct an appropriate amount of cottonseeds in water and apply the steam to the treatment area. Appropriate for the treatment of frostbite.

- Ginger Pepper Steam Treatment: Decoct equal amounts of fresh ginger and spicy pepper in water and apply the steam to the treatment area. When the water is merely warm use it to wash the treatment area. Appropriate for the treatment of frostbite.

- Wu Bei Zi Steam Treatment: Decoct 250g of Wu Bei Zi (Galla Chinensis Galla) and 10g of Bai Fan (Alumen) in water. Once the water is boiling pour it into a large wooden bucket. Instruct the patient to sit on the bucket and allow the steam to flow over the treatment area. Appropriate for the treatment of prolapse of the rectum.

- Jing Fang Steam Treatment: Decoct equal amounts of Jing Jie (Schizonepetae Herba), Fang Feng (Saposhnikoviae Radix), garlic (remove the skin), and Ai Ye (Artemisiae Argyi Folium) in water, then pour into a basin and apply the steam to the treatment area. Appropriate for the treatment of rheumatic arthritis and sciatica, for example.

- Wu Mei Steam Treatment: Decoct 60g of Wu Mei (Mume Fructus), 10g each of Wu Wei Zi (Schisandrae Fructus) and Shi Liu Pi (Granati Pericarpium) in water, then pour the water into a basin or large bucket and allow the steam to flow over the affected area. Appropriate for the treatment of prolapse of the uterus.

- Di Fu Zi Steam Treatment: Decoct 30g each of Di Fu Zi (Kochiae Fructus) and She Chuang Zi (Cnidii Fructus), 15g each of Ku Shen (Sophorae Flavescentis Radix) and Bai Xian Pi (Dictamni Cortex), 9g of Hua Jiao (Zanthoxyli Pericarpium), and 3g of Bai Fan (Alumen) in water. After decocting pour the water into a basin and allow the steam to flow over the treatment area. Appropriate for the treatment of eczema.

- Ba Xian Xiao Yao Steam Treatment: Decoct 18g each of Jing Jie (Schizonepetae Herba), Fang Feng (Saposhnikoviae Radix), Dang Gui (Angelicae Sinensis Radix), Huang Bai (Phellodendri Cortex) and Cang Zhu (Atractylodes), and 12g each of Dan Pi (Moutan Cortex) and Chuan Shao (Paeoniae Radix Alba Sichuanensis), 30g of Hua Jiao (Zanthoxyli Pericarpium), and 60g of Ku Shen (Sophorae Flavescentis Radix) in water. When finished decocting allow the steam to flow over the treatment area. Appropriate for the treatment of bone tuberculosis.

- Hai Tong Pi Steam Treatment: Decoct 30g each of Hai Tong Pi (Erythrinae Cortex) and Tou Gu Cao (Speranskiae seu Impatientis Herba), 9g each of Ru Xiang (Olibanum), Mo Yao (Myrrha), Chuan Jiao (Zanthoxyli Pericarpium), Hong Hua (Carthami Flos), Gan Cao (Glycyrrhizae Radix), and Wei Ling Xian (Clematidis Radix), 18g of Dang Gui (Angelicae Sinensis Radix), and 12g each of Chuan Xiao (Paeoniae Radix Alba Sichuanensis), Bai Zhi (Angelicae Dahuricae Radix) and Dan Pi (Moutan Cortex) in water. When finished decocting pour the water into a basin and allow the steam to flow over the treatment area. This method is also appropriate for the treatment of bone tuberculosis.

- Ba Dou Jiu Steam Treatment: Place 5–10 pieces of shelled Ba Dou (Crotonis Fructus) in 250ml of 50–60% alcohol Bai Jiu (Granorum Spiritus Incolor) and heat until boiling, then pour the alcohol into a bottle or small cup and steam Lao Gong (PC-8). Appropriate for treating facial paralysis.

- Ce Bai Ye Steam Treatment: Decoct 200–300g of Xian Ce Bai Ye (Platycladi Folium Recens) in water. Once the water is boiling, allow the steam to flow over the treatment area. Appropriate for treatment of 'goose-foot' wind (equivalent to tinea manuum).

Electrical Heating Device Moxa

When an electrical source of heat is used it is called electro-moxibustion, using, for example, specialized electromagnetic wave spectrum therapy devices (Teding Diancibo Pu, TDP). Usage is as follows: plug in and warm up a specialized electro-moxibustion device and direct it at the exposed treatment area. The device should be adjusted to a distance of approximately 30cm in order to maintain a constant temperature of approximately 40°C at the treatment area; a temperature that should feel comfortable to the patient. Moxibustion should be performed for 20–30 minutes once or twice per day. This method is applicable in the treatment of common diseases such as wind-cold-damp impediment, cold abdominal pain and diarrhoea.

Electro-warm-needle Moxa

Heat from an electrical source, rather than burning moxa, is applied to an acupuncture needle in order to treat disease. The acupoints chosen for needling will differ depending on the disease being treated. One method is as follows: eight acupuncture needles are placed in the body, and after obtaining qi, the needles are connected to the DWJ-I Electro-Warm-Needle Device (or the DWB-II device, or other electro-warm-needle treatment devices). Each treatment lasts 15–30 minutes. This method is used in cases of diseases such as cervical disease, bone spurs, nonsuppurative costo chondritis, arthritis, scapulohumeral periarthritis, coronary heart disease, hemiplegia, sciatica, bronchial asthma, pelvic inflammation and infertility.

Zhuang-style Medicated Thread Moxa

In this method a thread made of Zhu Ma (Boehmeria) that has undergone a medicinal soaking process is lit and applied directly to an acupoint or area on the surface of the body. This method has the effects of freeing impediment, stopping pain, alleviating itching, dispelling wind, reducing inflammation, activating blood and transforming stasis, dispersing swelling and dissipating knots. It can be used in the treatment of various types of internal organ and exterior pathologies.

The thread used in this method is 30cm long, and is one of three sizes: The diameter of the first thread (#1) is 1mm, and it is appropriate for use on acupoints on areas with thicker skin and in the treatment of tinea or similar diseases, and is generally used during the winter season. The second thread (#2), the diameter of which is 0.7mm, is the most commonly used, and is applicable in many different situations and disease patterns. The smallest thread (#3), with a diameter of 0.25mm, is appropriate for use on areas where the skin is quite delicate and thin, as well as in the treatment of children's conditions.

The principle for choosing acupoints is as follows:

- In all cases of eruption of papules with fear of cold, acupoints on the hands are most appropriate.

- In diseases involving heat effusion and an elevated body temperature, acupoints on the back are most appropriate.

- In the treatment of atrophy, drooping and paralysis, points on the affected muscle are appropriate.

- In the treatment of pain patterns, the painful area or nearby points are appropriate.

- In the case of numbness and insensitivity patterns, the centre point of the affected channel is chosen.

- In the case of all itching patterns, points on the itchy area are chosen.

- For treating swelling, local Mei Hua (Plum Blossom) points are chosen, for treating tinea and skin papule diseases local Lian Hua (Lotus Flower) or Kui Hua (Sunflower) points are chosen.

During the treatment session the patient can be sitting, prone or supine. The physician uses the thumb and forefinger to hold the thread approximately 1–2cm from the tip. The exposed tip is lit using a kerosene lamp (or alcohol lamp, candle, etc.). The flame should be extinguished leaving only an ember. The tip of the thread is pointed at an acupoint, and with a firm and nimble movement of the wrist and thumb, the tip of the thread is pressed directly onto the acupoint. Pressing once on each acupoint is usually adequate. A mild sensation of burning might be experienced. The following general rules for manipulation should be followed: when treating mild patterns, the length of time that the ember is in contact with the acupoint should be short, and the motion should be fast; when treating severe patterns, the ember should be pressed against the acupoint for a longer period of time, and the motion should be slow. Adult patients with skin diseases can be treated using #1 or #1 and #2 threads together; children, who have more tender skin and are more sensitive, can be treated using #3 threads; the palms and soles of the feet can be treated using #1 or #1 and #2 threads together; #2 threads should be used on the face area. If sensations of heat or itching are experienced after the treatment, the area should not be scratched with the fingers to prevent infection. This method should not be used on the eyes, and is contraindicated in the case of pregnancy and repletion heat patterns.

PART III

Clinical Applications

CHAPTER 6

Internal Medicine Conditions

1. Common Cold

Common cold is a disease caused by invasion of wind pathogens and characterized by a stuffy nose, cough, headache, an aversion to cold, fever and general malaise. The disease is often caused by weak general health allowing for invasion of wind. It can occur all year round, but is especially common in spring. It is known as 'wind damage' in TCM and is often seen in upper respiratory tract infection or acute infectious rhinitis.

Main Symptoms: Aversion to cold with fever, headache, nasal congestion and a runny nose, coughing, sneezing and a floating pulse. Accompanying symtoms can include a sore and swollen throat, expectoration of phlegm, thirst and oppression in the chest.

Acupoints:

- *Primary points:* Lie Que (LU-7), Feng Chi (GB-20), Da Zhui (DU-14), Fei Shu (BL-13), He Gu (LI-4).

- *Symptomatic points:* Nasal congestion: Ying Xiang (LI-20); Fever: Qu Chi (LI-11); Headache: Tai Yang (EX-HN-5), Yin Tang (EX-HN-3); Cough: Tian Tu (RN-22).

Moxibustion Method:

- Gentle Moxa: Moxa for 20–30 minutes per acupoint until local skin turns red. A course of treatment consists of one or two treatments a day for 3 days. (Figure 6.1.1)

- Moxa on Ginger: Apply moxa of 5–7 cones per acupoint. A course of treatment consists of two or three treatments a day for 3 days. (Figure 6.1.2)

- Cang Zhu Qiang Huo San Application: For headache without sweating, grind 30g of Cang Zhu (rhizoma atractylodis), 30g of Qiang Huo (Rhizoma seu Radix Notopterygii), and 10g of Ming Fan (alumen) into a fine powder, and then fry it with scallion white juice. Finally, apply the hot paste to Shen Que (RN-8). (Figure 6.1.3)

- Ba Jiao Gen Application: For cold with a high grade fever, mash 500g of Ba Jiao Gen (Musae Basjoo Caudex) with an appropriate amount of salt, and paste it on acupoints until the body temperature becomes normal. (Figure 6.1.4)

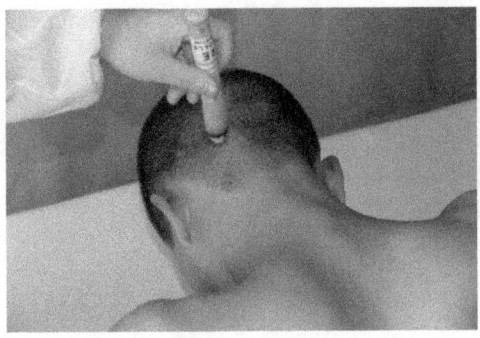

Figure 6.1.1 Gentle Moxa at Feng Chi (GB-20)

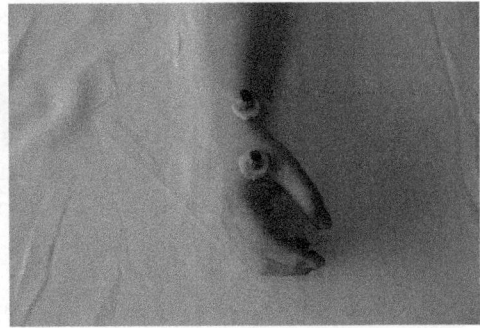

Figure 6.1.2 Moxa on Ginger at He Gu (LI-4) and Lie Que (LU-7)

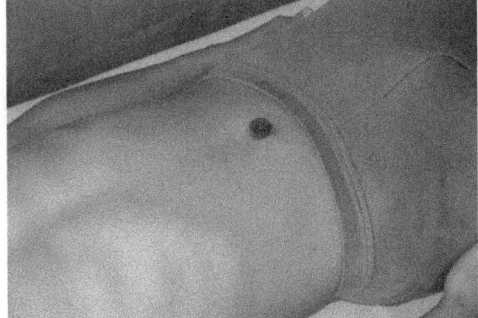

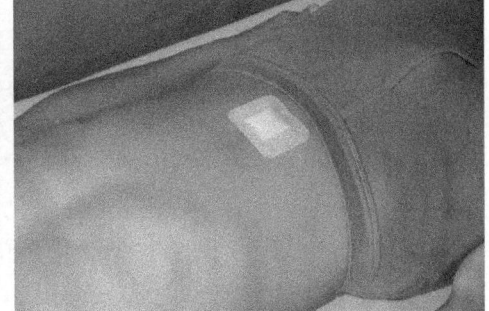

Figure 6.1.3 Cang Zhu Qiang Huo San Application at Shen Que (RN-8)

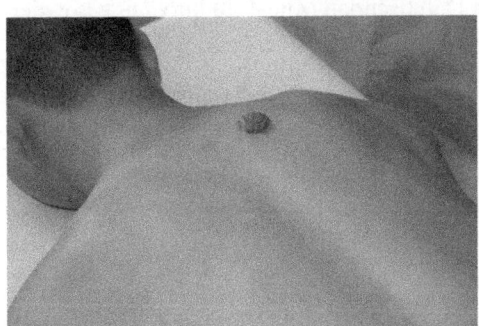

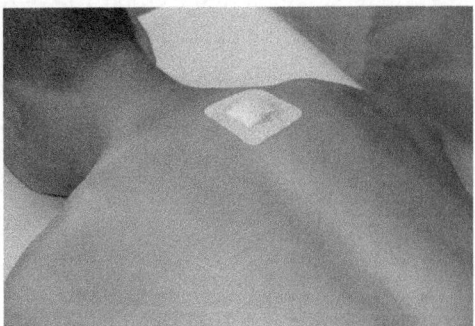

Figure 6.1.4 Ba Jiao Gen Application at Shen Que (RN-8)

2. Summer-Heat Stroke

Summer-heat stroke is a condition involving disorder of body temperature regulation induced by high temperatures or caloradiance. The key symptoms are dizziness, oppression in the chest, profuse sweating, tidal reddening of the face, scorching hot skin, weak limbs and impaired concentration; or, in severe cases, sudden coma and convulsions. This disease usually has the following causes: general deficiency, physical activity in a hot environment and lack of nutrition and water. It often occurs to older people and children. It is also commonly known as sunstroke, summer-heat damage, summer-heat wind and summer-heat epilepsy in TCM.

Main Symptoms: Dizziness, tinnitus, oppression in the chest, palpitations, nausea, vomiting, a flushed face, profuse sweating, scorching hot skin, weak limbs and impaired concentration; and, in severe cases, cold damp limbs, pale complexion, a drop in blood pressure, a fast pulse, sudden coma or convulsions.

Acupoints:

- *Primary points:* Da Zhui (DU-14), Bai Hui (DU-20), Guan Yuan (RN-4), Qi Hai (RN-6), Shen Que (RN-8).

- *Symptomatic points:* Spasms: Cheng Shan (BL-57), Yang Ling Quan (GB-34); Fever: Qu Chi (LI-11), He Gu (LI-4); Convulsions: Yong Quan (KI-1).

Moxibustion Method:

- Gentle Moxa: Apply moxa for 20–30 minutes per acupoint. A course of treatment consists of one treatment a day for 3 days. Scrub the body with warm water until the symptoms are relieved and slight sweating occurs. (Figure 6.2.1)

- Moxa on Ginger: Apply moxa of 5–7 cones per acupoint, twice or three times a day, or until the patient revives. (Figure 6.2.2)

- Moxa on Salt: Apply moxa on Shen Que (RN-8) and scrub the body with warm water or 30% alcohol until the patient revives. (Figure 6.2.3)

- Ren Dan Application: Grind 15g of Ren Dan (Rendan Mini-Pill) into a fine powder then apply the powder in the umbilicus and fix with gauze. (Figure 6.2.4)

- Tian Luo Application: Remove the shells of three large Tian Luo (freshwater snail; Cipangopaludina), and then mash with Qing Yan (Halitum) and apply on Qi Hai (RN-6). (Figure 6.2.5)

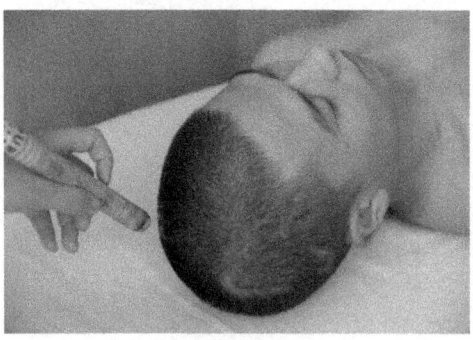
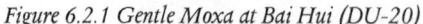
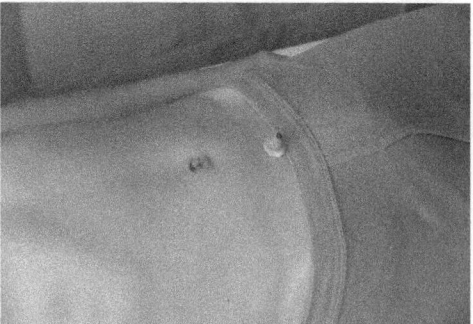

Figure 6.2.1 Gentle Moxa at Bai Hui (DU-20)   *Figure 6.2.2 Moxa on Ginger at Guan Yuan (RN-4)*

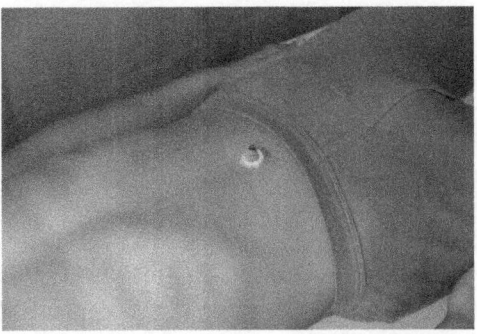

Figure 6.2.3 Moxa on Salt at Shen Que (RN-8)

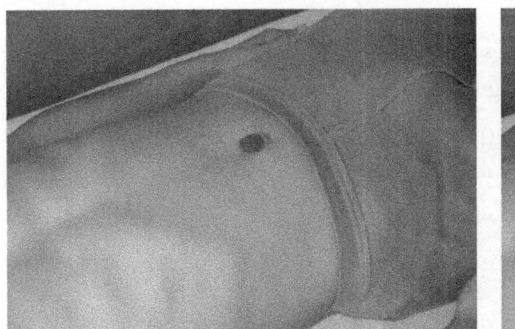 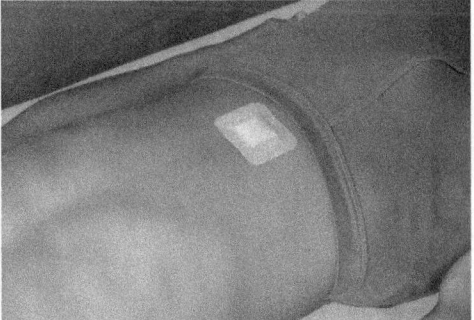

Figure 6.2.4 Ren Dan Application at Shen Que (RN-8)

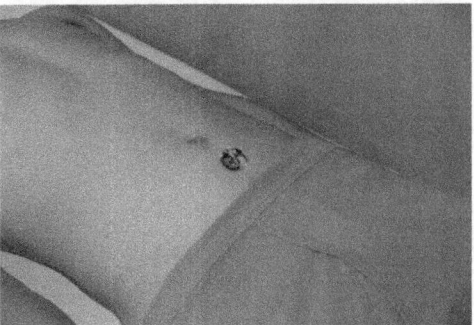

Figure 6.2.5 Tian Luo Application at Shen Que (RN-8)

3. Headache

Headache is a common subjective symptom encountered in clinic, and generally refers to the pain in the upper part of the head. It is characterized by distention and pain in the head, nape and neck, perhaps companied by dizziness and general malaise. The symptom usually has the following causes: malfunction of meridians in the head, disharmony of qi and blood, collateral blockage or the head being deprived of nourishment as a result of external contraction or internal damage. Headache occurs in hypertension, hemicranias, cluster headache, tension headache, infectious fever, cerebral trauma and ENT conditions.

Main Symptoms: Continuous or intermittent headache and tension radiating to the nape and neck that is aggravated by emotional stimulation, accompanied by dizziness, tinnitus, a red face and eyes.

Acupoints:

- *Primary points:* Bai Hui (DU-20), Feng Chi (GB-20), Da Zhui (DU-14), Tai Yang (EX-HN-5), Lie Que (LU-7).

- *Symptomatic points:* Dizziness: Tai Chong (LR-3); Red face: Qu Chi (LI-11); Heaviness in the head with the sensation of being swathed: Feng Long (ST-40); Tinnitus: Shen Shu (BL-23), Zu San Li (ST-36).

Moxibustion Method:

- Gentle Moxa: Moxa for 15–30 minutes per acupoint. A course of treatment consists of one treatment a day for 3 days. (Figure 6.3.1)

- Pecking Sparrow Moxa: Moxa for 6–20 minutes per acupoint. A course of treatment consists of one or two treatments a day for 3 days. (Figure 6.3.2)

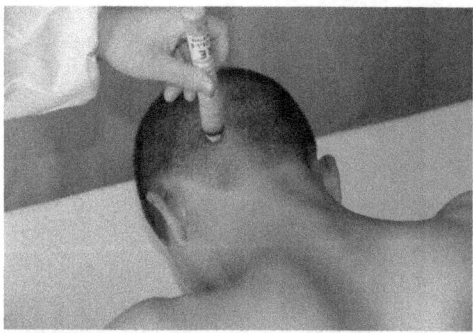

Figure 6.3.1 Gentle Moxa at Feng Chi (GB-20)

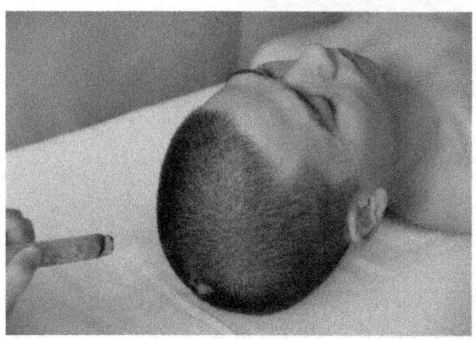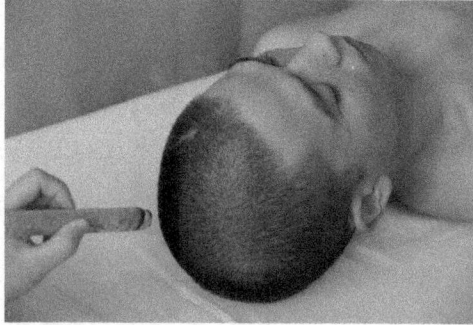

Figure 6.3.2 Pecking Sparrow Moxa at Bai Hui (DU-20)

- Moxa on Garlic: Apply 5–7 cones per acupoint. A course of treatment consists of one or two treatments a day for 3 days. (Figure 6.3.3)

- Ginger Application: Wind-cold headache or phlegm-damp headache: Mash an appropriate amount of ginger (retaining the ginger juice), and apply it on Tai Yang (EX-HN-5), once daily, 1–2 hours each time. (Figure 6.3.4)

- Peppermint Leaf Application: Wind-heat headache or liver yang headache: Mash an appropriate amount of peppermint leaves and apply it on the acupoints once daily, 1–2 hours each time. (Figure 6.3.5)

- Juncibustion:* Kidney deficiency headache: Choose 1–3 acupoints to apply juncibustion once. In severe cases, repeat 3–5 days later. A course of treatment consists of 3 days. (Figure 6.3.6)

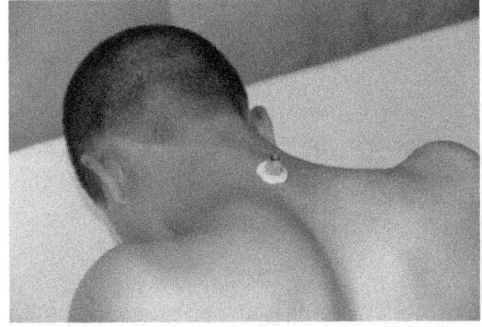

Figure 6.3.3 Moxa on Garlic at Da Zhui (DU-14)

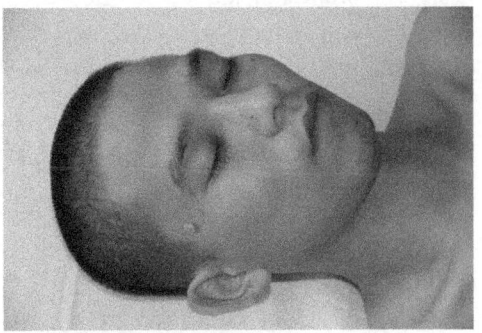

Figure 6.3.4 Ginger Application at Tai Yang (M-HN-9)

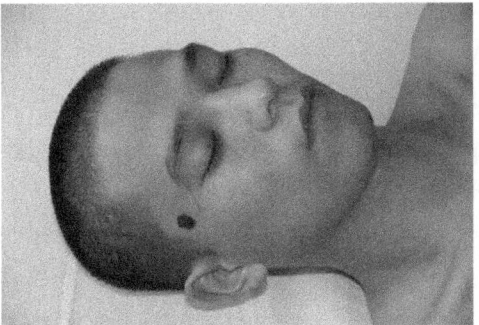

Figure 6.3.5 Peppermint Leaf Application at Tai Yang (M-HN-9)

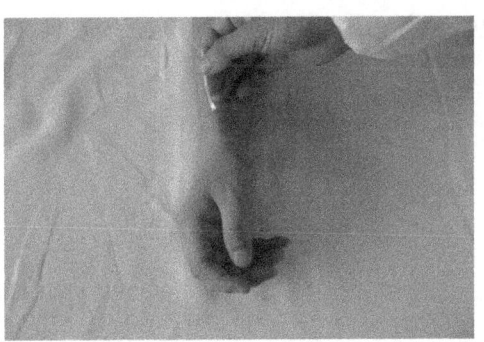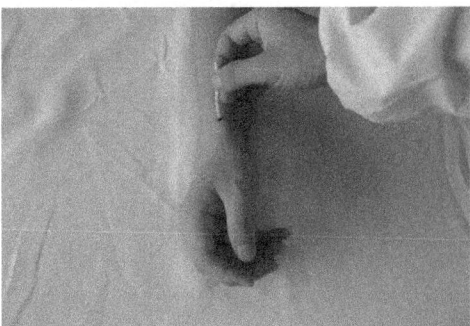

Figure 6.3.6 Juncibustion at Lie Que (LU-7)

4. Hypertension

Hypertension is a chronic general vascular disease characterized by rising systolic and/or diastolic pressure ($\geq$140/90 mmHg). The key symptoms are dizziness, tinnitus, blurred vision, a heavy cumbersome body, red face and eyes, palpitations, rashness, impatience, and irascibility. The disease is usually caused by anxiety and anger, mental stress, dietary irregularities, indulgence in alcohol and fatty foods. It can induce vascular disease of the heart, cerebrum and kidney. It often occurs in people over 40 years old, but recently there has been an increase in cases occurring in young people. It falls within the scope of dizziness, liver wind, headache, and wind-stroke in TCM.

Main Symptoms: Dizziness, tinnitus, vertigo, a red face and eyes, rashness, impatience, irascibility, palpitations, string like pulse, accompanied by a bitter taste in the mouth and dry pharynx, heavy head as if swathed, heavy cumbersome body and numbness of the limbs.

Acupoints:

- *Primary points:* Feng Chi (GB-20), Bai Hui (DU-20), Tai Yang (EX-HN-5), Gan Shu (BL-18), Shen Shu (BL-23).

- *Symptomatic points:* Glomus and oppression in the chest and epigastric region: Nei Guan (PC-6); Palpitations and insomnia: Shen Men (HT-7); Numbness of the limbs: Qu Chi (LI-11), Yang Ling Quan (GB-34).

Moxibustion Method:

- Gentle Moxa: Apply moxa for 20–30 minutes per acupoint. A course of treatment consists of one treatment a day for 10 days. (Figure 6.4.1)

- Moxa on Ginger: Apply 5–7 cones per acupoint. A course of treatment consists of one treatment every other day for 10 days. (Figure 6.4.2)

- Moxa on Celery Root: Apply 5–7 cones per acupoint. A course of treatment consists of one treatment every other day for 10 days. (Figure 6.4.3)

- Warm Needle Moxa: Apply acupuncture for 20–30 minutes per acupoint. A course of treatment consists of one treatment every other day for 10 days. (Figure 6.4.4)

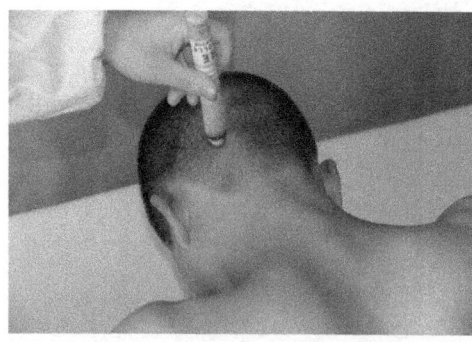

Figure 6.4.1 Gentle Moxa at Feng Chi (GB-20)

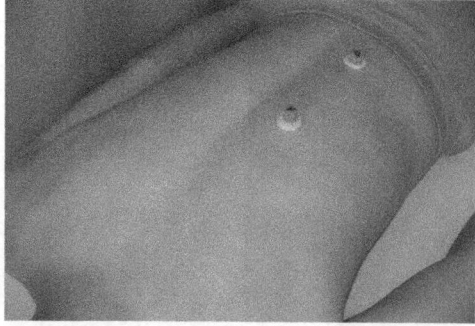

Figure 6.4.2 Moxa on Ginger at Gan Shu (BL-18) and Shen Shu (BL-23)

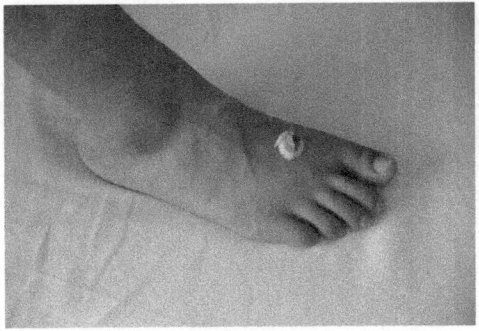
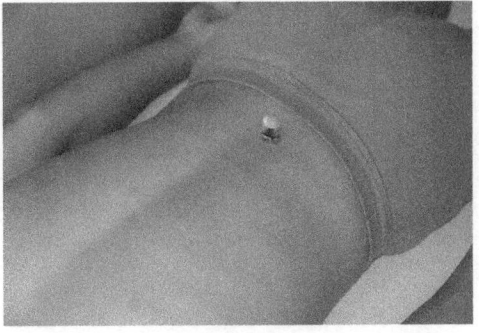

Figure 6.4.3 Moxa on Celery Root at Tai Chong (LR-3)   *Figure 6.4.4 Warm Needle Moxa at Shen Shu (BL-23)*

- Tao Ren Compound Application: Ingredients: 12g each of Tao Ren (Persicae Semen) and Xing Ren (Armeniacae Semen), 3g of Zhi Zi (Gardeniae Fructus), 7 grains of Hu Jiao (Piperis Fructus), and 14 grains of Nuo Mi (Oryzae Glutinosae Semen). Mash the above drugs and mix with an egg white. Apply the compound medicine on unilateral Yong Quan (KI-1) alternately at bedtime, 6 days for a treatment course. (Figure 6.4.5)

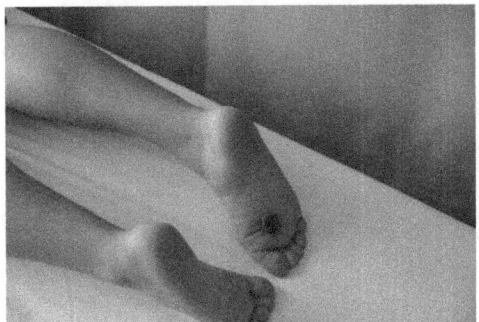
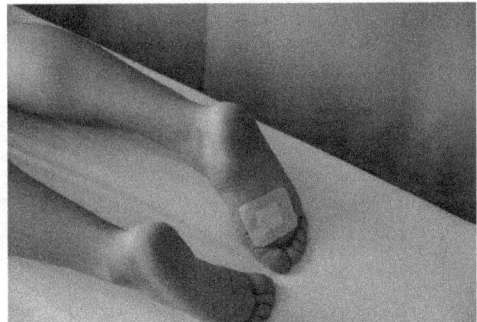

Figure 6.4.5 Tao Ren Compound Application at Yong Quan (KI-1)

- Wu Zhu Yu Compound Application: Ingredients: 100g of Wu Zhu Yu (Evodiae Fructus) prepared with pig's bile, 50g of Long Dan Cao (Gentianae Radix), 50g of Ming Fan (Alumen), 20g of Liu Huang (Sulphur), and 15g of Zhu Sha (Cinnabaris). Grind the above drugs into a fine powder, and then mix with a Xiao Ji Gen Zhi (Cirsii Herbae seu Radicis Succus) and apply the compound medicine on Shen Que (RN-8). Change the medicine every 2 days, and continue for 10 days for one course of treatment. (Figure 6.4.6)

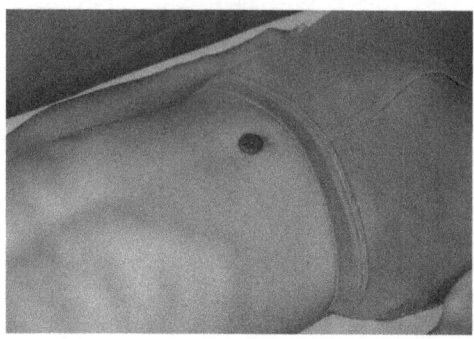 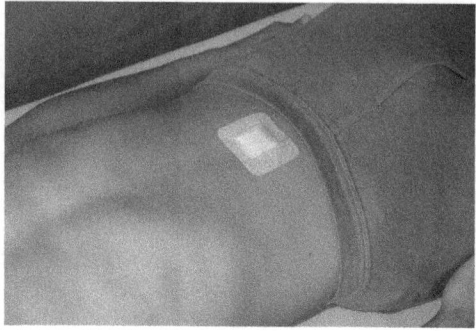

Figure 6.4.6 Wu Zhu Yu Compound Application at Shen Que (RN-8)

5. Hypotension

Hypotension is a set of symptoms caused by a reduction in blood pressure, manifesting as dizziness, a lack of strength, confusion, a withered-yellow facial complexion and devitalized essence-spirit. The condition is usually caused by a weak constitution, deficiency of qi and yin. It often occurs mainly in women between the age of 20–50 and older people, and falls within the scope of vacuity detriment (severe chronic insufficiency), dizziness, and syncope in TCM.

Main Symptoms: Dizziness, headache, weakness, cold sweating, confusion, shortness of breath, and even oliguria, fainting or shock; accompanied by a withered-yellow facial complexion, indigestion, devitalized essence-spirit, aversion to cold and cold limbs.

Acupoints:

- *Primary points:* Bai Hui (DU-20), Shen Que (RN-8), Guan Yuan (RN-4), Shen Shu (BL-23).

- *Symptomatic points:* Dizziness: Tou Wei (ST-8), Jue Yin Shu (BL-14); Fainting: Yong Quan (KI-1); Palpitations: Xin Shu (BL-15), Nei Guan (PC-6); Orthostatic hypotension: Zhong Wan (RN-12), Pi Shu (BL-20), Gan Shu (BL-18).

Moxibustion Method:

- Gentle Moxa: Apply moxa for 15–30 minutes per acupoint. Combine with digital compression: press hard with the thumb on Yong Quan (KI-1) for 6 seconds while exhaling. Press and relax 20 times. A course of treatment consists of one treatment every day for 10 days. (Figure 6.5.1)

- Pecking Sparrow Moxa: Moxa for 6–20 minutes per acupoint. A course of treatment consists of one treatment every other day for 10 days. (Figure 6.5.2)

- Non-scarring Cone Moxa: Apply 5–7 cones per acupoint. A course of treatment consists of one treatment every other day for 10 days. (Figure 6.5.3)

- Moxa on Fu Zi Cake: Apply 5–7 cones per acupoint. A course of treatment consists of one treatment every other day for 10 days. (Figure 6.5.4)

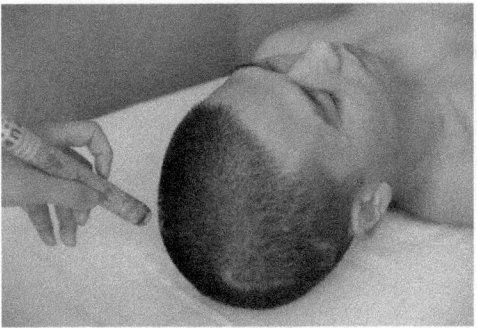

Figure 6.5.1 Gentle Moxa at Bai Hui (DU-20)

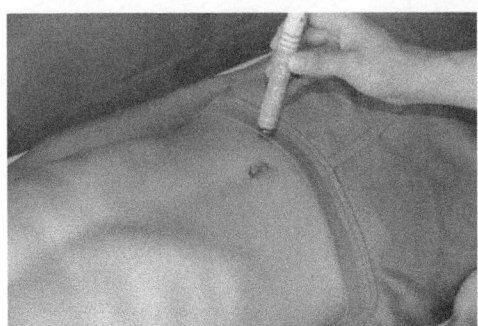

Figure 6.5.2 Pecking Sparrow Moxa at Shen Que (RN-8)

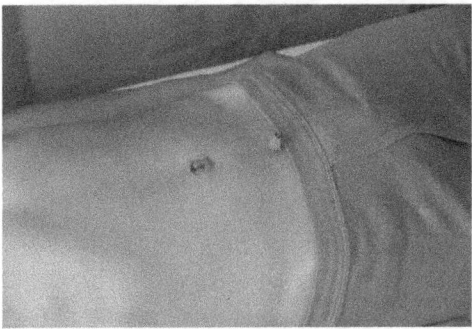

Figure 6.5.3 Non-scarring Cone Moxa at Guan Yuan (RN-4)

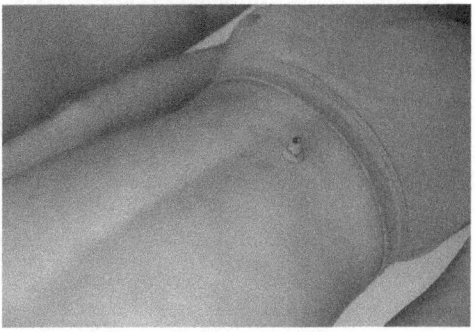

Figure 6.5.4 Moxa on Fu Zi Cake at Shen Shu (BL-23)

6. Hyperlipidemia

Hyperlipidemia is a disease that manifests as increased cholesterin and/or triglyceride levels in serum and is characterized by atherosclerosis. The disease usually has the following causes: constitutional spleen deficiency resulting in exuberant phlegm; dietary irregularities such as excessive consumption of fatty and sweet foods; phlegm accumulation and blood stasis caused by debility in old age and decreased visceral qi, which leads to the formation of fat turbidity. It often occurs in the elderly and falls within the scope of phlegm pattern, deficiency detriment, damp obstruction and obesity in TCM.

Main Symptoms: Obesity, palpitations, dizziness, glomus and fullness in the chest and stomach duct, abdominal distension, intake of turbid food, fatigue and a lack of strength, nausea, drooling from the mouth, thirst with no desire to drink, a pale tongue, oily tongue coating and a soggy pulse. Further symptoms may include heart vexation and a clouded mind, increased food intake, frequent and rapid hunger sensations, a red facial complexion, a dry and bitter mouth, a red tongue, oily yellow tongue coating, and a string-like and slippery pulse.

Acupoints:

- *Primary points:* Yang Chi (SJ-4), San Jiao Shu (BL-22), Zu San Li (ST-36), Tai Chong (LR-3), Fu Liu (KI-7).

- *Symptomatic points:* Di Ji (SP-8), Ming Men (DU-4), San Yin Jiao (SP-6), Da Zhui (DU-14), Pi Shu (BL-20), Gan Shu (BL-18), Feng Long (ST-40), Nei Guan (PC-6).

Moxibustion Method:

- Gentle Moxa: Apply moxa for 20–30 minutes per acupoint. A course of treatment consists of one treatment every day for one month. (Figure 6.6.1)

- Moxa on Ginger: Apply 5–7 cones per acupoint. A course of treatment consists of one treatment every other day for one month. (Figure 6.6.2)

- Scarring Cone Moxa:* Apply moxa unilaterally on Zu San Li (ST-36) and Xuan Zhong (GB-39) alternately, once a week for 10 weeks. Usually one course of treatment is sufficient. (Figure 6.6.3)

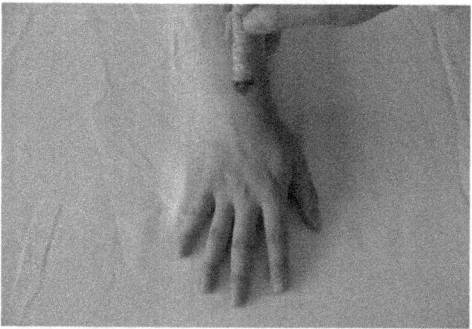

Figure 6.6.1 Gentle Moxa at Yang Chi (SJ-4)

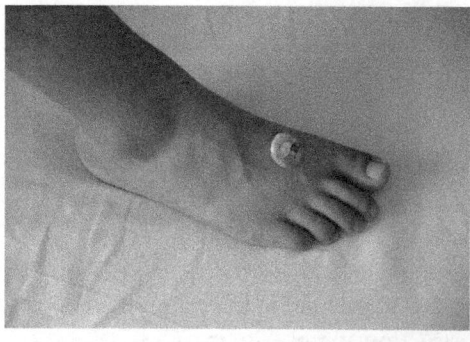

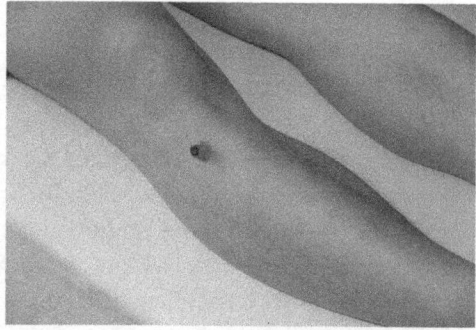

Figure 6.6.2 Moxa on Ginger at Tai Chong (LR-3)   *Figure 6.6.3 Scarring Cone Moxa at Zu San Li (ST-36)*

7. Sequelae of Wind Stroke

Sequelae of wind stroke is a series of symptoms occurring after acute cerebral vascular diseases, such as cerebral haemorrhage and cerebral infarction. The key symptoms are hemianopia, hemiplegia, allolalia, dysphagia, disgnosia, daily activity disorder, and bowel and urinary disturbances. The disease is usually caused by one of the following: constitutional debilitation, emotional depression, liver-kidney yin deficiency, hyperactive heart-fire and liver-yang resulting in difficulty in recovering the body's functions after stroke. It often occurs in older people in winter and falls in the categories of wind-stroke, hemi-lateral atrophy and vacuity taxation in TCM.

Main Symptoms: Unconsciousness, deviated eyes and mouth, a stiff tongue and impeded speech, hemiplegia, a red tongue and a string-like pulse. Accompanying symptoms include hemianopia, disgnosia, daily activity disorder, dysphagia, bowel and urinary disturbances.

Acupoints:

- *Primary points:* Bai Hui (DU-20), Tian Chuang (SI-16), Xuan Zhong (GB-39), Yang Ling Quan (GB-34), Zu San Li (ST-36).

- *Symptomatic points:* Deviated mouth: Di Cang (ST-4), Jia Che (ST-6); Numb limbs: Yin Bai (SP-1), Shen Ting (DU-24); Upper limbs dysfunction: Jian Yu (LI-15), Qu Chi (LI-11); Lower limbs dysfunction: Huan Tiao (GB-30); Strephenopodia: Qiu Xu (GB-40); Flaccid paralysis: Qi Hai (RN-6), Gan Shu (BL-18), Pi Shu (BL-20); Spastic paralysis: Zhong Wan (RN-12), Ju Que (RN-14), Gan Shu (BL-18).

Moxibustion Method:

- Gentle Moxa: Apply moxa for 20–30 minutes per acupoint. A course of treatment consists of one or two treatments per day for one month. (Figure 6.7.1)

- Pecking Sparrow Moxa: Apply moxa for 6–20 minutes per acupoint. A course of treatment consists of one treatment every other day for one month. (Figure 6.7.2)

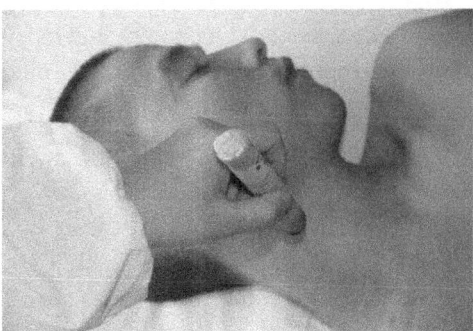

Figure 6.7.1 Gentle Moxa at Tian Chuang (SI-16)

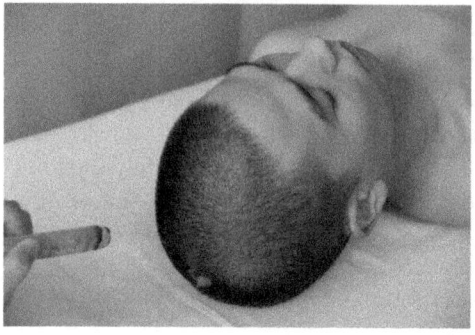
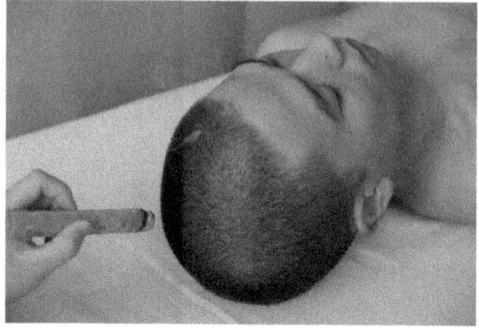

Figure 6.7.2 Pecking Sparrow Moxa at Bai Hui (DU-20)

- Moxa on Ginger: Apply 5–7 cones per acupoint, once every other day. A course of treatment consists of one treatment every other day for one month. (Figure 6.7.3)

- Moxa on Salt: Apply 5–7 cones per acupoint. A course of treatment consists of one treatment every other day for 10 days. (Figure 6.7.4)

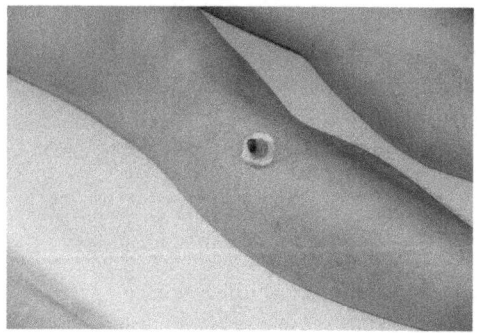
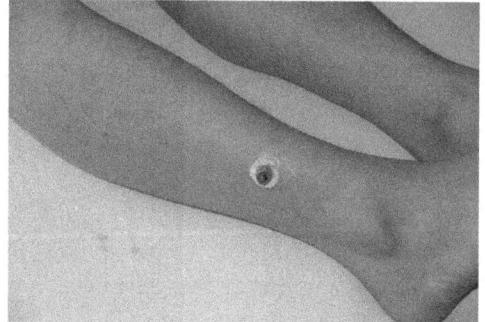

Figure 6.7.3 Moxa on Ginger at Zu San Li (ST-36)   *Figure 6.7.4 Moxa on Salt at Xuan Zhong (GB-39)*

- Scarring Cone Moxa:* Choose 2–3 acupoints and apply moxa. A course of treatment consists of one treatment every other day for one month. (Figure 6.7.5)

- Tan Huan Cake Application: Ingredients: 60g of Chuan Shan Jia (Manis Squama), 60g of Da Chuan Wu Tou (Aconiti Radix), and 60g of Hong Hai Ha (Meretricis seu Cyclinae Concha). Grind the above medicinals into a fine powder, then mix 1.5g of the powder with scallion white juice and form it into small cakes. Finally paste the cakes on Yong Quan (KI-1), Yang Ling Quan (GB-34), Zu San Li (ST-32), Qu Chi (LI-11) and He Gu (LI-4). Change the cakes after 3 days, and repeat until the patient recovers. (Figure 6.7.6)

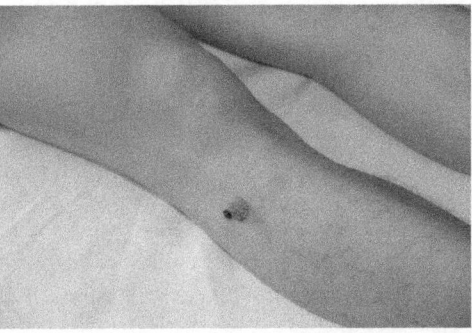

Figure 6.7.5 Scarring Cone Moxa at Yang Ling Quan (GB-34)

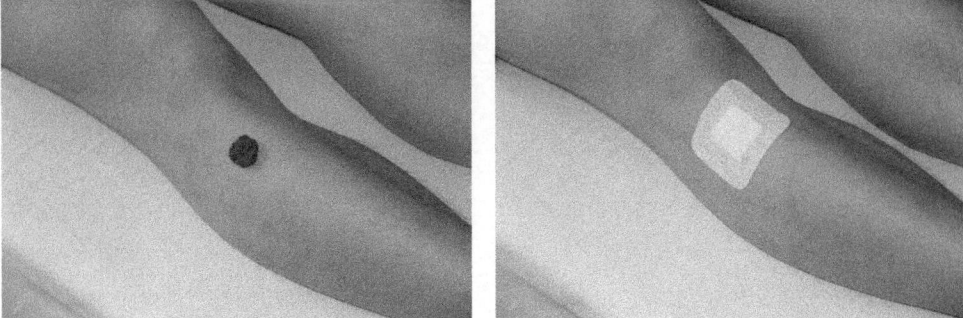

Figure 6.7.6 Tan Huan Cake Application at Zu San Li (ST-36)

8. Dizziness

Dizziness is characterized by a whirling sensation in the head and visual distortion. In mild cases, a transient attack is relieved after lying down for a moment. In severe cases, the patient feels as if they are on a moving boat or bus, and can even become unstable; this sensation can be accompanied by nausea and vomiting. It can be of varying intensity, accompanied by other patterns, and occurs repeatedly. The condition usually has the following causes: depression and anger harassing the clear orifices; indulgence in rich fatty foods clouding the clear orifices; overwork leading to insufficient bone marrow; qi and blood deficiency resulting in malnourishment of the clear orifices. It often occurs as a symptom in hypertension, cerebral arteriosclerosis, cervical spondylopathy, anaemia, neurasthenic and otogenic disease.

Main Symptoms: Dizziness and blurred vision, vertigo, possible relief after lying down for a short period of time, or a sensation of being on a moving boat or bus.

Acupoints: Bai Hui (DU-20), Feng Chi (GB-20), Tou Wei (ST-8), Shen Ting (DU-24).

Moxibustion Method:

- Gentle Moxa: Apply moxa for 15–20 minutes per acupoint. A course of treatment consists of one treatment per day for 15 days. (Figure 6.8.1)

- Non-scarring Cone Moxa: Apply 5–7 cones per acupoint. A course of treatment consists of one treatment every other day for 5 days. (Figure 6.8.2)

- Moxa on Ginger: Apply 5–7 wheat kernel-sized cones per acupoint. A course of treatment consists of one treatment every one or two days for 6–15 days. (Figure 6.8.3)

- Moxa on Celery Root: Slice the celery root into pieces 0.2cm thick, then put wheat kernel-sized moxa cones on it. Apply 3–5 cones per acupoint. A course of treatment consists of one treatment per day for 10 days. (Figure 6.8.4)

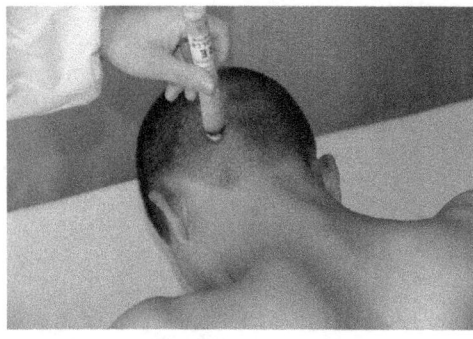
Figure 6.8.1 Gentle Moxa at Feng Chi (GB-20)

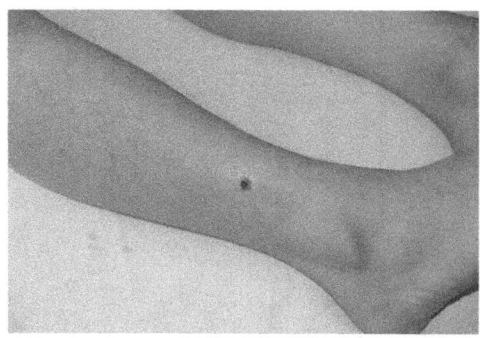
Figure 6.8.2 Non-scarring Moxa at Xuan Zhong (GB-39)

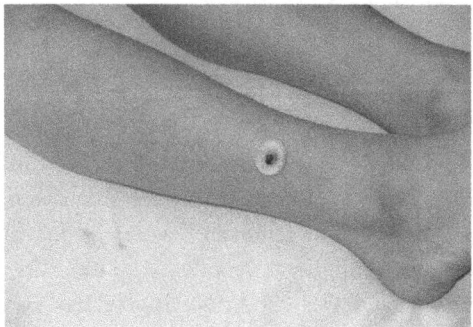
Figure 6.8.3 Moxa on Ginger at Xuan Zhong (GB-39)

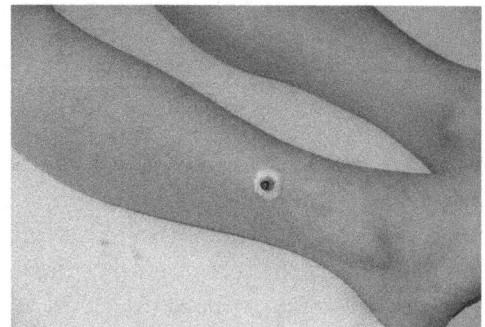
Figure 6.8.4 Moxa on Celery Root at Xuan Zhong (GB-39)

- Wu Zhu Yu Application: Grind Wu Zhu Yu (Evodiae Fructus) into a powder, then mix with vinegar, paste the compound medicine on the centre of the sole of the foot. A course of treatment consists of one treatment per day for 7 days. (Figure 6.8.5)

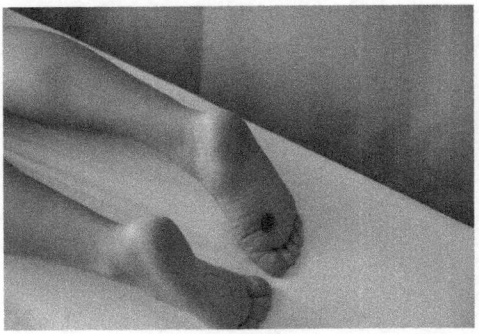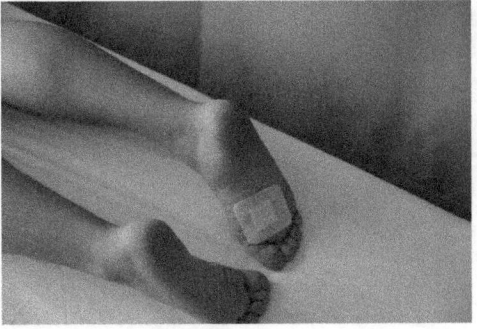

Figure 6.8.5 Wu Zhu Yu Application on Yong Quan (KI-1)

9. Coronary Heart Disease (CHD)

Coronary heart disease, also known as coronary atherosclerosis, is a myocardial dysfunctional and (or) organic disease caused by coronary artery stenosis and circulation insufficiency. It is also known as ischemic cardiomyopathy and manifests as heart pain stretching through to the back, accompanied by hasty panting with an inability to lie down. This disease usually has the following causes: insufficient heart-yang, congealing cold in the blood vessels causing vasoconstriction; indulgence in rich fatty foods resulting in phlegm-damp harassing the heart; seven-affect binding depression causing qi stagnation and blood stasis. It often occurs in older people and falls within the category of chest impediment and true heart pain in TCM.

Main Symptoms: Heart pain radiating through to the back, or intermittent dull pain in the chest, a red tongue, string-like and rough pulse or a bound, intermittent and skipping pulse. Accompanying symptoms include distension and oppression in the stomach duct and abdomen, expectorating phlegm-drool, shortness of breath and a lack of strength.

Acupoints:

- *Primary points:* Nei Guan (PC-6), Xin Shu (BL-15), Dan Zhong (RN-I7), Jue Yin Shu (BL-14), Qu Ze (PC-3).

- *Symptomatic points:* Tian Tu (RN-22), Qi Hai (RN-6); Zhong Wan (RN-12), Zu San Li (ST-36); Shen Tang (BL-44), Jiu Wei (RN-15); Qi Men (LR-14), Tai Chong (LR-3).

Moxibustion Method:

- Gentle Moxa: Apply moxa for 6–15 minutes per acupoint. A course of treatment consists of one treatment per day for 10 days. (Figure 6.9.1)

- Direct Moxa: Use wheat kernel-sized moxa cones. Apply 6–50 cones. The symptoms can be relieved with just treatment. (Figure 6.9.2)

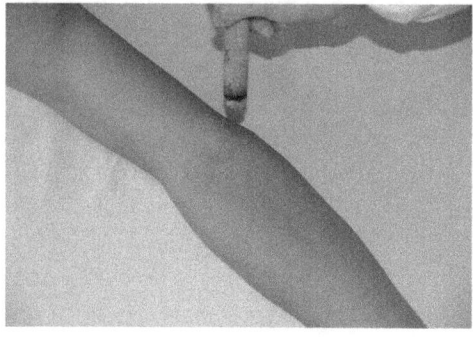

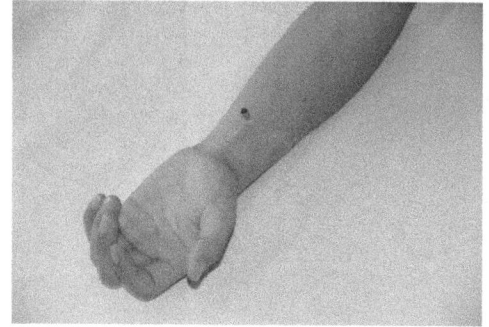

Figure 6.9.1 Gentle Moxa at Qu Ze (PC-3)   *Figure 6.9.2 Direct Moxa at Nei Guan (PC-6)*

- Scarring Cone Moxa:* Apply moxa on 2–3 acupoints every other day, for 10 consecutive days. (Figure 6.9.3)

- Moxa on Fu Zi Cake: Apply 5–7 cones per acupoint every other day, for 10 consecutive days. (Figure 6.9.4)

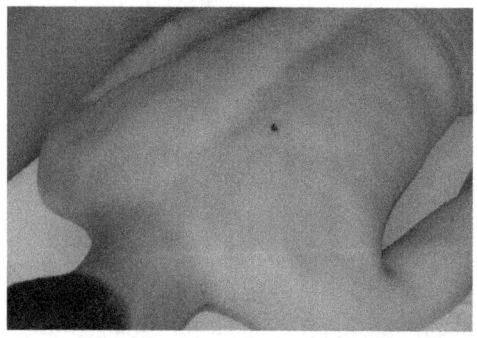

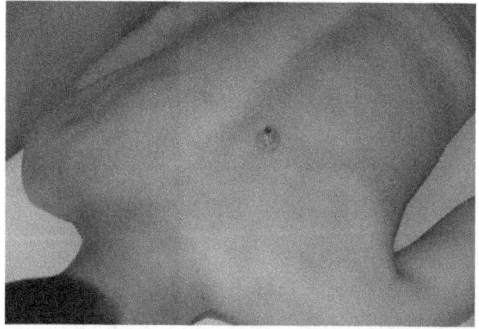

Figure 6.9.3 Scarring Cone Moxa at Xin Shu (BL-15)   *Figure 6.9.4 Moxa on Fu Zi Cake at Jue Yin Shu (BL-14)*

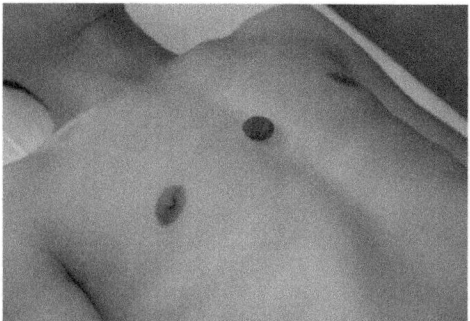

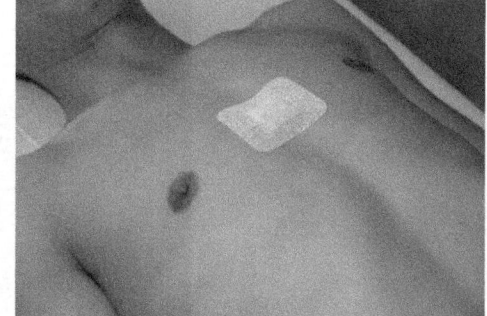

Figure 6.9.5 Chuan Xiong Application at Dan Zhong (RN-17)

- Chuan Xiong Application: Apply Chuan Xiong (Chuanxiong Rhizoma) on Dan Zhong (RN-17) and Nei Guan (PC-6) for 6–15 min. Continue for a month to complete one course of treatment. (Figure 6.9.5)

- Juncibustion:* A course of treatment consists of one treatment daily for 15 days. (Figure 6.9.6)

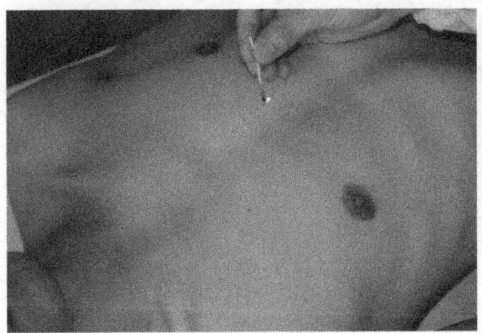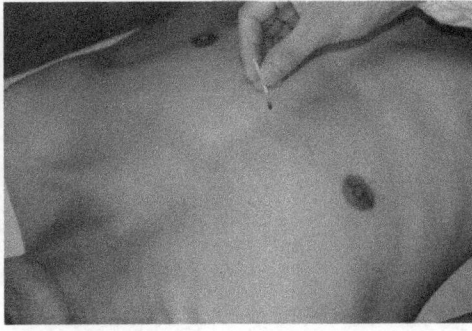

Figure 6.9.6 Juncibustion at Dan Zhong (RN-17)

10. Pulmonary Heart Disease

Pulmonary heart disease is induced by pulmonary hypertension. It is often caused by chronic bronchitis, emphysema pulmonum or pulmonary vascular disease. Acute respiratory infection is the common incentive. The disease often occurs in winter or spring in people over the age of 40. It falls within the category of cough and panting, accumulation of fluid in the body and oedema in TCM.

Main Symptoms: Cough and panting, expectoration of phlegm, palpitations, dyspnoea, aggravated by movement, shortness of breath, and a deep and fine pulse; accompanied by turning blue, lack of strength, poor food intake, oedema and scanty urine. In severe cases, coma, profuse sweating, haemorrhage and bloody stools may occur.

Acupoints:

- *Primary points:* Fei Shu (BL-13), Shen Shu (BL-23), Tian Tu (RN-22), Zhong Fu (LU-1), Dan Zhong (RN-17), Ju Que (RN-14).

- *Symptomatic points:* Shortness of breath: Qi Hai (RN-6); Chi Ze (LU-5); Palpitations: Nei Guan (PC-6), Shen Men (HT-7); Copious phlegm: Zu San Li (ST-36), Feng Long (ST-40).

Moxibustion Method:

- Non-scarring Moxa: Apply 5–7 cones per acupoint. Repeat once daily for 10 days to complete one course of treatment. (Figure 6.10.1)

- Gentle Moxa: Apply 6–15 minutes per acupoint. Repeat once daily for 10 days to complete one course of treatment. (Figure 6.10.2)

- Moxa on Salt: Apply 5–7 cones on Shen Que (RN-8) once daily to relieve the symptoms of an acute attack. (Figure 6.10.3)

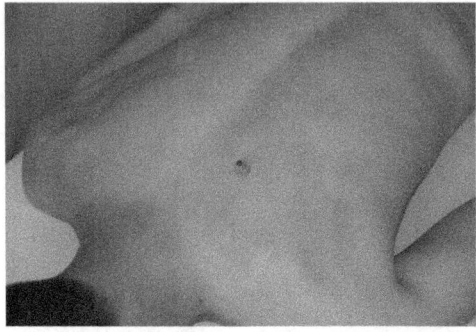

Figure 6.10.1 Non-scarring Moxa at Fei Shu (BL-13)

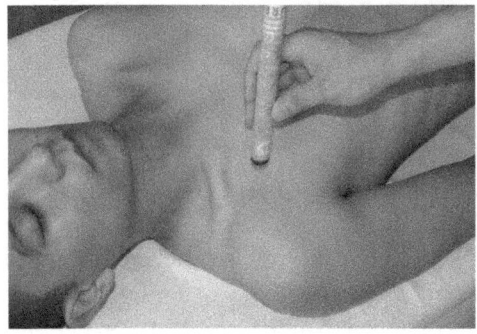

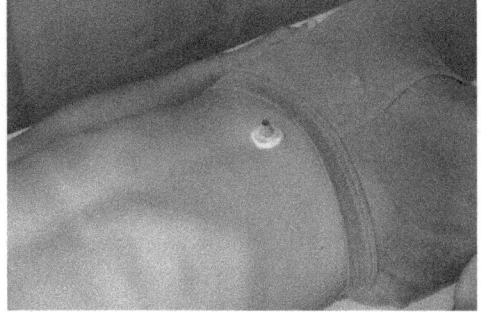

Figure 6.10.2 Gentle Moxa at Zhong Fu (LU-1)   *Figure 6.10.3 Moxa on Salt at Shen Que (RN-8)*

- Moxa on Ginger: Apply 5–7 cones on Bai Hui (DU-20) once daily to relieve the symptoms of an acute attack. Alternatively apply 5–7 cones on 3–5 acupoints and repeat once daily for 10 days to complete one course of treatment. (Figure 6.10.4)

- Moxa on Fu Zi Cake: Choose 3–5 acupoints and apply 5–7 cones per acupoint. Repeat once daily for 10 days to complete one course of treatment. (Figure 6.10.5)

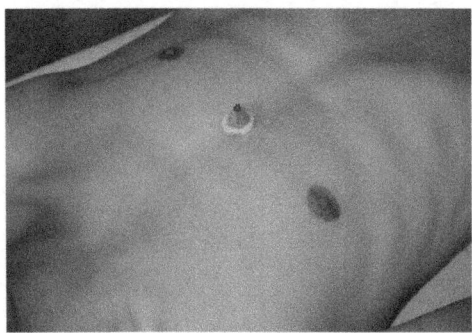

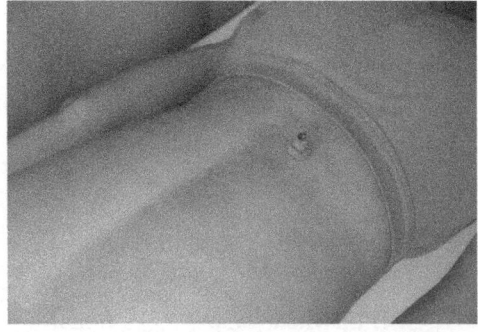

Figure 6.10.4 Moxa on Ginger at Dan Zhong
(RN-17)

Figure 6.10.5 Moxa on Fu Zi Cake at Shen Shu
(BL-23)

11. Arrhythmia (Palpitations)

Arrhythmia, also known as palpitations, is often found in various kinds of organic heart disease, especially in CHD, myocardiosis and rheumatic heart disease. It is characterized by a subjective sensation of an accelerated heart rate and precordial discomfort. This disease usually has the following causes: malnourishment of the heart, inhibited blood flow in the heart vessels caused by a weak constitution, taxation damage, internal damage by the seven affects, qi stagnation and blood stasis. It falls in the category of fright palpitations and fearful throbbing in TCM.

Main Symptoms: Palpitations and shortness of breath, fatigued spirit and spontaneous sweating, insomnia, profuse dreaming, dizziness, blurred vision, and a fine and weak pulse. In extreme cases susceptibility to fright and agitation when sitting or lying. Accompanying symptoms include a sombre white or withered-yellow facial complexion, poor food intake, a lack of strength, tinnitus, aching lumbar region and oppression in the chest.

Acupoints:

- *Primary points:* Xin Shu (BL-15), Ju Que (RN-14), Nei Guan (PC-6), Xi Men (PC-4), Shen Men (HT-7).

- *Symptomatic points:* Susceptibility to fright: Da Lin (PC-7), Dan Shu (BL-19); Spontaneous sweating and shortness of breath: Zu San Li (ST-36), Fu Liu (KI-7); Profuse dreaming: Shen Shu (BL-23), Tai Xi (KI-3); Red face: Lao Gong (PC-8).

Moxibustion Method:

- Non-scarring Moxa: Apply 5–7 cones per acupoint. A course of treatment consists of one treatment per day for 10 days. (Figure 6.11.1)

- Gentle Moxa: Apply 6–15 minutes per acupoint. A course of treatment consists of one treatment per day for 10 days. (Figure 6.11.2)

- Warm Needle Moxa: Apply 6–15 minutes per acupoint. A course of treatment consists of one treatment per day for 10 days. (Figure 6.11.3)

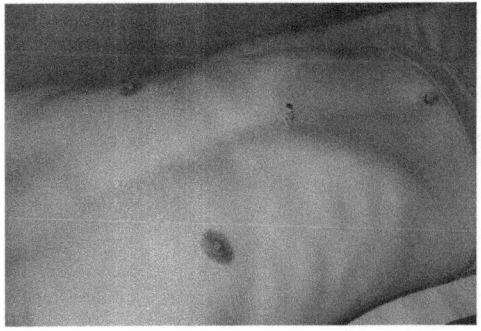

Figure 6.11.1 Non-scarring Moxa at Ju Que (RN-14)

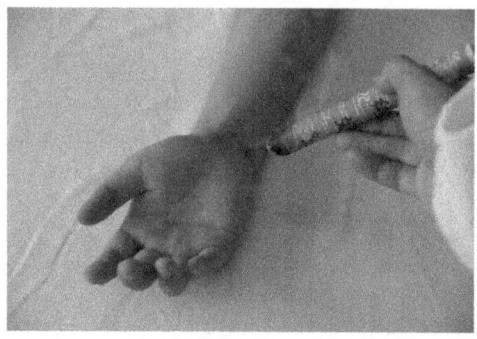

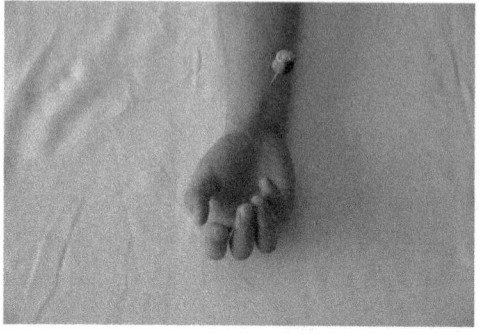

Figure 6.11.2 Gentle Moxa at Shen Men (HT-7)   *Figure 6.11.3 Warm Needle Moxa at Nei Guan (PC-6)*

- Juncibustion:* Apply 6–15 minutes per acupoint. A course of treatment consists of one treatment every 3 days for 5 treatments in total. (Figure 6.11.4)

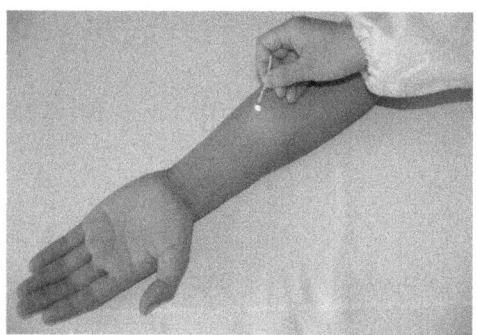

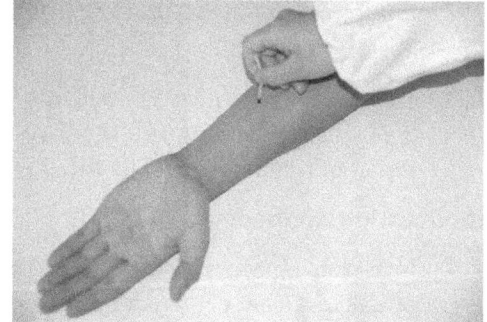

Figure 6.11.4 Juncibustion at Xi Men (PC-4)

- Moxa on Fu Zi Cake: Choose 3–5 acupoints and apply 5–7 cones per acupoint, performed once daily or every other day for 7 treatments in total. (Figure 6.11.5)

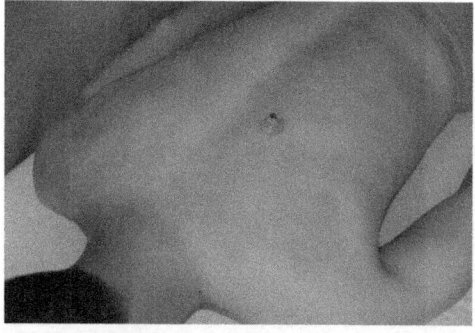

Figure 6.11.5 Moxa on Fu Zi Cake at Xin Shu (BL-15)

12. Bronchitis

Bronchitis is a common clinical respiratory disease. It is characterized by long-term recurrent cough, expectoration of phlegm or panting. It is often caused by externally contracted wind-cold, wind-heat or wind-dryness and attacks in autumn and winter. It falls within the category of cough, accumulation of fluid in the body, and panting rale in TCM.

Main Symptoms: Long-term recurrent cough, expectoration of phlegm, panting, aggravated in the morning or evening, copious white or sticky phlegm; accompanied by fever or headache.

Acupoints:

- *Primary points:* Ding Chuan (EX-B-1), Feng Men (BL-12), Da Zhui (DU-14), Fei Shu (BL-13), He Gu (LI-4).

- *Symptomatic points:* Qi deficiency: Qi Hai (RN-6), Tian Tu (RN-22); Chest pain: Dan Zhong (RN-17); Copious phlegm: Feng Long (ST-40).

Moxibustion Method:

- Gentle Moxa: Apply for 20–30 minutes per acupoint. Repeat once or twice a day for 5 days to complete a course of treatment. (Figure 6.12.1)

- Moxa on Ginger: Apply 5–7 cones per acupoint. Repeat once or twice a day for 7 days to complete a course of treatment. (Figure 6.12.2)

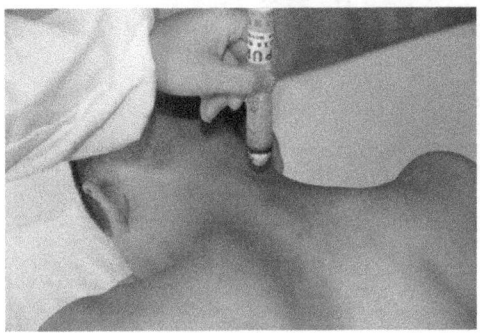
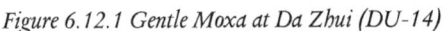

Figure 6.12.1 Gentle Moxa at Da Zhui (DU-14)

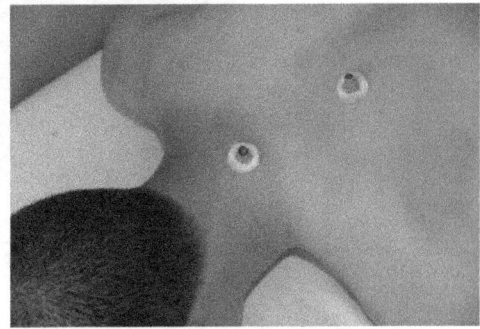

Figure 6.12.2 Moxa on Ginger at Fei Shu (BL-13) and Ding Chuan (EX-B-1)

- Moxa on Garlic: Apply 5–7 cones per acupoint. Repeat once or twice a day for 5 days to complete a course of treatment. (Figure 6.12.3)

- Warm Needle Moxa: Apply 5–7 cones per acupoint. Repeat once or twice a day for 7 days to complete a course of treatment. (Figure 6.12.4)

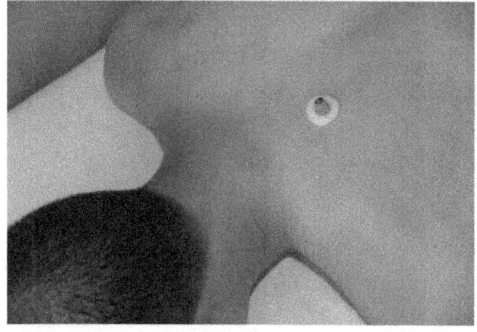 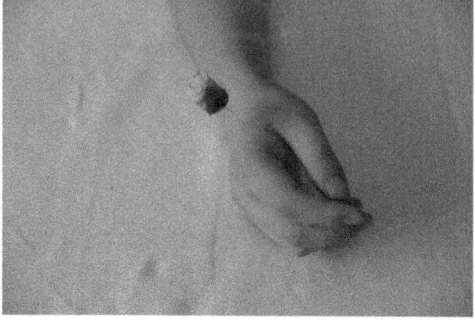

Figure 6.12.3 Moxa on Garlic at Feng Men (BL-12)   *Figure 6.12.4 Warm Needle Moxa at He Gu (LI-4)*

- Moxa on Ginger with Medicinal Application: Ingredients: 3g of Bai Jie Zi (Sinapis Albae Semen), 3g of Ban Xia (Pinelliae Rhizoma), 0.5g of Gong Ding Xiang (Caryophylli Flos), 5g of Ma Huang (Ephedrae Herba), 2g of Xi Xin (Asari Herba), and a small amount of She Xiang (Moschus). Grind the above into a fine powder, apply to the umbilicus and cover with a piece of ginger. Apply 5–7 large cones per acupoint. Repeat once daily for 10 days to complete a course of treatment. (Figure 6.12.5)

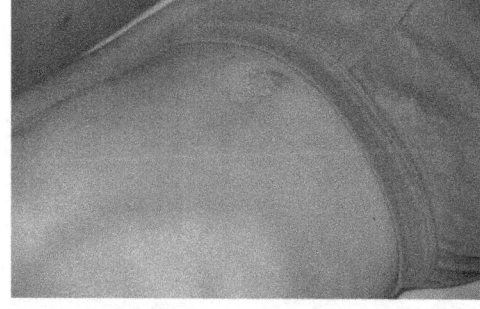

Figure 6.12.5 Moxa on Ginger with Medicinal Application at Shen Que (RN-8)

13. Chronic Asthmatic Bronchitis

Chronic asthmatic bronchitis is a common clinical disease characterized by long-term reduplicated cough, panting aggravated in the evening, copious phlegm, oppression in the chest, rapid breathing with an inability to lie down. This disease usually has the following causes: weak health, deep-lying phlegm in the lung, weather changes, dietary irregularities, or physicochemical irritations such as bacteria or virus. It can occur all the year round, especially in winter and spring. It falls in the category of cough, phlegm-rheum, panting and pulmonary distension in TCM.

Main Symptoms: Long-term reduplicated cough aggravated in the evening, oppression in the chest, rapid breathing with an inability to lie down, short and rapid inhalation, long and rapid exhalation, copious white or sticky phlegm; accompanied, in severe cases by a phlegm rale in the throat and cyanosis.

Acupoints:

- *Primary points:* Fei Shu (BL-13), Lie Que (LU-7), Qi Hai (RN-6), Feng Men (BL-12), Da Zhui (DU-14), Shen Shu (BL-23).

- *Symptomatic points:* Severe panting: Tian Tu (RN-22); Deficiency of heart-qi: Xin Shu (BL-15), Dan Zhong (RN-17); Weak health: Gao Huang (BL-43).

Moxibustion Method:

- Gentle Moxa: Apply 20–30 minutes per acupoint. Repeat once daily for 10 days to complete a course of treatment. (Figure 6.13.1)

- Moxa on Ginger: Apply 5–7 cones per acupoint. Repeat once daily for 7–10 days to complete a course of treatment. (Figure 6.13.2)

- Scarring Moxa:* Apply moxa on 3–5 acupoints until suppurative blisters appear, once a year, and repeat for 3 years. (Figure 6.13.3)

- Indirect Moxa: Put a piece of kohlrabi on an acupoint, then add some mashed garlic, and finally apply moxa cones until the skin turns purplish-red. Repeat once daily for 7 days to complete a course of treatment. (Figure 6.13.4)

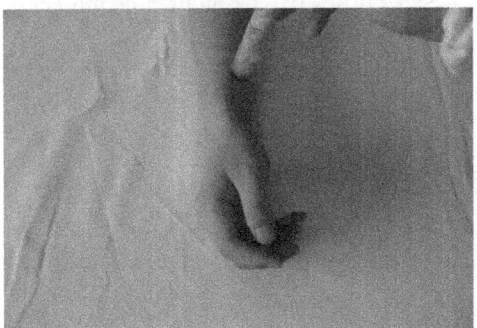

Figure 6.13.1 Gentle Moxa at Lie Que (LU-7)

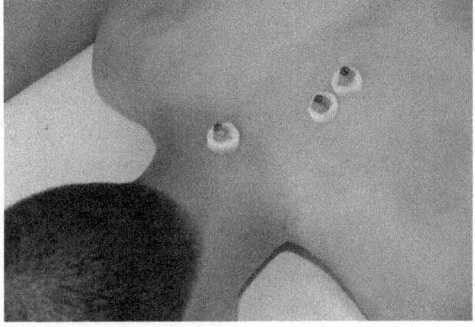

Figure 6.13.2 Moxa on Ginger at Fei Shu (BL-13), Feng Men (BL-12), and Da Zhui (DU-14)

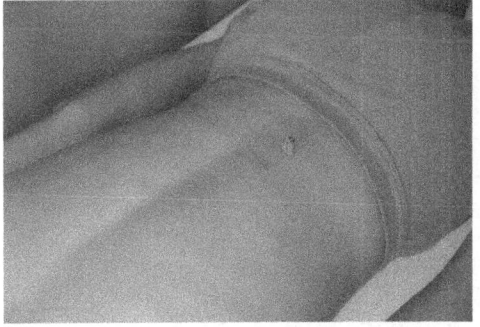

Figure 6.13.3 Scarring Moxa at Shen Shu (BL-23)

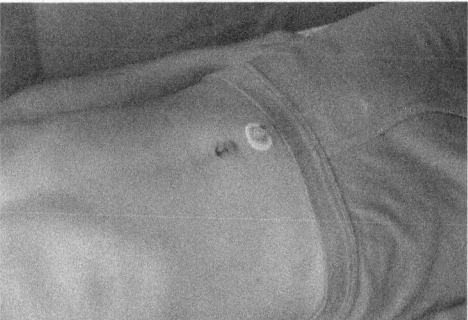

Figure 6.13.4 Indirect Moxa at Qi Hai (RN-6)

14. Bronchial Asthma

Bronchial asthma is a common clinical disease characterized by recurrent panting, hasty breathing, oppression in the chest and cough attacking at night or before dawn. The disease is often caused by constitutional deficiency, deep-lying phlegm in the lung, externally contracted wind-cold, mental over-stimulation, sudden environmental changes and inhalation of dust. It can occur all year round, but is especially common in winter or when the climate suddenly changes. It falls within the scope of asthma and rapid panting in TCM.

Main Symptoms: Sudden onset, hasty rapid breathing, gaping mouth and raised shoulders, flaring nostrils, thoracic oppression, wheezing in the throat, rapid breathing with an inability to lie down (often paroxysmal); accompanied by vexation, agitation, fatigued spirit, a lack of strength and a sombre white or purple facial complexion.

Acupoints:

- *Primary points:* Da Zhui (DU-14), Ding Chuan (EX-B-1), Fei Shu (BL-13), Feng Men (BL-12), Zhong Fu (LU-1).

- *Symptomatic points:* Oppression in the chest: Tian Tu (RN-22), Dan Zhong (RN-17); Deficiency pattern: Shen Shu (BL-23), Zu San Li (ST-36); Copious phlegm: Feng Long (ST-40), Pi Shu (BL-20).

Moxibustion Method:

- Gentle Moxa or Circling Moxa: Apply 20–30 minutes per acupoint. Repeat once daily for 10 days to complete a course of treatment. (Figure 6.14.1)

- Moxa on Ginger: Apply 5–7 cones per acupoint. Repeat once daily for 7–10 days to complete a course of treatment. (Figure 6.14.2)

- Scarring Moxa:* Apply moxa on 3–5 acupoints until suppurative blisters appear. Repeat once every other day. (Figure 6.14.3)

- Mao Lang Ye Application: Apply moxa on Da Zhui (DU-14) until blisters appear. Repeat once every ten days 3 times in total to complete a course of treatment. (Figure 6.14.4)

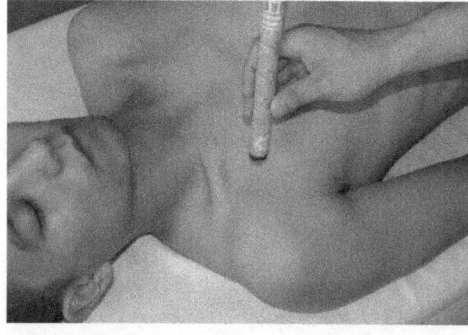

Figure 6.14.1 Gentle Moxa or Circling Moxa at Zhong Fu (LU-1)

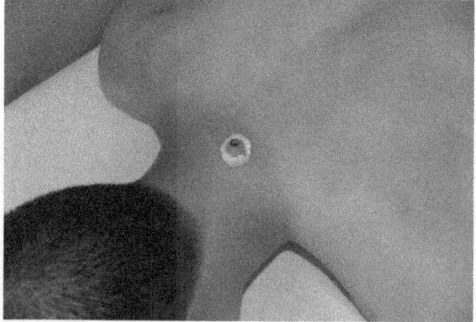

Figure 6.14.2 Moxa on Ginger at Ding Chuan (EX-B-1)

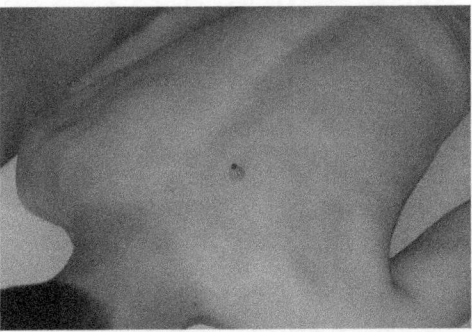

Figure 6.14.3 Scarring Moxa at Fei Shu (BL-13)

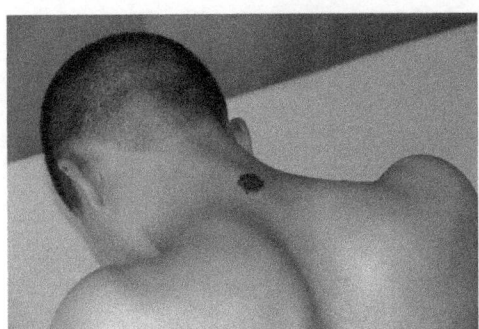 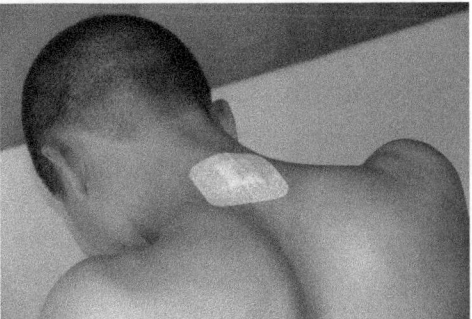

Figure 6.14.4 Mao Lang Ye Application at Da Zhui (DU-14)

- Medicinal Scarring Cone Moxa:* Ingredients: 500g of Chen Ai Ye (aged Artemisiae Argyi Folium), 30g of Liu Huang (Sulfur); 15g each of Ma Huang (Ephedrae Herba), Gui Zhi (Cinnamomi Ramulus), Rou Gui (Cinnamomi Cortex), Qiang Huo (Notopterygii Rhizoma et Radix), Du Huo (Angelicae Pubescentis Radix), Ru Xiang (Olibanum), Mo Yao (Myrrha), Xi Xin (Asari Herba), Gan Jiang (Zingiberis Rhizoma), Ding Xiang (Caryophylli Flos), Bai Zhi (Angelicae Dahuricae Radix), Chuan Jiao (Zanthoxyli Pericarpium), Cang Zhu (Atractylodis Rhizoma), Fang Feng (Saposhnikoviae Radix), Guang Mu Xiang (Aucklandiae Radix), Ban Xia Qu (Pinelliae Massa Fermentata); 9g each of Su Zi (Perillae Fructus), Ya Zao (Gleditsiae Fructus Abnormalis), Wu Yao (Linderae Radix), Chuan Wu (Aconiti Radix), Chang Pu (Acori Tatarinowii Rhizoma), Chen Pi (Citri Reticulatae Pericarpium), Gan Cao (Glycyrrhizae Radix), Pao Jia Pian (stir-baked Manis Squama), and 1g of She Xiang (Moschus). Grind the above medicinals into a fine powder and mix with moxa. Make the compound medicine into moxa cones (0.6–0.8cm in diameter and 1cm in height). Choose 3–5 acupoints and apply 5–9 cones per acupoint. Apply skin disinfectant or local anaesthesia with procaine and garlic juice on acupoints before performing moxa, once a year or twice every three years. Apply moxa 3 times for adults but once for children. (Figure 6.14.5)

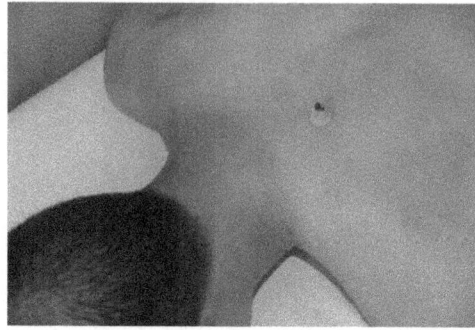

Figure 6.14.5 Medicinal Scarring Cone Moxa at Feng Men (BL-12)

15. Pulmonary Tuberculosis

Pulmonary tuberculosis is a chronic infectious disease induced by tubercle bacillus, and characterized by a progressive aggravating cough, tidal fever, haemoptysis, night sweating and emaciation. The disease is often induced by constitutional weakness, unclean food and long-term contact with dust or tuberculosis patients. It falls within the category of pulmonary consumption and consumptive disease in TCM.

Main Symptoms: Long-term low-grade fever, fatigue and a lack of strength, reduced appetite, aggravated cough, postmeridian tidal fever, reddening of the cheeks, red lips, dry mouth, expectoration of blood, night sweats, emaciation and a rapid heart rate. Accompanying symptoms include chest pain, dyspnoea, nocturnal emission in men and amenorrhoea in women.

Acupoints:

- *Primary points:* Fei Shu (BL-13), Dan Zhong (RN-17), Gao Huang (BL-43), Guan Yuan (RN-4), Zu San Li (ST-36).

- *Symptomatic points:* Tidal fever and night sweating: Yin Xi (HT-6), Tai Xi (KI-3); Haemoptysis: Kong Zui (LU-6); Nocturnal emissions: Shen Shu (BL-23); Severe cough: Feng Men (BL-12).

Moxibustion Method:

- Gentle Moxa or Circling Moxa: Apply 20–30 minutes per acupoint. Repeat once daily for 10 days to complete a course of treatment. (Figure 6.15.1)

- Moxa on Ginger: Apply 5–7 cones per acupoint. Repeat once daily for 7–10 days to complete a course of treatment. (Figure 6.15.2)

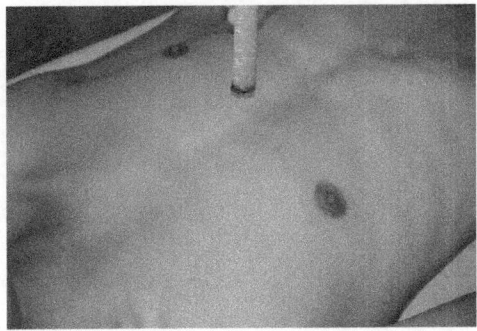

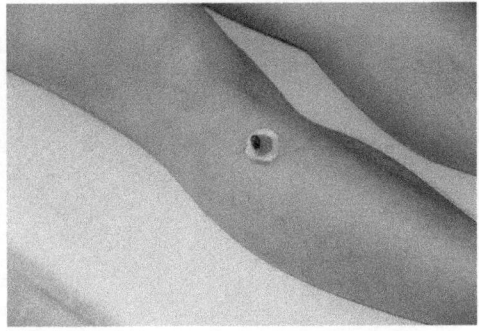

Figure 6.15.1 Gentle Moxa or Circling Moxa at
Dan Zhong (RN-17)

Figure 6.15.2 Moxa on Ginger at Zu San Li
(ST-36)

- Moxa on Garlic: Apply 5–7 cones per acupoint. Repeat once daily for 7–10 days to complete a course of treatment. (Figure 6.15.3)

- Wu Bei Zi Application: Grind some Wu Bei Zi (Galla Chinensis Galla) into fine powder, then put 1g of the powder in the umbilicus and fix with gauze before sleeping. It is effective for obvious night sweating. (Figure 6.15.4)

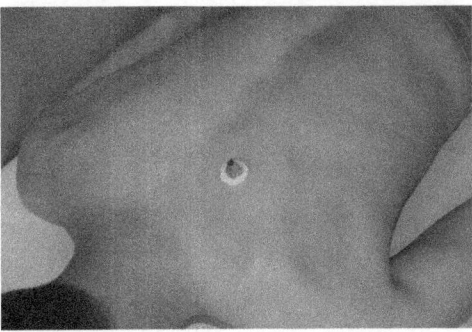

Figure 6.15.3 Moxa on Garlic at Fei Shu (BL-13)

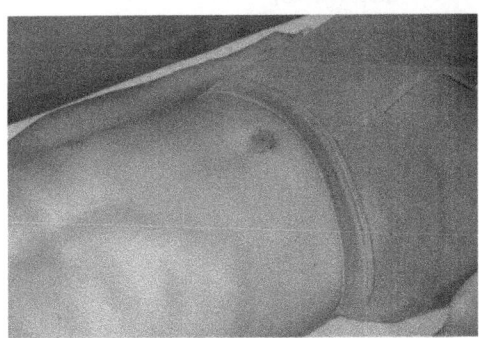

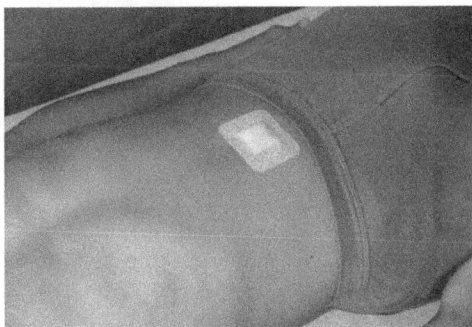

Figure 6.15.4 Wu Bei Zi Application at Shen Que (RN-8)

- Bai Jie Zi Application: Grind some Bai Jie Zi (Sinapis Albae Semen) into a fine powder and mix with rice vinegar. Apply the compound medicine on acupoints for 1–3 hours. Repeat every 4–5 days, and continue for 3 months. (Figure 6.15.5)

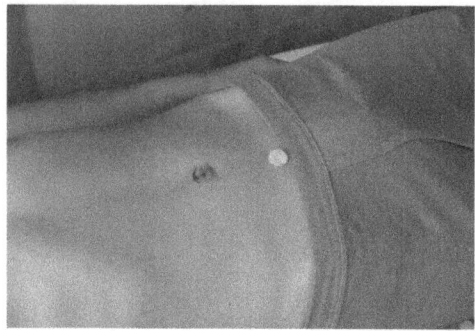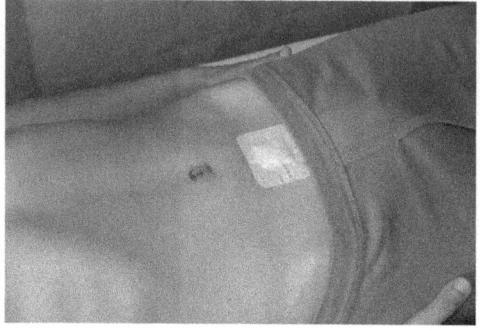

Figure 6.15.5 Bai Jie Zi Application at Guan Yuan (RN-4)

16. Emphysema

Emphysema is a chronic disease induced by air-filled expansions of the lung. It often develops from chronic bronchitis and bronchial breathing. When it attacks, it manifests as very difficult breathing, and is aggravated by slight movements. It often occurs in older people and is challenging to treat and cure. It is known as lung distension in TCM.

Main Symptoms: Shortness of breath during labour or sports in the early stage. As the state of the illness develops, symptoms of dyspnoea⊠cough and panting appear, accompanied by pale skin, a lack of strength, weight loss, reduced appetite, distension and fullness in the upper abdomen. Symptoms of congestive heart failure emerge in the end-stages.

Acupoints:

- *Primary points:* Fei Shu (BL-13), Da Zhui (DU-14), Xin Shu (BL-15), Dan Zhong (RN-17), Shen Shu (BL-23), Gao Huang (BL-43).

- *Symptomatic points:* Lung qi deficiency: Qi Hai (RN-6); Kidney qi deficiency: Guan Yuan (BL-26); Lung-kidney qi deficiency: Tai Yuan (LU-9), Tai Xi (KI-3).

Moxibustion Method:

- Gentle Moxa or Circling Moxa: Apply 20–30 minutes per acupoint. Repeat once daily for 10 days to complete a course of treatment. (Figure 6.16.1)

- Moxa on Ginger: Apply 5–7 cones per acupoint. Repeat once daily for 7–10 days to complete a course of treatment. (Figure 6.16.2)

- Non-scarring Moxa: Apply 5–7 cones per acupoint. Repeat once or twice a day for 10 days to complete a course of treatment. (Figure 6.16.3)

- Warm Needle Moxa: Choose 3–5 acupoints each treatment, and apply acupuncture and 3 moxa cones (approximately 6–15 min) per acupoint. Repeat once daily or every other day for a total of 10 times to complete a course of treatment. Repeat a treatment course after 7 days. (Figure 6.16.4)

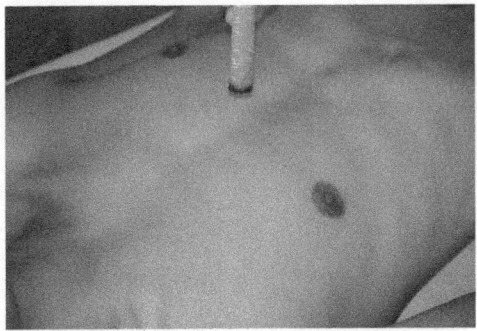

Figure 6.16.1 Gentle Moxa or Circling Moxa at Dan Zhong (RN-17)

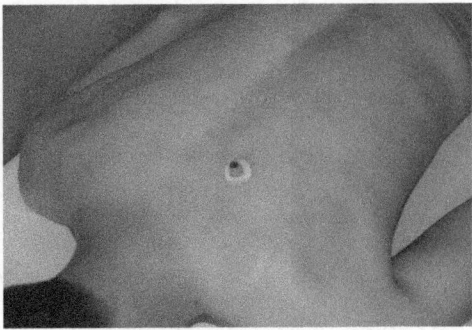

Figure 6.16.2 Moxa on Ginger at Fei Shu (BL-13)

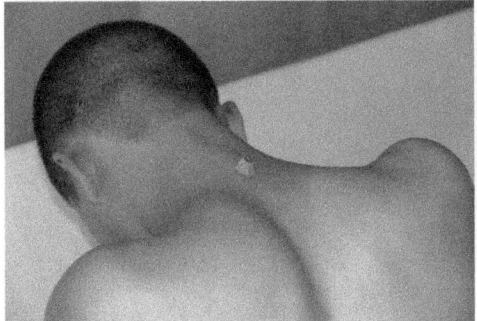

Figure 6.16.3 Non-scarring Moxa at Da Zhui (DU-14)

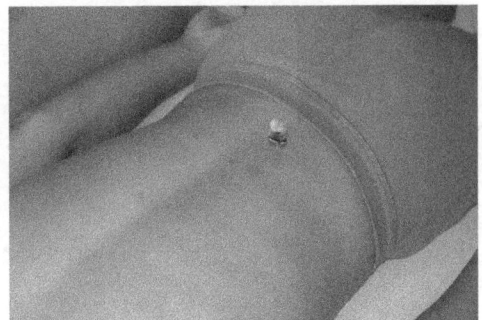

Figure 6.16.4 Warm Needle Moxa at Shen Shu (BL-23)

17. Stomach Pain

The main symptom of stomach pain, also known as epigastric pain, involves paroxysmal repeated pain in the upper abdomen, aggravated by hunger or fullness. Stomach pain is usually caused by weakness of the spleen and stomach and is related to changes in food, drink, emotions and climate; it may therefore appear rhythmically. Stomach pain is categorized into cardialgia, gastropathic stomach ache and epigastric pain in Chinese medicine. This condition is often seen in cases of acute or chronic gastritis, peptic ulcers and gastroneurosis.

Main Symptoms: Epigastric pain or a dull pain in the gastric cavity, a fatigued spirit and a lack of strength; accompanied by hydroptysis.

Acupoints:

- *Primary points:* Pi Shu (BL-20), Wei Shu (BL-21), Zhong Wan (RN-12), Zu San Li (ST-36).

- *Symptomatic points:* Cold pathogens invading the stomach: Wei Shu (BL-21); Qi stagnation and blood stasis: Ge Shu (BL-17); Dyspeptic retention: Liang Men (ST-21), Xia Wan (RN-10); Liver qi invading the stomach: Tai Chong (LR-3).

Moxibustion Method:

- Gentle Pole Moxa: Apply moxa to each point for 15–20 minutes. Perform treatment once per day. Ten treatments comprise one course of treatment. (Figure 6.17.1)

- Moxa on Ginger: Apply moxa to each point using 5–7 cones. Perform treatment once per day. Ten treatments comprise one course of treatment. (Figure 6.17.2)

- Moxa on Salt: Apply moxa to Shen Que (RN-8) for 5–7 cones. Perform treatment once per day. Seven treatments comprise one course of treatment. (Figure 6.17.3)

- Moxa on Fu Zi Cake: Apply moxa to 3–5 points, 5–7 cones per point. Perform treatment once per day. Seven treatments comprise one course of treatment. (Figure 6.17.4)

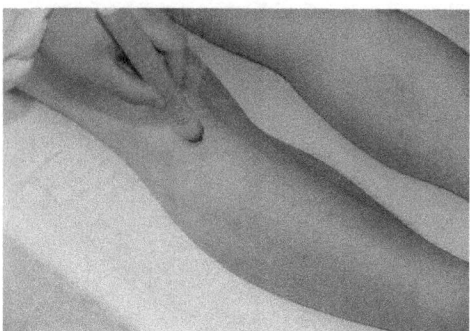

Figure 6.17.1 Gentle Pole Moxa at Zu San Li (ST-36)

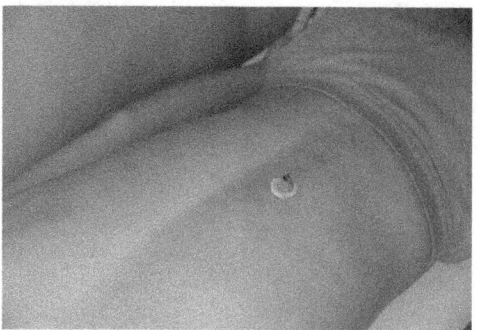

Figure 6.17.2 Moxa on Ginger at Pi Shu (BL-20)

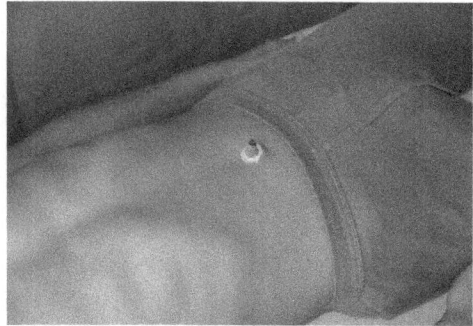

Figure 6.17.3 Moxa on Salt at Shen Que (RN-8)

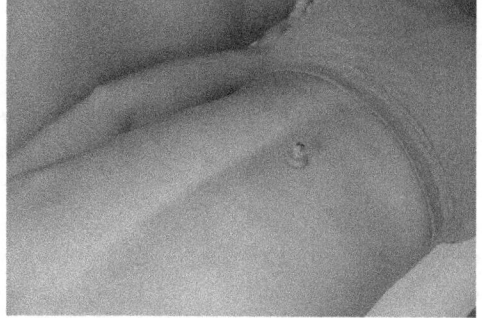

Figure 6.17.4 Moxa on Fu Zi Cake at Wei Shu (BL-21)

- Non-scarring Moxa: Apply moxa to each point for 5–7 cones until the area reddens. Perform treatment once per day or every other day. Ten treatments comprise one course of treatment. (Figure 6.17.5)

- Wu Zhu Yu Compound Application: Apply Wu Zhu Yu (Evodiae Fructus) to Shen Que (RN-8) for 3–6 hours. Perform treatment once or twice per day. (Figure 6.17.6)

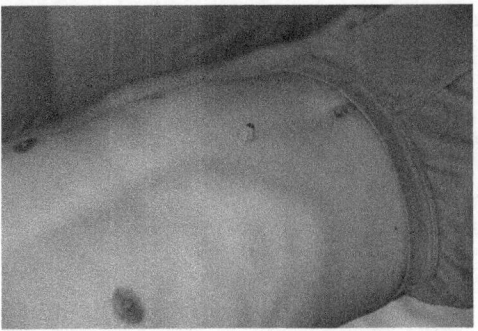

Figure 6.17.5 Non-scarring Moxa at Zhong Wan (RN-12)

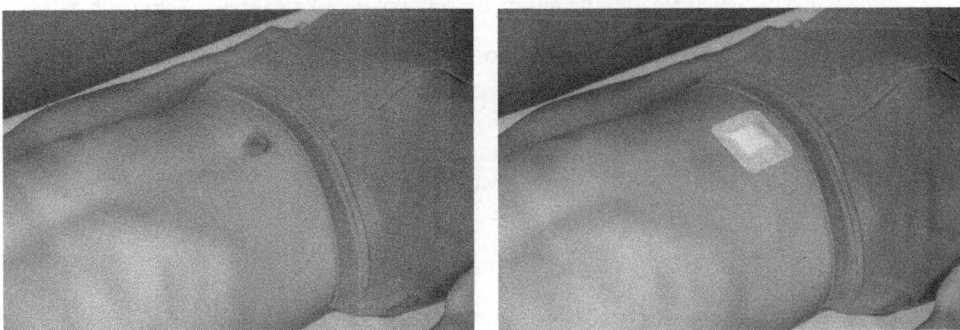

Figure 6.17.6 Wu Zhu Yu Compound Application at Shen Que (RN-8)

18. Gastroptosis

Gastroptosis is a common chronic disease, the diagnostic criterion of which involves the lower border of the stomach reaching the pelvic cavity, and the arc of the lesser curvature of the stomach being below the line connecting the iliac crests. Gastroptosis is usually caused by one of the following: weakness of the spleen and stomach, binge overeating or chronic hunger, eating and drinking without temperance, leading to impairment of the spleen and stomach; or correlated with emotion. It is more commonly seen in slim and thin patients. Gastroptosis is categorized into stomach atony, gastric upset and belching in Chinese medicine.

Main Symptoms: The upper abdomen is concave while the lower abdomen bulges. The stomach has a feeling of fullness and prolapse; belching and nausea, vomiting, rugitus, a dull pain in the abdomen and accompanying constipation, diarrhoea, dizziness, debilitation, palpitations, insomnia and excessive dreams.

Acupoints:

- *Primary points:* Zhong Wan (RN-12), Liang Men (ST-21), Qi Hai (RN-6), Guan Yuan (RN-4), Zu San Li (ST-36).

- *Symptomatic points:* Hepaptosia: Qi Men (LR-14), Gan Shu (BL-18); Nephroptosis: Shen Shu (BL-23), Jing Men (GB-25); Gastric and duodenal ulcer: Gong Sun (SP-4), Nei Guan (PC-6).

Moxibustion Method:

- Gentle Pole Moxa: Apply moxa to each point for 20–30 minutes. Perform treatment once per day. Ten treatments comprise one course of treatment. (Figure 6.18.1)

- Moxa on Ginger: Apply moxa to each point using 5–7 cones. Perform treatment once per day. Ten treatments comprise one course of treatment. (Figure 6.18.2)

- Moxa on Salt: Apply moxa to Shen Que (RN-8) in 5–7 cones. Perform treatment once per day. Seven treatments comprise one course of treatment. (Figure 6.18.3)

- Moxa on Fu Zi Cake: Apply moxa to 3–5 points, 5–7 cones per point. Perform treatment once per day. Seven treatments comprise one course of treatment. (Figure 6.18.4)

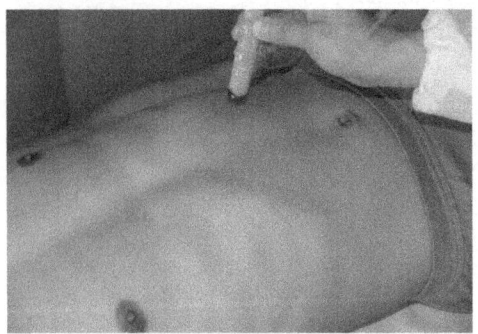

Figure 6.18.1 Gentle Pole Moxa at Liang Men (ST-21)

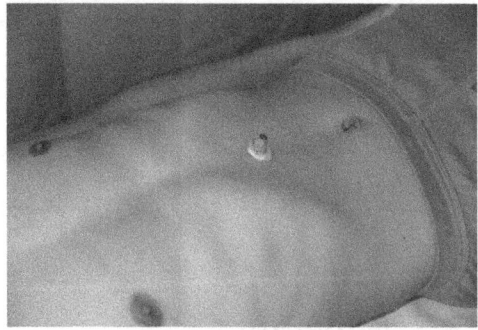

Figure 6.18.2 Moxa on Ginger at Zhong Wan (RN-12)

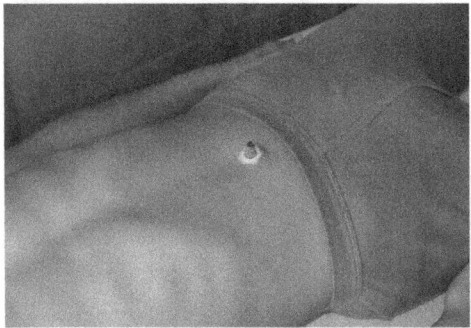

Figure 6.18.3 Moxa on Salt at Shen Que (RN-8)

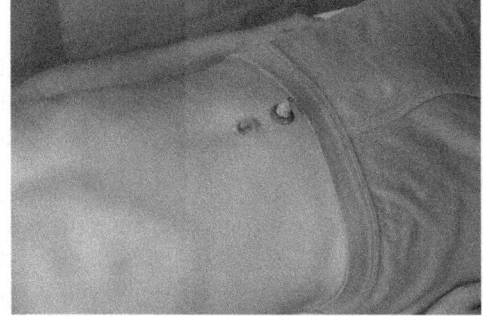

Figure 6.18.4 Moxa on Fu Zi Cake at Qi Hai (RN-6)

- Non-scarring Moxa: Apply moxa to 2–3 points, 3–5 cones per point. Perform treatment once every 7–14 days. (Figure 6.18.5)

- Mao Gen Gen Application: Mash Mao Gen Gen (Ranunculi Japonici Radix) into a paste and form the paste into a coin-like cake. Apply moxa to each point for

20 minutes. Perform treatment once per day. Seven treatments comprise one course of treatment. (Figure 6.18.6)

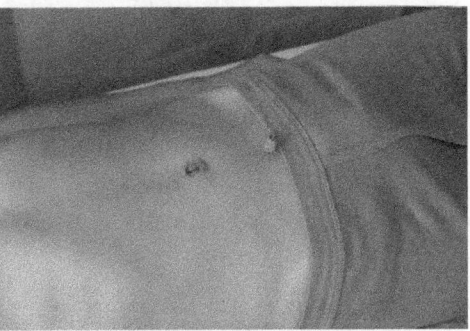

Figure 6.18.5 Non-scarring Moxa at Guan Yuan (RN-4)

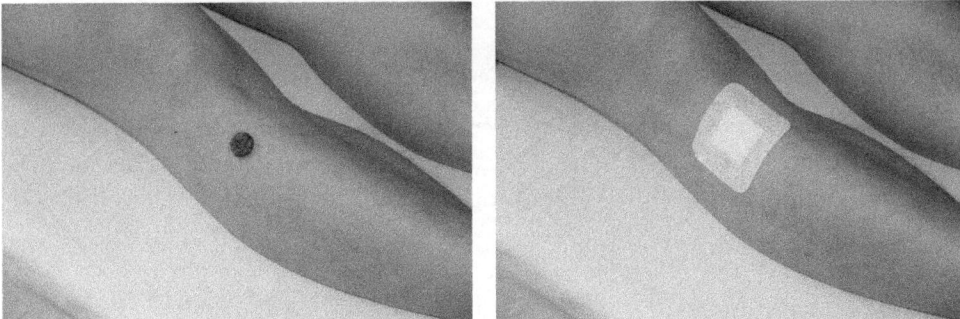

Figure 6.18.6 Mao Gen Gen Application at Zu San Li (ST-36)

- Warm Needle Moxa: Apply moxa to 3–5 points, 3 cones or 6–15 minutes per point. Perform treatment once per day or every other day. Ten treatments comprise one course of treatment, with an interval of seven days between treatment courses. (Figure 6.18.7)

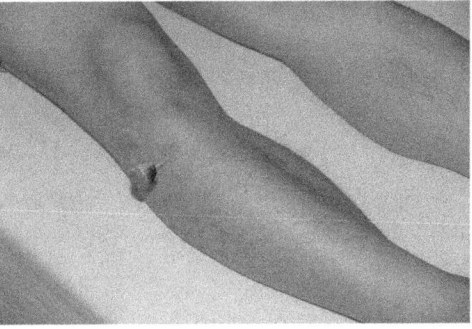

Figure 6.18.7 Warm Needle Moxa at Zu San Li (ST-36)

19. Vomiting

Vomiting refers to a type of symptom that involves nausea, vomiting, spitting and dry retching. Vomiting substances accompanied by retching sounds is known as 'vomiting', vomiting substances noiselessly is called 'spitting', vomiting without substances but accompanied by loud sounds is called 'dry retching'. Vomiting is usually caused by impaired harmonious down bearing of the stomach causing ascending counter flow of stomach qi or eating and drinking without temperance which impairs the spleen and stomach. This disease can be seen in every age group and gender, and is often seen in the case of acute gastritis, gastroectasia, pylorospasm, gastroneurosis, cholecystitis and pancreatitis.

Main Symptoms: Nausea, vomiting, specific discomfort in the upper abdomen, often accompanied by symptoms of dizziness, dribbling, a slow pulse and low blood pressure. Chronic and violent vomiting can cause water-electrolyte disturbances.

Acupoints:

- *Primary points:* Nei Guan (PC-6), Zu San Li (ST-36), Zhong Wan (RN-12).

- *Symptomatic points:* Cold vomiting: Wei Shu (BL-21), Shang Wan (RN-13); Hot vomiting: He Gu (LI-4); Dyspeptic retention: Liang Men (ST-21), Tian Shu (ST-25); Rugitus: Pi Shu (BL-20), Da Chang Shu (BL-25); Pantothen: Gong Sun (SP-4).

Moxibustion Method:

- Gentle Pole Moxa or Circling Moxa: Apply moxa to each point for 15–20 minutes. Perform treatment once per day. Seven treatments comprise one course of treatment. (Figure 6.19.1)

- Moxa on Ginger: Apply moxa to each point using 5–7 cones. Perform treatment once per day, 7 treatments comprise one course of treatment. (Figure 6.19.2)

- Moxa on Salt: Apply moxa to Shen Que (RN-8) using 5–7 cones. Perform treatment once per day. There should be obvious warmth in the abdomen, which spreads to the abdominal cavity. This treatment applies to the pattern of spleen-stomach vacuity cold. (Figure 6.19.3)

- Non-scarring Moxa: Apply moxa to each point using 5–7 cones until the skin turns red. Perform treatment once per day or every other day. Ten treatments comprise one course of treatment. (Figure 6.19.4)

- Warm Needle Moxa: Apply moxa to 3–5 points, 3 cones or 6–15 minutes per point. Perform treatment once per day or every other day. Seven treatments comprise one course of treatment. (Figure 6.19.5)

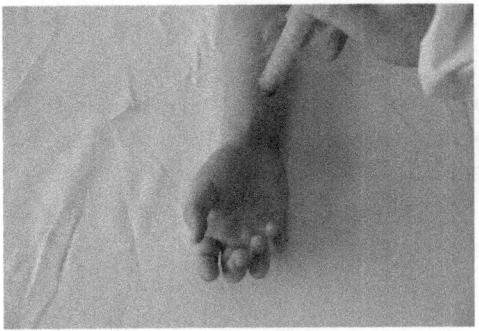

Figure 6.19.1 Gentle Pole Moxa or Circling Moxa at Nei Guan (PC-6)

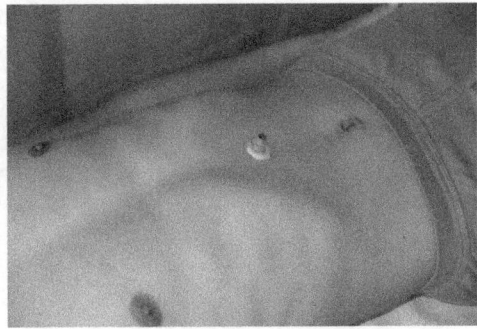

Figure 6.19.2 Moxa on Ginger at Zhong Wan (RN-12)

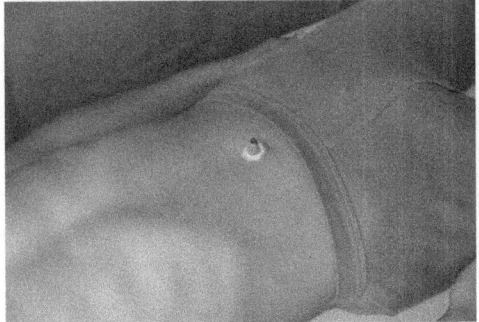

Figure 6.19.3 Moxa on Salt at Shen Que (RN-8)

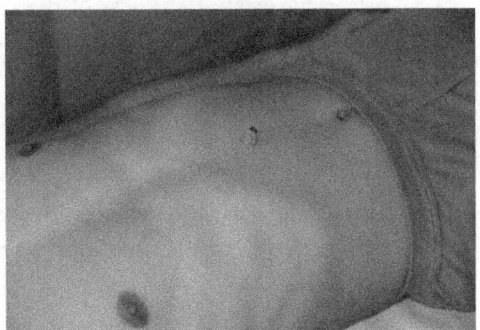

Figure 6.19.4 Non-scarring Moxa at Zhong Wan (RN-12)

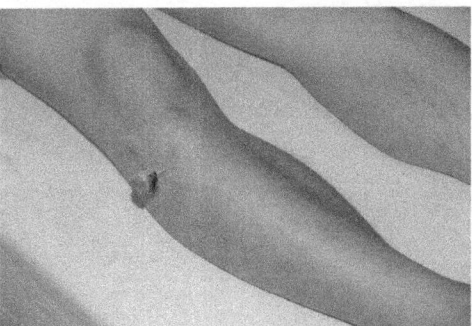

Figure 6.19.5 Warm Needle Moxa at Zu San Li (ST-36)

20. Chronic Ulcerative Colitis

Chronic ulcerative colitis refers to a type of agnogenic superficial nonspecific inflammation of the rectal and colonic mucosa. The main symptoms are abdominal pain, hemafecia and tenesmus. The condition of the disease can be prolonged, mild or severe. This disease is usually caused by one of the following: invasion of exogenous pathogens, drinking and eating irregularly, and spiritual excitement. The age of onset is often between 20–50 years.

Chronic ulcerative colitis is categorized into enduring diarrhoea, dysentery or intestinal wind and visceral toxins in Chinese medicine.

Main Symptoms: Diarrhoea, mucous stools with pus and blood, abnormal stool consistency, dull pain or abdominal angina, hemafecia, tenesmus and heat, accompanied by fatigued spirit and lack of strength, abdominal fullness and rugitus, depressed emotions, abdominal pain radiating to the sides of the ribs or dull aching in the lumbar region and knees and early morning diarrhoea.

Acupoints:

- *Primary points:* Tian Shu (ST-25), Qi Hai (RN-6), Guan Yuan (RN-4), Zu San Li (ST-36), Shang Ju Xu (ST-37).

- *Symptomatic points:* Weakness of the spleen and stomach: Pi Shu (BL-20), Wei Shu (BL-21), Da Chang Shu (BL-25), Gong Sun (SP-4); Liver depression: Gan Shu (BL-18), Zu San Li (ST-36); Insufficiency of kidney yang: Shen Shu (BL-23), Ming Men (DU-4).

Moxibustion Method:

- Gentle Pole Moxa or Circling Moxa: Apply moxa to each point for 30 minutes. Perform treatment once per day; 10 treatments comprise one course of treatment. (Figure 6.20.1)

- Moxa on Ginger: Apply moxa to each point using 5–7 cones. Perform treatment once per day; 10 treatments comprise one course of treatment. (Figure 6.20.2)

- Scarring Cone Moxa:* Apply moxa to Zu San Li (ST-36), Shang Ju Xu (ST-37) in 5–7 cones. Perform treatment once monthly. (Figure 6.20.3)

- Moxa on Salt: Apply moxa to Shen Que (RN-8) in 5–7 cones. Perform treatment once every other day. Ten treatments comprise one course of treatment. (Figure 6.20.4)

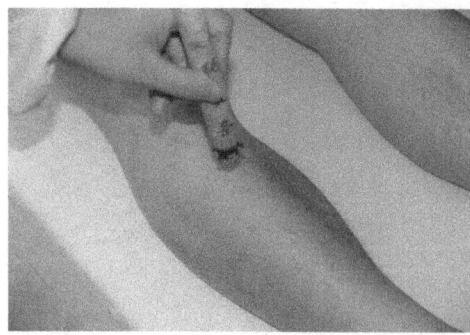

Figure 6.20.1 Gentle Pole Moxa or Circling Moxa at Shang Ju Xu (ST-37)

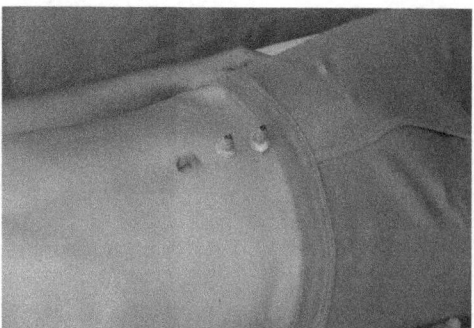

Figure 6.20.2 Moxa on Ginger at Qi Hai (RN-6) and Guan Yuan (RN-4)

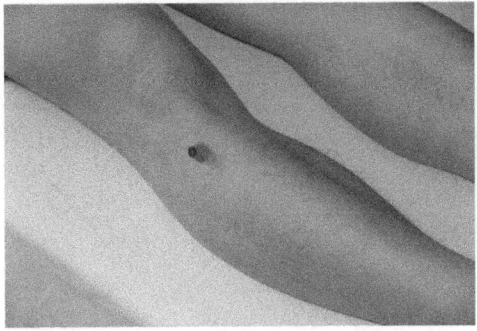

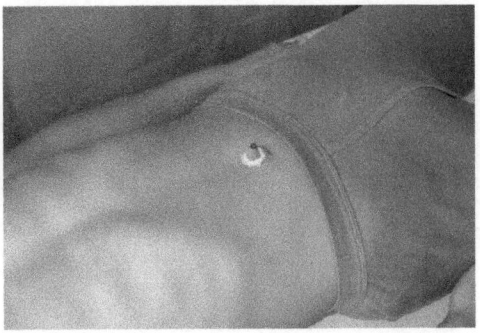

Figure 6.20.3 Scarring Cone Moxa at Zu San Li (ST-36)

Figure 6.20.4 Moxa on Salt at Shen Que (RN-8)

21. Abdominal Pain

Abdominal pain occurs below the epigastric region and above the symphysis pubis. This condition is usually caused by one of the following: externally contracted wind, cold, summer-heat, damp; or eating and drinking without temperance, emotional depression, qi stagnation or blood stasis. This condition can be seen in every age group and gender, and is often seen in diseases of the internal organs, especially digestive system and gynaecological pathologies.

Main Symptoms: Acute abdominal pain is characterized by an acute onset, severe pain, distension-fullness that increases with pressure, often accompanied by abdominal distension, rugitus and incessant belching. Chronic abdominal pain is characterized by long-term disease and non-specific pain, accompanied by a lack of warmth in the limbs, excessive excretion of clear urine, a thin, pale tongue, and a deep fine pulse.

Acupoints:

- *Primary points:* Zhong Wan (RN-12), Tian Shu (ST-25), He Gu (LI-4), Zu San Li (ST-36), San Yin Jiao (SP-6).

- *Symptomatic points:* Cold accumulation: Shen Que (RN-8), Guan Yuan (RN-4); Humid heat: Yin Ling Quan (SP-9), Nei Ting (ST-44); Qi stagnation and blood stasis: Xue Hai (SP-10), Tai Chong (LR-3).

Moxibustion Method:

- Gentle Pole Moxa: Apply moxa to each point for 20–30 minutes. Perform treatment once per day. Ten treatments comprise one course of treatment. (Figure 6.21.1)

- Moxa on Ginger: Apply moxa to each point using 5–7 cones. Perform treatment once per day. Ten treatments comprise one course of treatment. (Figure 6.21.2)

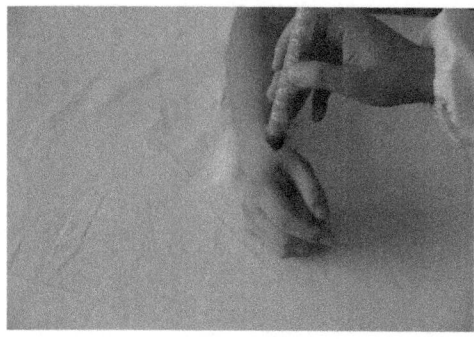

Figure 6.21.1 Gentle Pole Moxa at He Gu (LI-4)

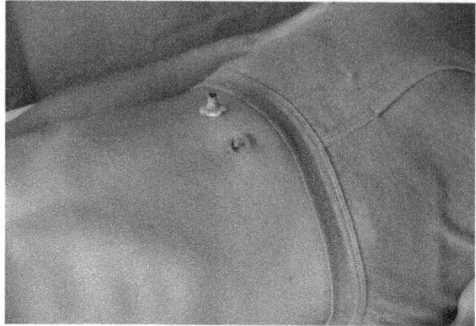

Figure 6.21.2 Moxa on Ginger at Tian Shu (ST-25)

- Moxa on Salt: Apply moxa to Shen Que (RN-8) using 5–7 cones. Perform treatment once per day. Seven treatments comprise one course of treatment. This treatment applies to the pattern of vacuity cold. (Figure 6.21.3)

- Non-scarring Moxa: Apply moxa to each point using 5–7 cones until reddened. Perform treatment once per day or every other day. Ten treatments comprise one course of treatment. (Figure 6.21.4)

- Moxa on Fu Zi Cake: Apply moxa to 3–5 points, using 5–7 cones per point. Perform treatment once per day. Seven treatments comprise one course of treatment. (Figure 6.21.5)

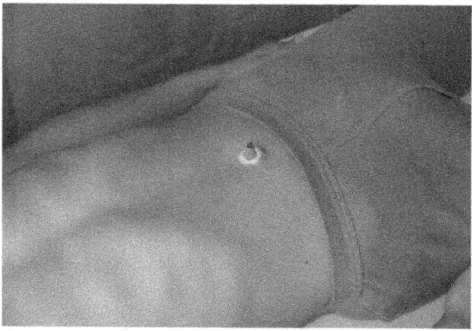

Figure 6.21.3 Moxa on Salt at Shen Que (RN-8)

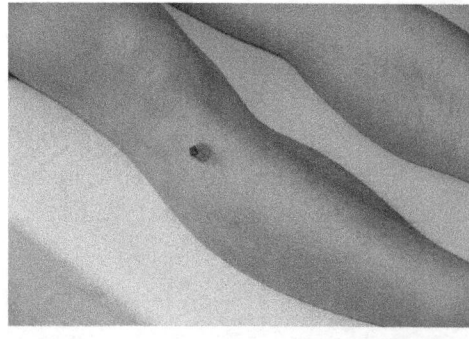

Figure 6.21.4 Non-scarring Moxa at Zu San Li (ST-36)

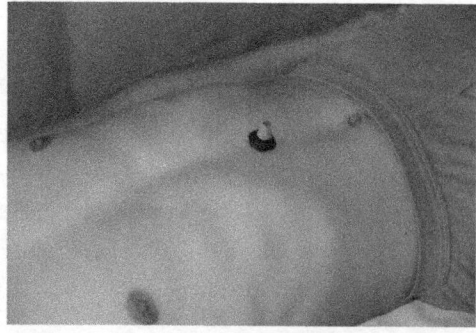

Figure 6.21.5 Moxa on Fu Zi Cake at Zhong Wan (RN-12)

22. Abdominal Distension

Abdominal distension refers to a type of symptom involving excess gas in the intestinal tract. Its main manifestation is meteorism and gas retention in the abdomen. Abdominal distension is usually caused by one of the following: damp-heat, food accumulation, qi stagnation, as well as an abiding ailment or deficient distension caused by post-operative invalidism. This disease is often seen in the case of chordapsus, hepatopathy, gastropathy, malnutritional stagnation and post-operative invalidism.

Main Symptoms: Abdominal discomfort, constrained bloating, mild or severe abdominal distension, which may be more severe after eating. These symptoms may be more severe with emotion changes, alleviated after passing gas and accompanied by hyperactive bowel sounds or abdominal pain.

Acupoints:

- *Primary points:* Zhong Wan (RN-12), Wei Shu (BL-21), Pi Shu (BL-20), Da Chang Shu (BL-25), Xiao Chang Shu (BL-27).

- *Symptomatic points:* Cold: Guan Yuan (RN-4), Zu San Li (ST-36); Heat: Yin Ling Quan (SP-9); Qi stagnancy: Tai Chong (LR-3); Liver depression: Xuan Zhong (GB-39).

Moxibustion Method:

- Gentle Pole Moxa or Circling Moxa: Apply moxa to each point for 30 minutes. Perform treatment once per day. Ten treatments comprise one course of treatment. (Figure 6.22.1)

- Moxa on Ginger: Apply moxa to each point using 5–7 cones. Perform treatment once per day. Ten treatments comprise one course of treatment. (Figure 6.22.2)

- Scarring Cone Moxa:* Apply moxa to Zu San Li (ST-36) and Shang Ju Xu (ST-37) using 5–7 cones. Perform treatment once monthly. (Figure 6.22.3)

- Moxa on Scallion and Salt: Take 90g of scallion white and 30g of salt, and grind them together to form a small cake. Apply moxa to Tian Shu (ST-25) and Shang Ju Xu (ST-37) using 5–7 cones. Perform treatment once or twice every other day. The course of treatment is determined by the condition of the disease. (Figure 6.22.4)

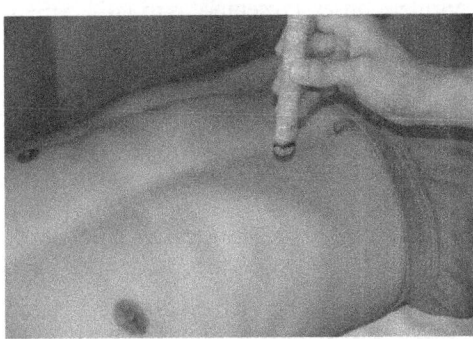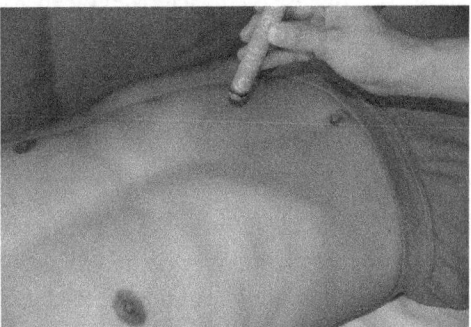

Figure 6.22.1 Gentle Pole Moxa or Circling Moxa at Zhong Wan (RN-12)

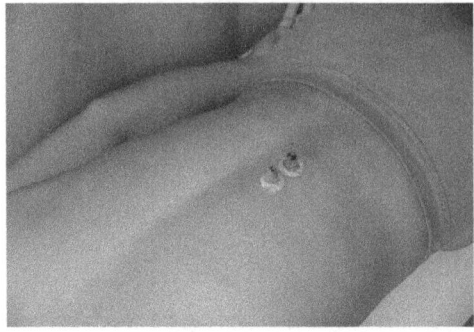

Figure 6.22.2 Moxa on Ginger at Pi Shu (BL-20) and Wei Shu (BL-21)

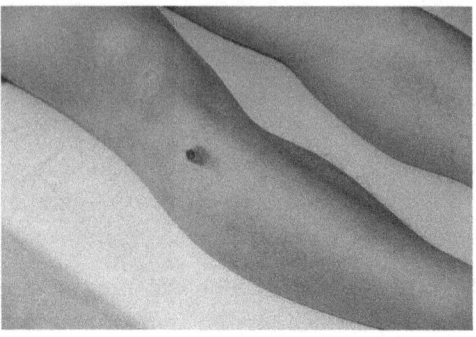

Figure 6.22.3 Scarring Cone Moxa at Zu San Li (ST-36)

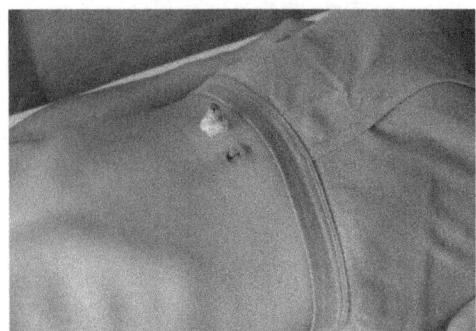

Figure 6.22.4 Moxa on Scallion and Salt at Tian Shu (ST-25)

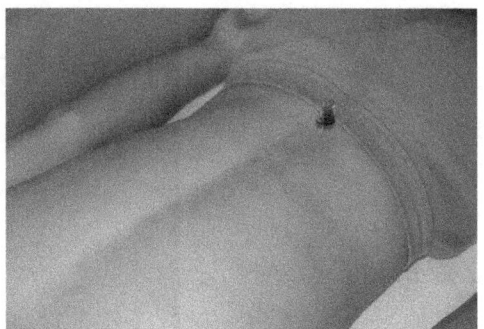

Figure 6.22.5 Warm Needle Moxa at Da Chang Shu (BL-25)

- Warm Needle Moxa: Apply moxa to 3–5 points, using 3 cones or for 6–15 minutes per point. Perform treatment once per day or every other day. Ten treatments comprise one course of treatment. (Figure 6.22.5)

23. Dysentery

Dysentery is an intestinal infectious disease common in summer and autumn. Its main manifestation is abdominal pain and diarrhoea, tenesmus and stools containing pus and blood. This disease is characterized by an acute, virulent onset. Dysentery is usually caused by one of the following: infection with summer hygrosis and toxic heat causing injury to the spleen and stomach; or a vacuous constitution with external contraction of cold leading to chronic dysentery. It is also called stagnant diarrhoea and intestinal afflux in Chinese medicine. This disease is often seen in the case of acute bacillary dysentery, toxic dysentery and amoebic dysentery.

Main Symptoms: An increase in the frequency of defecation, mucous stools containing pus and blood, abdominal pain, tenesmus, accompanied by diarrhoea, a burning sensation in the anus and short voiding of reddish urine. Damp-heat dysentery presents with an aversion to cold with heat, heart vexation, thirst, a red tongue with an oily yellow tongue coating, and a slippery, rapid pulse. Cold-damp dysentery presents with diarrhoea containing pus and blood and adhesive freezing, fullness in the stomach, a desire for warmth and an aversion to cold, an oily white tongue coating, and a fine, weak pulse.

Acupoints:

- *Primary points:* Xia Wan (RN-10), Shang Ju Xu (ST-37), Tian Shu (ST-25), Guan Yuan (RN-4), He Gu (LI-4).

- *Symptomatic points:* Cold: Zhong Wan (RN-12), Qi Hai (RN-6); Damp-heat: Qu Chi (LI-11), Nei Ting (ST-44); Lingering dysentery: Pi Shu (BL-20), Shen Shu (BL-23); Archocele: Qi Hai (RN-6), Chang Qian (DU-1).

Moxibustion Method:

- Gentle Pole Moxa: Apply moxa to each point for 20–30 minutes. Perform treatment once per day. Ten treatments comprise one course of treatment. (Figure 6.23.1)

- Moxa on Ginger or Garlic: Apply moxa to each point using 5–7 cones. Perform treatment once per day. Ten treatments comprise one course of treatment. (Figure 6.23.2)

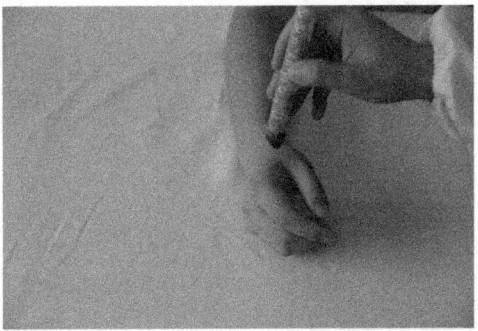

Figure 6.23.1 Gentle Pole Moxa at He Gu (LI-4)

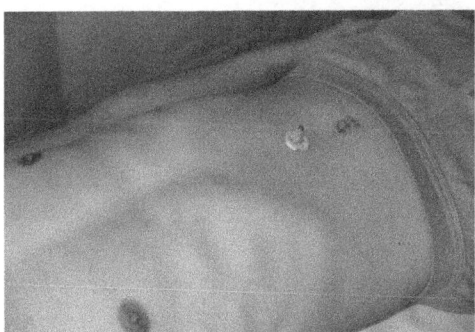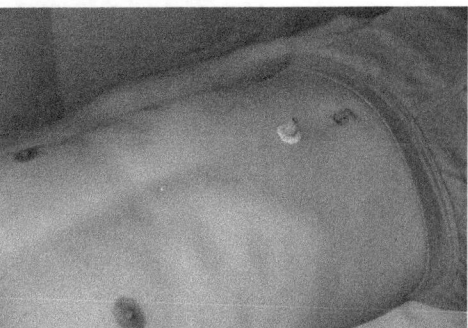

Figure 6.23.2 Moxa on Ginger or Garlic at Xia Wan (RN-10)

- Moxa on Salt: Apply moxa to Shen Que (RN-8) and Chang Qian (DU-1) using 5–7 cones. Perform treatment once per day. Seven treatments comprise one course of treatment. (Figure 6.23.3)

- Non-scarring Moxa: Apply moxa to each point using 5–7 cones until the skin turns red. Perform treatment once per day or every other day. Ten treatments comprise one course of treatment. (Figure 6.23.4)

- Tai Yi Amazing Needle: Apply moxa to each point 5–7 times. Perform treatment once every other day or every 3 days. (Figure 6.23.5)

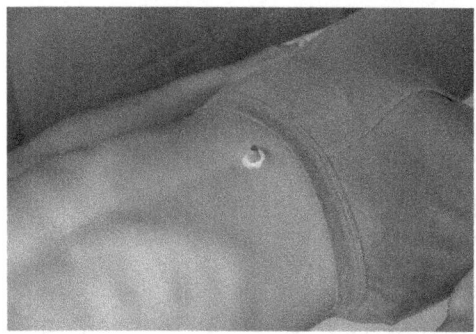 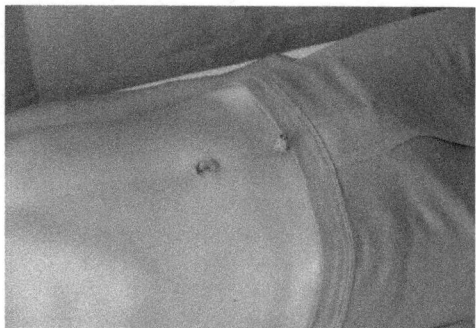

Figure 6.23.3 Moxa on Salt at Shen Que (RN-8)   *Figure 6.23.4 Non-scarring Moxa at Guan Yuan (RN-4)*

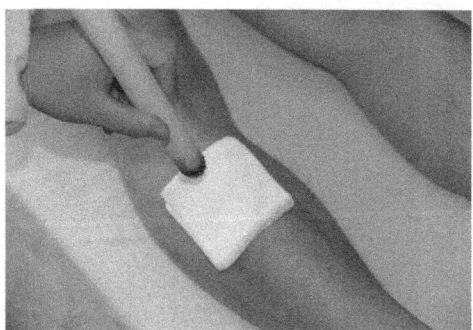 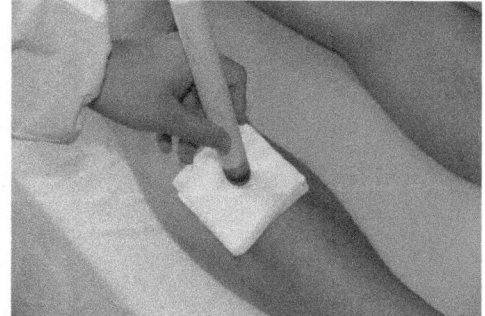

Figure 6.23.5 Tai Yi Amazing Needle at Shang Ju Xu (ST-37)

24. Diarrhoea

Diarrhoea is a common disease, the clinical symptom of which mainly involves an increase in the frequency of defecation, and tenuous or watery stools. This disease is usually caused by one of the following: eating and drinking without temperance, deficiency of the spleen and kidney, and contraction of exogenous damp; all of which cause functional disorders of the spleen and stomach. It can occur regardless of the individual constitution or season. Diarrhoea is often seen in cases of acute or chronic enteritis, gastrointestinal dysfunction, enteritis anaphylactica, colitis gravis and enterophthisis.

Main Symptoms: Abdominal pain, rugitus, an increase in the frequency of defecation to several times a day, loose or watery stools, defecation without pus or blood and tenesmus. The tongue is red with an oily yellow tongue coating, accompanied by distension and fullness in the chest and sides or dull aching of the lumbar region and knees.

Acupoints:

- *Primary points:* Tian Shu (ST-25), Shang Ju Xu (ST-37), Shen Que (RN-8), Guan Yuan (RN-4).

- *Symptomatic points:* Damp-heat: Nei Ting (ST-44); Dyspeptic retention: Zhong Wan (RN-12); Spleen vacuity: Pi Shu (BL-20), Tai Bai (SP-3); Liver depression: Tai Chong (LR-3); Kidney vacuity: Shen Shu (BL-23), Ming Men (DU-4).

Moxibustion Method:

- Gentle Pole Moxa: Apply moxa to each point for 20–30 minutes. Perform treatment once per day. Ten treatments comprise one course of treatment. (Figure 6.24.1)

- Moxa on Ginger: Apply moxa to each point using 5–7 cones. Perform treatment once per day. Ten treatments comprise one course of treatment. (Figure 6.24.2)

- Moxa on Salt: Apply moxa to Shen Que (RN-8) using 5–7 cones. Perform treatment once per day. Seven treatments comprise one course of treatment. (Figure 6.24.3)

- Moxa on Fu Zi Cake: Apply moxa to 3–5 points, using 5–7 cones per point. Perform treatment once per day. Seven treatments comprise one course of treatment. (Figure 6.24.4)

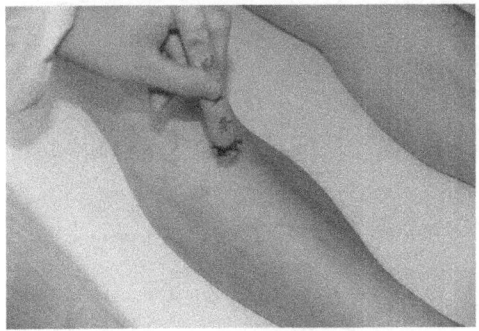

Figure 6.24.1 Gentle Pole Moxa at Shang Ju Xu (ST-37)

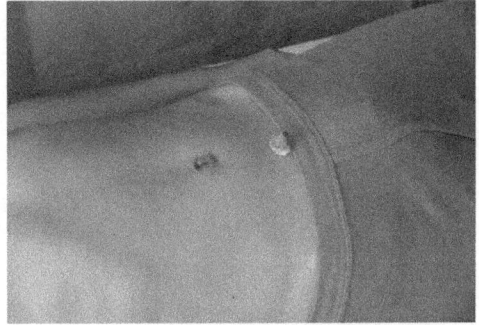

Figure 6.24.2 Moxa on Ginger at Guan Yuan (RN-4)

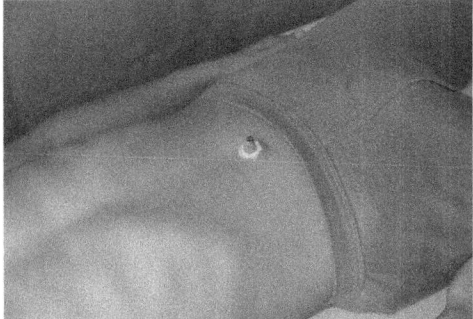

Figure 6.24.3 Moxa on Salt at Shen Que (RN-8)

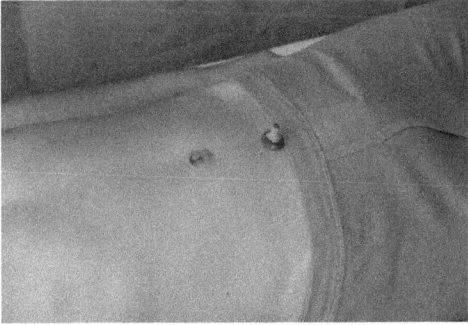

Figure 6.24.4 Moxa on Fu Zi Cake at Guan Yuan (RN-4)

- Moxa on Pepper Cake: Apply moxa to 3–5 points, using 5–7 cones per point. Perform treatment once per day. Seven treatments comprise one course of treatment. (Figure 6.24.5)

- Warm Needle Moxa: Apply moxa to 3–5 points, using 3 cones or for 6–15 minutes per point. Perform treatment once per day or every other day. Ten treatments comprise one course of treatment, with a 7-day interval between the courses. (Figure 6.24.6)

- Juncibustion:* Apply moxa to Tian Shu (ST-25), Chang Qian (DU-1) and Yin Bai (SP-1). Perform treatment once every 3 days. This method applies to deficiency-type diarrhoea. (Figure 6.24.7)

- Tai Yi Amazing Needle: Apply moxa to 3–5 points, using 5–7 times each point. Perform treatment once every other day or every 3 days. This method applies to deficiency-type diarrhoea. (Figure 6.24.8)

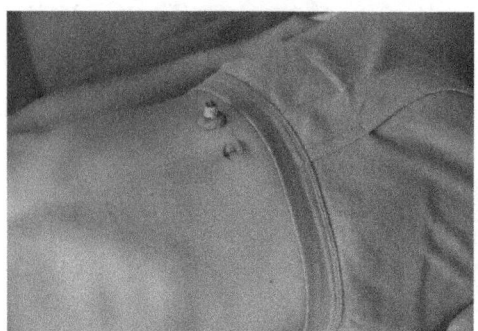 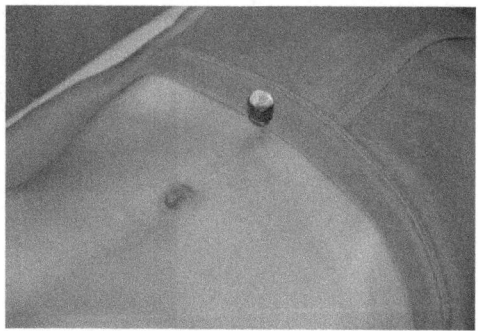

Figure 6.24.5 Moxa on Pepper Cake at Tian Shu (ST-25)   Figure 6.24.6 Warm Needle Moxa at Guan Yuan (RN-4)

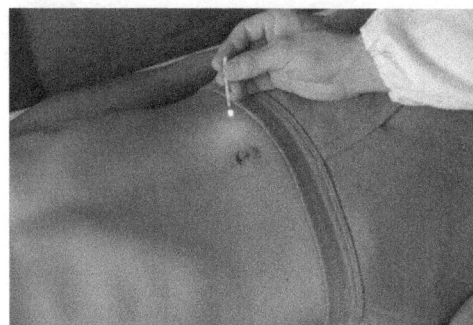 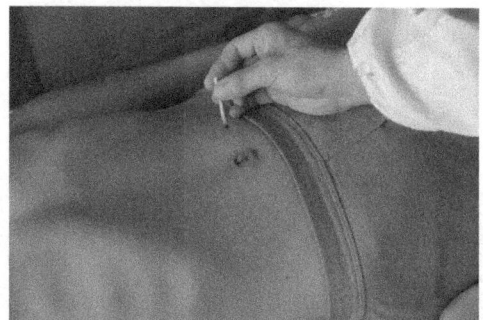

Figure 6.24.7 Juncibustion at Tian Shu (ST-25)

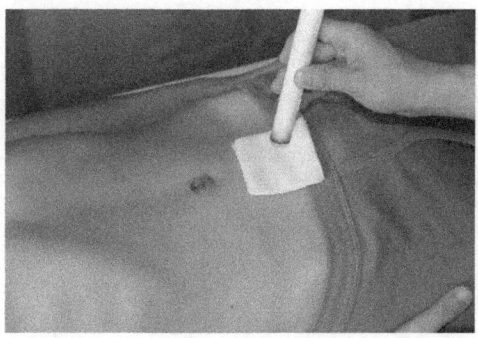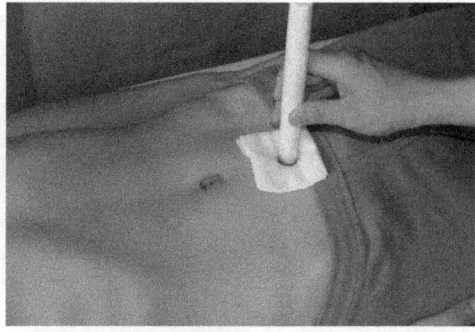

Figure 6.24.8 Tai Yi Amazing Needle at Guan Yuan (RN-4)

25. Constipation

Constipation refers to a common symptom that involves dry, bound stools and a prolonged period between each defecation; or difficulty in defecating with dry hard stools but with a normal period between defecations; or experiencing a strong desire to defecate while having difficulty evacuating non-hard stools. This is accompanied by symptoms that involve abdominal distension, abdominal pain, a decreased appetite, eructation, regurgitation and bloody stool. Constipation is usually caused by one of the following: accumulated heat in the intestine and stomach causing damage to the fluids; depression and stagnation of qi leading to a failure of freeflow; a deficiency of yin-fluids and blood causing the intestinal tract to become dry and astringent; congealing yin cold causing constipation of the intestinal tract. This condition is often seen in cases of functional constipation, irritable bowel syndrome, drug-induced constipation, constipation caused by diseases of the rectum and anus, endocrine secretion and metabolism, and impairment of muscle strength.

Main Symptoms: Constipation of the stools and difficulty defecating, or difficult evacuation of non-hard stools.

Acupoints: Tian Shu (ST-25), Shen Que (RN-8), Fei Shu (BL-13), Da Chang Shu (BL-25), Zu San Li (ST-36), Zhi Gou (SJ-6).

Moxibustion Method:

- Gentle Pole Moxa: Apply moxa to each point for 6–15 minutes. Ten treatments comprise one course of treatment, with an interval of 5 days between each course. (Figure 6.25.1)

- Moxa on Salt: Fill the umbilicus with salt and cover it with a ginger slice. Apply 5–10 cones of moxa or until the skin reddens. Perform treatment once per day or every other day. Ten treatments comprise one course of treatment. (Figure 6.25.2)

- Moxa on Garlic: Apply moxa to each point using 3–5 cones once per day. Ten treatments comprise one course of treatment, with a 5-day interval between each course. (Figure 6.25.3)

- Scallion and Fermented Soybean Paste Application: Using 3 stems of scallion, 12 grains of fermented soybean, 10g of ginger and 3g of salt, grind them into a powder and form the paste into a medicinal cake. Warm it and apply it on Shen Que (RN-8). (Figure 6.25.4)

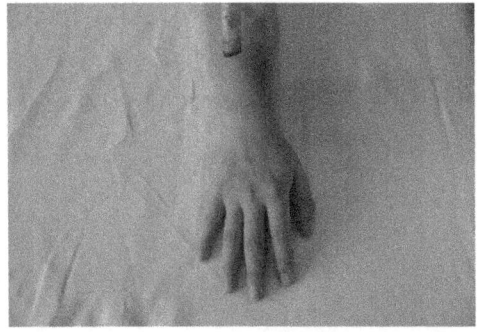 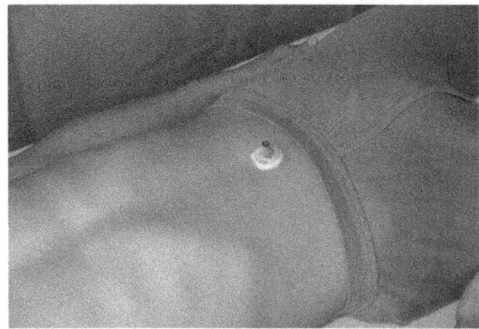

Figure 6.25.1 Gentle Pole Moxa at Zhi Gou (SJ-6)   *Figure 6.25.2 Moxa on Salt at Shen Que (RN-8)*

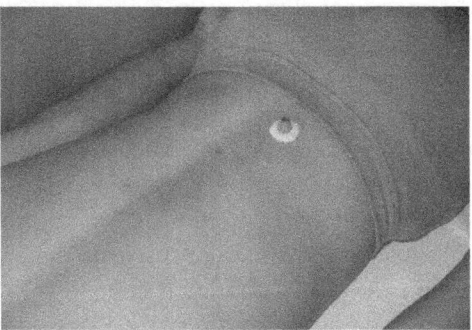

Figure 6.25.3 Moxa on Garlic at Da Chang Shu (BL-25)

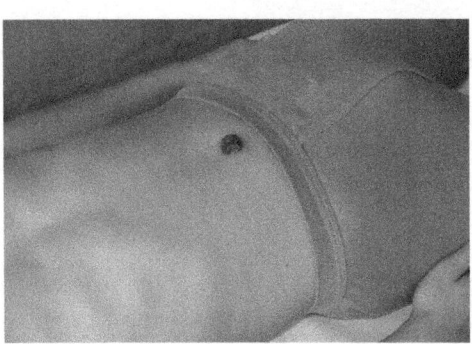 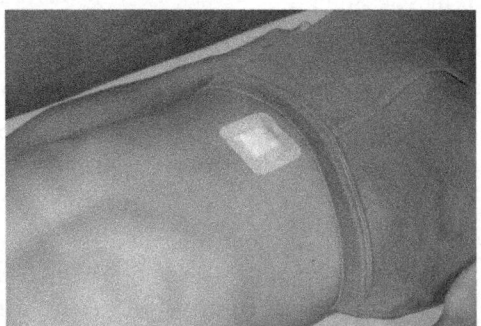

Figure 6.25.4 Scallion and Fermented Soybean Paste Application at Shen Que (RN-8)

- Fu Zi Ding Xiang Application: Use a herbal concoction including 25g each of Fu Zi (Aconiti Radix Lateralis Praeparata) and Ding Xiang (Caryophylli Flos), 15g each of Chuan Wu (Aconiti Radix), Bai Zhi (Angelicae Dahuricae Radix) and Zhu Ya Zao (Gleditsiae Fructus Abnormalis), a single clove of garlic (10g) and 5g of pepper. Grind the ingredients into a coarse powder, warm and wrap with a cloth and apply to the lower abdomen. Perform for 30 minutes, once or twice per day. (Figure 6.25.5)

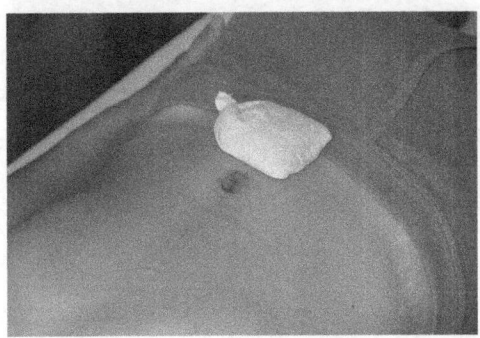 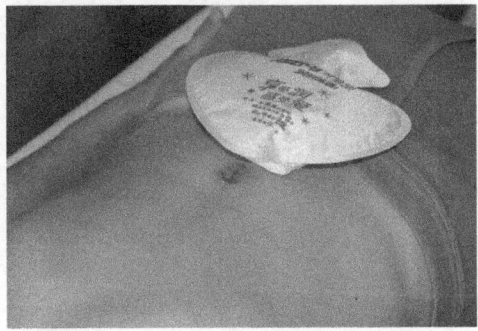

Figure 6.25.5 Fu Zi Ding Xiang Application on the Lower Abdomen

26. Chronic Hepatitis

Chronic hepatitis refers to a type of chronic liver inflammation with several causes and a disease course of over half a year. It includes the subcategories of chronic persistent hepatitis and chronic active hepatitis. In Chinese medicine, chronic hepatitis is referred to as hypochondriac pain and is closely associated with the liver, gallbladder, spleen and stomach. It is usually caused by one of the following: stagnation of qi due to depression of the liver; static blood causing obstruction and stagnation; endoretention of damp-heat or deficiency of liver-blood.

Main Symptoms: A decreased appetite, fatigue and weakness, abdominal distension and diarrhoea, pain in the hepatic region and a low-grade fever.

Acupoints: Gan Shu (BL-18), Dan Shu (BL-19), San Yin Jiao (SP-6), Zu San Li (ST-36), Tai Chong (LR-3), Yang Ling Quan (GB-34).

Moxibustion Method:

- Gentle Pole Moxa: Apply moxa to each point for 10 minutes. Perform treatment once per day. Seven treatments comprise one course of treatment. (Figure 6.26.1)

- Cone Moxa: Apply moxa to each point using 3–5 cones. Perform treatment once or twice per day. Seven treatments comprise one course of treatment. (Figure 6.26.2)

- Juncibustion:* Perform treatment once per day or every other day until the condition recovers. (Figure 6.26.3)

- Warm Needle Moxa: Retain needles for 20–25 minutes. Perform treatment once per day. Ten treatments comprise one course of treatment. (Figure 6.26.4)

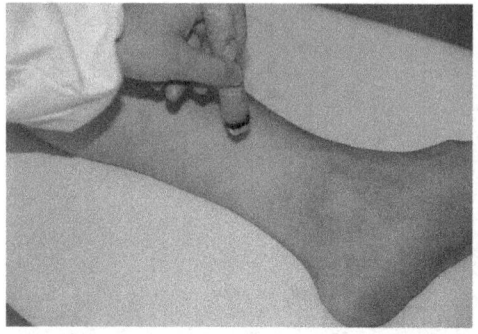

Figure 6.26.1 Gentle Pole Moxa at San Yin Jiao (SP-6)

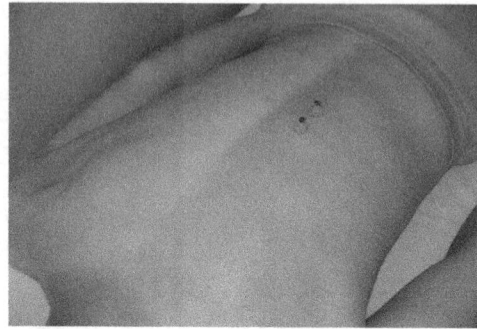

Figure 6.26.2 Cone Moxa at Gan Shu (BL-18) and Dan Shu (BL-19)

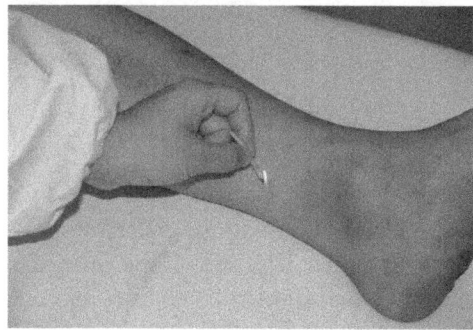

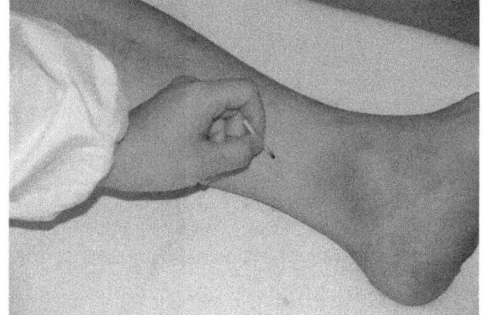

Figure 6.26.3 Juncibustion at San Yin Jiao (SP-6)

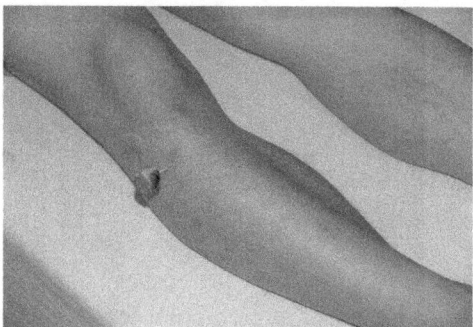

Figure 6.26.4 Warm Needle Moxa at Zu San Li (ST-36)

27. Hepatic Cirrhosis

Hepatic cirrhosis refers to a type of chronic, aggressive liver disease due to various etiological factors that repeatedly impair the liver. It involves extensive degeneration, necrosis and irregular regeneration of liver cells, accompanied by hyperplasia and fibrosis of connective tissue. The normal hepatic lobules disorganize and are replaced by pseudolobules with abnormal organization and function, resulting in deformation, hardening and severe functional disorder of the liver. In Chinese medicine, hepatic cirrhosis is referred to as tympanite, simple abdominal distension or conglomerations and accumulations. It is usually caused by one of the following: dyssplenism, stagnation of the liver with deficiency of the spleen or a lack of coordination between the liver and spleen causing retention of dampness due to stagnation of qi; stagnation of qi inhibiting the flow of blood, vessel and network stasis obstruction causing blood stasis of the liver and spleen; or stagnation of the liver with deficiency of the spleen, inhibiting the waterways of the triple-burner causing water-damp to collect internally.

Main Symptoms: A severely distended abdomen like a drum holding water accompanied by a sombre yellow discoloration of the skin and prominent veins on the abdominal wall, coupled with emaciated limbs.

Acupoints: Zhi Yang (DU-9), Gan Shu (BL-18), Zhang Men (LR-13), Qi Men (LR-14), Shui Fen (RN-9), San Yin Jiao (SP-6).

Moxibustion Method:

- Scarring Cone Moxa:* Apply moxa to each point using 7–9 cones. Perform treatment once per day. Five treatments comprise one course of treatment. (Figure 6.27.1)

- Moxa on Ginger: Apply moxa to each point using 5–7 cones. Perform treatment once per day. Ten treatments comprise one course of treatment, with a 5-day interval between each course. (Figure 6.27.2)

- Gentle Pole Moxa: Apply moxa to each point for 6–15 minutes. Perform treatment twice per day. Twenty treatments comprise one course of treatment, with a 5-day interval between each course. (Figure 6.27.3)

- Warm Needle Moxa: Apply moxa to each point for 6–30 minutes. Perform treatment once per day or every other day. Ten treatments comprise one course of treatment, with a 5-day interval between each course. (Figure 6.27.4)

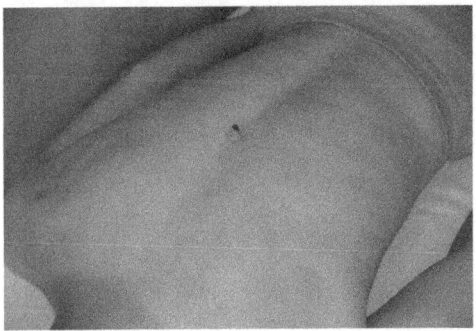

Figure 6.27.1 Scarring Cone Moxa at Zhi Yang (DU-9)

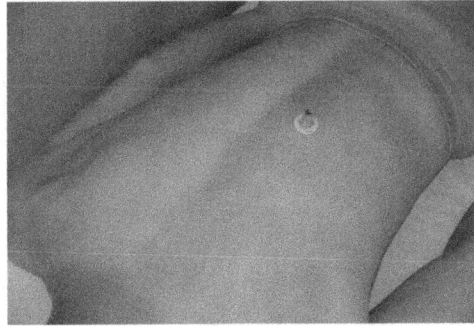

Figure 6.27.2 Moxa on Ginger at Gan Shu (BL-18)

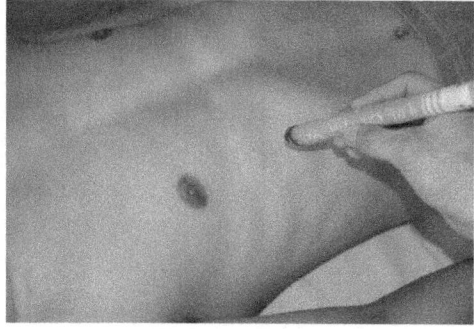
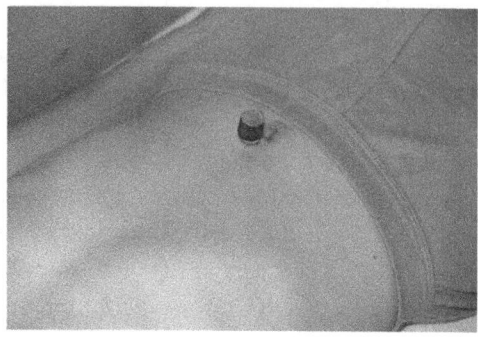

Figure 6.27.3 Gentle Pole Moxa at Qi Men (LR-14)   *Figure 6.27.4 Warm Needle Moxa at Shui Fen (RN-9)*

- Chuan Jiao Compound Application: Use the herbal concoction that includes 100g of Chuan Jiao (Zanthoxyli Pericarpium), 15g each of E Wei (Ferulae Resina), San Leng (Sparganii Rhizoma), Bai Zhu (Atractylodis Macrocephalae Rhizoma) and Zhi Bie Jia (mix-fried Trionycis Carapax). Grind the ingredients into a fine powder and mix with distillate spirit. Parch heat, wrap with a cloth and apply it to the hepatic region, and Shen Que (RN-8), in the case of abdominal dropsy. Maintain the warmth with a hot water bottle. Perform treatment once daily for 30–60 minutes. (Figure 6.27.5)

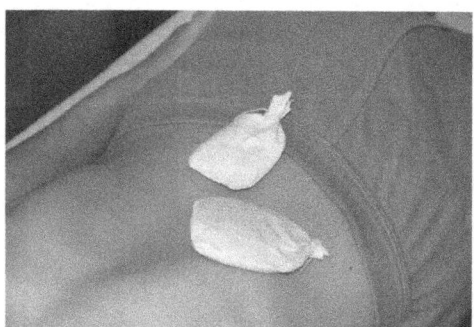
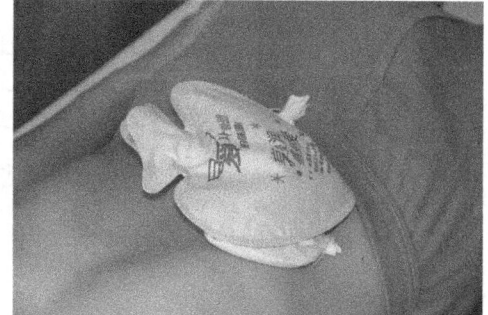

Figure 6.27.5 Chuan Jiao Compound Application at Shen Que (RN-8)

28. Adiposis Hepatica

Adiposis hepatica refers to a common type of diffuse hepatic disease involving adipose accumulation in the liver cells. In Chinese medicine, adiposis hepatica is usually caused by one of the following: stagnation of liver-qi causing disharmony between the liver and stomach; damp abundance due to splenic asthenia causing internal phlegm-damp obstruction; deficiency of the liver and kidney, dyssplenism; or qi-stagnation and blood stasis causing blockage of phlegm and further blood stasis.

Main Symptoms: A gassy pain in the hepatic region, distension of the right ribcage, a decreased appetite, tiredness and debility.

Acupoints: Gan Shu (BL-18), Zhang Men (LR-13), Zhong Wan (RN-12), San Yin Jiao (SP-6), Shen Shu (BL-23), Zu San Li (ST-36).

Moxibustion Method:

- Gentle Pole Moxa: Apply moxa to each point for 6–15 minutes. Perform treatment once per day. Ten treatments comprise one course of treatment. (Figure 6.28.1)

- Moxa on Ginger: Apply moxa to each point using 5–7 cones. Perform treatment once per day or every other day. Ten treatments comprise one course of treatment. (Figure 6.28.2)

- Non-scarring Moxa: Using moxa cones the size of a grain of wheat; apply moxa to each point using 3–5 cones. Perform treatment once per day or every other day. Ten treatments comprise one course of treatment. (Figure 6.28.3)

- Warm Needle Moxa: Apply moxa to each point for 6–15 minutes. Perform treatment once per day or every other day. Ten treatments comprise one course of treatment. (Figure 6.28.4)

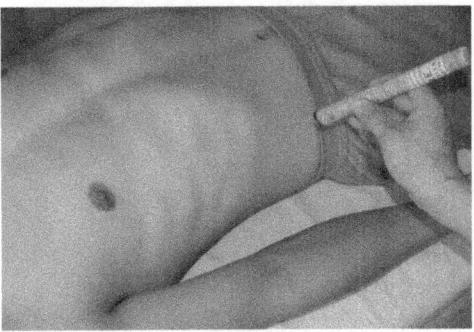

Figure 6.28.1 Gentle Pole Moxa at Zhang Men (LR-13)

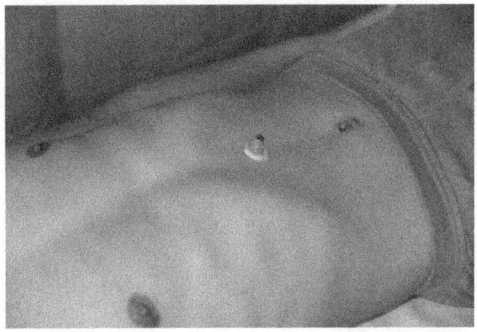

Figure 6.28.2 Moxa on Ginger at Zhong Wan (RN-12)

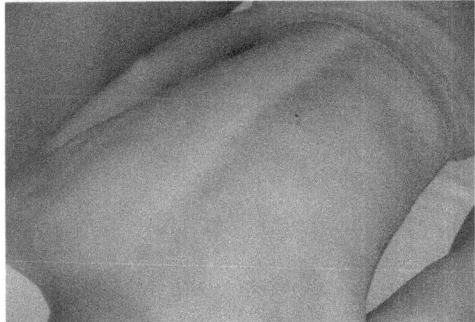

Figure 6.28.3 Non-scarring Moxa at Gan Shu (BL-18)

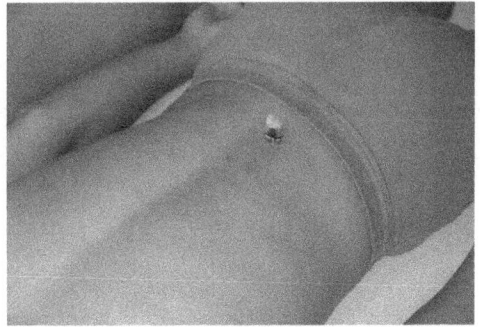

Figure 6.28.4 Warm Needle Moxa at Shen Shu (BL-23)

29. Dropsy

Dropsy refers to a type of condition that involves water retention overflowing the muscles and skin causing dropsy in the face, eyelids, limbs, abdomen, back or even throughout the body. In severe cases it is accompanied by pleural fluid and abdominal dropsy. Dropsy is usually caused by one of the following: wind pathogens assailing the outer body causing failure of the lung to regulate the waterways; spleen-lung impairment resulting in spreading of damp-toxins; flooding of water-dampness encumbering spleen-qi; exuberant internal damp-heat causing San Jiao stagnation; an improper diet and exhaustion causing spleen-stomach impairment or over-indulgence in sexual activities causing impairment of the kidney. This condition is often related to acute and chronic nephritis, chronic congestive cardiac failure, hepatic cirrhosis, anaemia, endocrine disturbances and dystrophia.

Main Symptoms: Puffiness of the face, eyelids, limbs, abdomen, back or throughout the body.

Acupoints:

- *Primary points:* Shen Shu (BL-23), Zhong Wan (RN-12), Guan Yuan (RN-4), Shui Fen (RN-9).

- *Symptomatic points:* Yang oedema: Fei Shu (BL-13), San Jiao Shu (BL-22), Yin Ling Quan (SP-9); Yin oedema: Pi Shu (BL-20), Fu Liu (KI-7), Qi Hai (RN-6).

Moxibustion Method:

- Gentle Pole Moxa: Apply moxa to each point for 15–20 minutes. Perform treatment once per day. Ten treatments comprise one course of treatment. (Figure 6.29.1)

- Cone Moxa: Apply 3–5 cones of moxa to each point. Perform treatment once per day. Ten treatments comprise one course of treatment. (Figure 6.29.2)

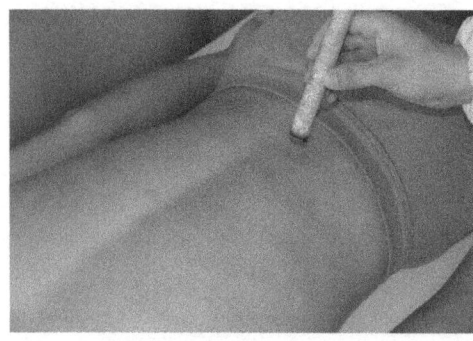

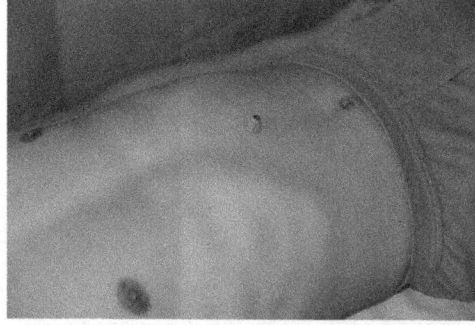

Figure 6.29.1 Gentle Pole Moxa at Shen Shu (BL-23)   *Figure 6.29.2 Cone Moxa at Zhong Wan (RN-12)*

- Moxa on Fu Zi Cake: Apply 3–5 cones of moxa to each point. Perform treatment once per day. Ten treatments comprise one course of treatment. (Figure 6.29.3)

- Juncibustion:* Use Ming Deng Bao juncibustion method on each point for yang oedema; perform treatment once per day until recovery is achieved. Use Zhuo juncibustion method on each point for yin oedema; perform treatment once per day until recovery is achieved. (Figure 6.29.4)

- Cone Moxa on Chi Xiao Dou: For oedema of the lower extremities, grind Chi Xiao Dou (Phaseoli Semen) into a powder, mix with diluted salt-water and form the paste into a small cake. Apply 6–8 cones of moxa to each point. Perform treatment once per day. (Figure 6.29.5)

- Various Applications: Tian Luo Application for Yang oedema: Strip shells from four Tian Luo (freshwater snail; Cipangopaludina) and grind with five cloves of garlic and 10g of Che Qian Zi (Plantaginis Semen), and plaster the paste onto the umbilical region for 8 hours. Perform treatment once per day. Lou Gu Application for Yin oedema: Grind five live Lou Gu (mole cricket; Gryllotalpa) and plaster the paste onto the umbilical region. Perform treatment once per day. Shang Lu Compound Application: Use a herbal concoction which includes 6g each of Shang Lu (Phytolaccae Radix), Yuan Hua (Genkwa Flos), Gan Sui (Kansui Radix), Hei Bai Chou (Pharbitidis Semen) and Bing Pian (Borneolum). Grind them into a fine powder, mix with fistular onion stalk and plaster onto the umbilical region. Perform treatment once per day. (Figure 6.29.6)

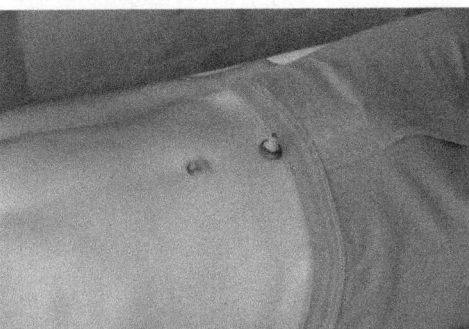

Figure 6.29.3 Moxa on Fu Zi Cake at Guan Yuan (RN-4)

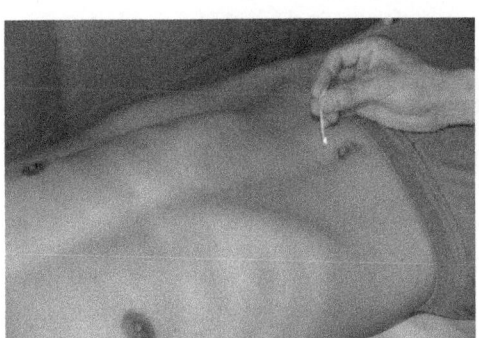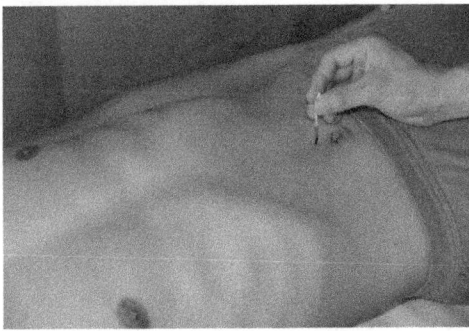

Figure 6.29.4 Juncibustion at Shui Fen (RN-9)

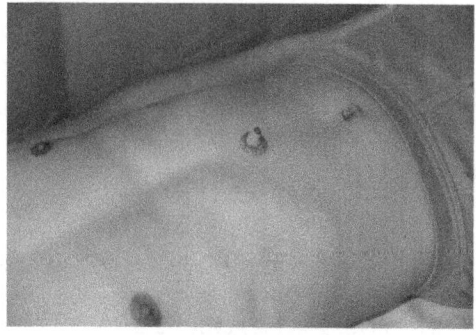

Figure 6.29.5 Cone Moxa on Chi Xiao Dou at Zhong Wan (RN-12)

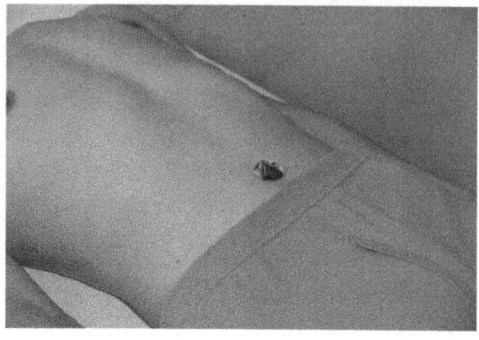

Figure 6.29.6 Various Applications at Shen Que (RN-8)

30. Urinary System Infection

Urinary system infection refers to the propagation of pathogenic bacterium in the urinary tract resulting in infection of the urinary canal, bladder, ureter and renal pelvis. It is often seen in cystitis and nephropyelitis. Urinary system infection is considered to be a strangury pattern in TCM and is usually caused by one of the following: external pathogenic invasion causing damp-heat to brew and bind in the lower Jiao or impair bladder qi transformation.

Main Symptoms: Frequent urination, urgency and odynuria.

Acupoints: Bai Hui (DU-20), Shen Shu (BL-23), Pang Guang Shu (BL-28), Zhong Ji (RN-3), San Yin Jiao (SP-6), Qi Hai (RN-6).

Moxibustion Method:

- Gentle Pole Moxa: Apply moxa to each point for 15–20 minutes. Perform treatment 2–3 times per day during the acute stage, once per day in the chronic stage. Seven treatments comprise one course of treatment. (Figure 6.30.1)

- Non-scarring Moxa: Apply moxa to each point using 5–10 cones. Perform treatment once per day or every other day. Seven treatments comprise one course of treatment, with a 3-day interval between courses. (Figure 6.30.2)

- Cone Moxa on Shan Yao: Slice fresh Shan Yao (Dioscoreae Rhizoma Crudum) into 0.2cm pieces after soaking in saline solution for 10 minutes. Apply 4–8 cones of moxa to each point. Perform treatment once per day. (Figure 6.30.3)

- Warm Needle Moxa: Apply moxa to each point for 6–15 minutes. Perform treatment once per day or every other day. Seven treatments comprise one course of treatment. (Figure 6.30.4)

- Tian Luo Compound Application: Strip shells from 7 Tian Luo (freshwater snail; Cipangopaludina), and grind with 10 fermented soybeans, 30g of fresh Che Qian Cao (Plantaginis Herba), 3 stems of onion bulbs and 1g of salt. Plaster the paste onto the umbilical region and secure with a bandage. Perform treatment once per day. (Figure 6.30.5)

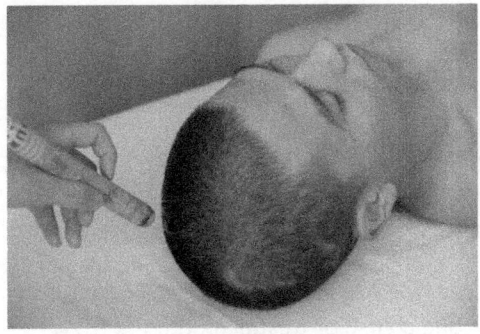

Figure 6.30.1 Gentle Pole Moxa at Bai Hui (DU-20)

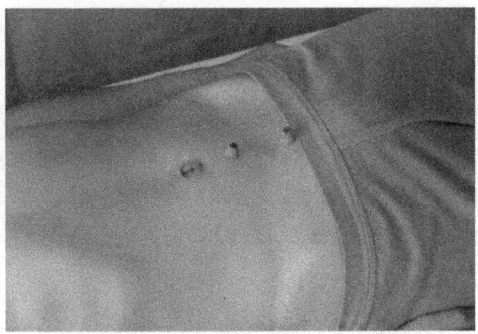

Figure 6.30.2 Non-scarring Moxa at Qi Hai (RN-6) and Zhong Ji (RN-3)

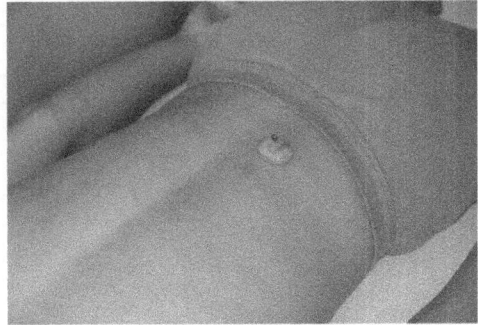

Figure 6.30.3 Cone Moxa on Shan Yao at Shen Shu (BL-23)

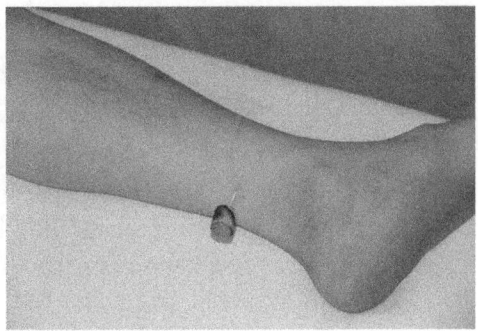

Figure 6.30.4 Warm Needle Moxa at San Yin Jiao (SP-6)

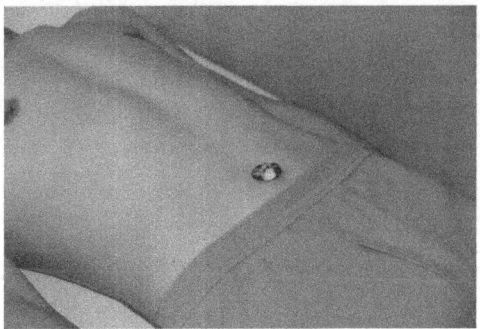

Figure 6.30.5 Tian Luo Compound Application at Shen Que (RN-8)

31. Anischuria

Anischuria refers to a kind of disease involving uncontrolled urination while in a state of alertness. It can be divided into five categories: overflow, nonresistance, reflectivity, urgency and stress incontinence. Anischuria is considered to be urinary incontinence in TCM and is usually caused by one of the following: taxation damage, worry, qi vacuity after illness and kidney depletion in old age causing insecurity of the lower orifice and a lack of control of the urinary bladder. This disease is often seen in cases of cerebrovascular disease, encephalitis, cerebral trauma, epileptic paroxysm and myeleterosis.

Main Symptoms: A lack of control of urination when in a state of alertness.

Acupoints: Zu San Li (ST-36), Pang Guang Shu (BL-28), Shen Shu (BL-23), Guan Yuan (RN-4), San Yin Jiao (SP-6), Zhong Ji (RN-3).

Moxibustion Method:

- Gentle Pole Moxa: Apply moxa to each point for 20–30 minutes. Perform treatment once per day. Seven treatments comprise one course of treatment. (Figure 6.31.1)

- Moxa on Ginger: Use moxa cones half the size of a jujube seed. Apply 5–10 cones per acupoint, once or twice per day, 3–5 treatments comprise one course of treatment. (Figure 6.31.2)

- Moxa on Salt: Use moxa cones half the size of a jujube seed. Apply 3–5 cones on Shen Que (RN-8) once or twice per day, 3–5 treatments comprise one course of treatment. (Figure 6.31.3)

- Moxa on Onion Cake: Using an appropriate amount of fistular onion stalk, grind it into paste and form a small cake. Place it on points, with the option of adding a ginger slice. Apply moxa to each point using 3–5 cones once or twice per day until recovery is achieved. (Figure 6.31.4)

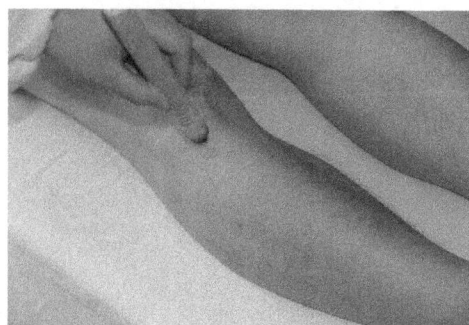

Figure 6.31.1 Gentle Pole Moxa at Zu San Li (ST-36)

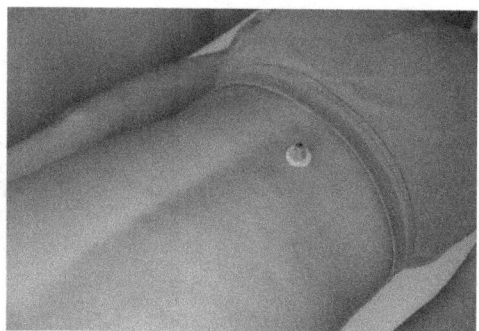

Figure 6.31.2 Moxa on Ginger at Shen Shu (BL-23)

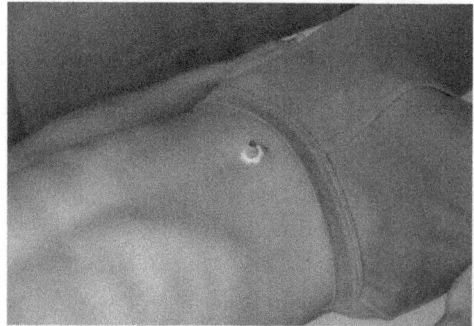

Figure 6.31.3 Moxa on Salt at Shen Que (RN-8)

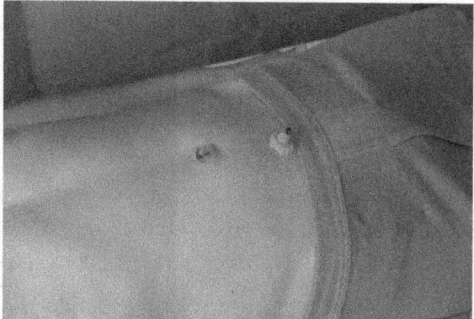

Figure 6.31.4 Moxa on Onion Cake at Guan Yuan (RN-4)

- Warm Needle Moxa: Apply moxa to each point for 6–15 minutes. Perform treatment once per day until recovery. (Figure 6.31.5)

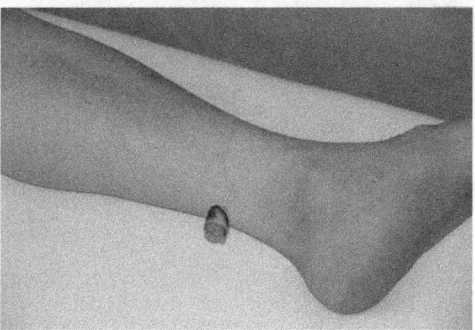

Figure 6.31.5 Warm Needle Moxa at San Yin Jiao (SP-6)

32. Urinary Retention

Urinary retention refers to a common symptom involving an inability to evacuate a large quantity of urine. It can be divided into three categories: reflexive, innervative-disorder and obstruction. Urinary retention is considered to be dribbling urinary block in TCM and is usually caused by one of the following: inhibited qi transformation of San Jiao causing difficult micturition; trauma causing damage to meridian-qi, deficiency of kidney-yang causing debilitation of the life gate fire.

Main Symptoms: An inability to evacuate a large quantity of urine.

Acupoints: Shen Que (RN-8), Guan Yuan (RN-4), San Yin Jiao (SP-6), Zu San Li (ST-36), Zhong Ji (RN-3), San Jiao Shu (BL-22).

Moxibustion Method:

- Gentle Pole Moxa: Apply moxa to each point for 6–20 minutes. Perform treatment once per day. Three treatments comprise one course of treatment. (Figure 6.32.1)

- Moxa on Ginger: Apply 5–10 cones of moxa to each point once or twice per day. Three treatments comprise one course of treatment. (Figure 6.32.2)

- Xian Qing Gao Application: Mash 200–300g of Xian Qing Hao (Artemisiae Annuae Herba), maintaining the juices, and plaster on Shen Que (RN-8), strapping it first with a 25×30cm piece of plastic membrane and then a piece of absorbent gauze. Keep the plaster in place until urination occurs. (Figure 6.32.3)

- Long Bi San Application: Grind 15g of Gan Sui (Kansui Radix) into a fine powder, and additionally decoct 10g of Gan Sui. Grind 3g of ginger with scallion white and form into a plaster. Place it on Shen Que (RN-8) after putting 6g of Gan Sui powder on the point. Bandage with an absorbent gauze; finally drink the Gan Sui decoction. (Figure 6.32.4)

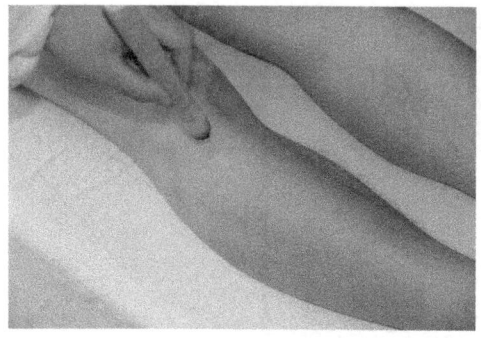

Figure 6.32.1 Gentle Pole Moxa at Zu San Li (ST-36)

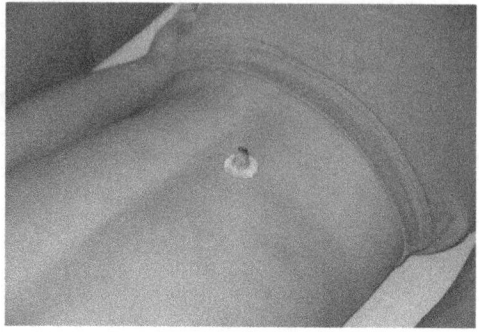

Figure 6.32.2 Moxa on Ginger at San Jiao Shu (BL-22)

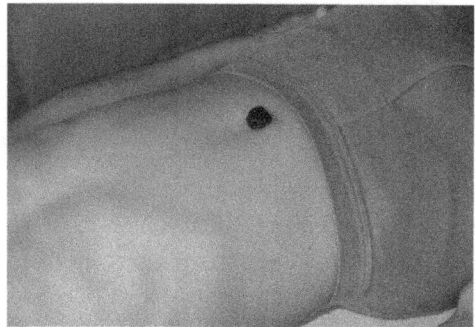

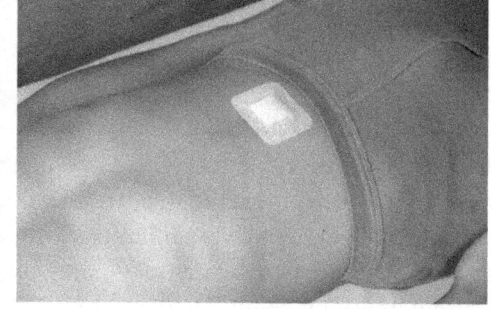

Figure 6.32.3 Xian Qing Gao Application at Shen Que (RN-8)

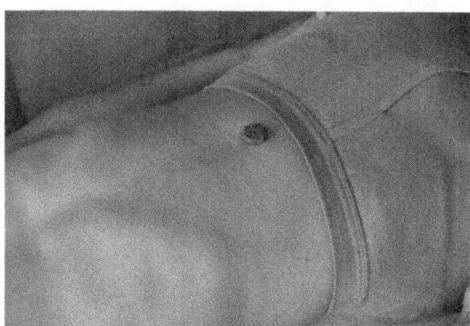

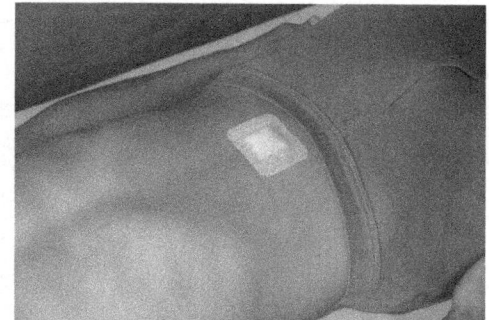

Figure 6.32.4 Long Bi San Application at Shen Que (RN-8)

- Zhu Shui San Application: Grind 5g each of Ci Shi (Magnetitum) and Shang Lu (Phytolaccae Radix) into a fine powder and mix with 0.1g of She Xiang (Moschus). Divide the powder into two parts and apply to Shen Que (RN-8) and Guan Yuan (RN-4) with a plastic membrane. Perform treatment once per day until urination occurs. (Figure 6.32.5)

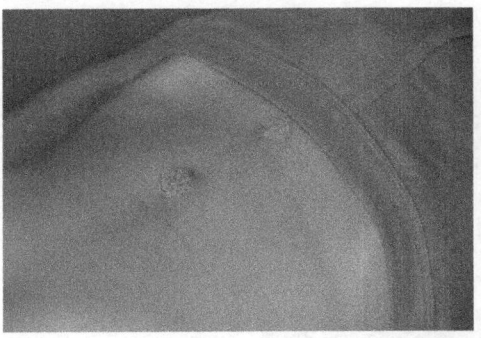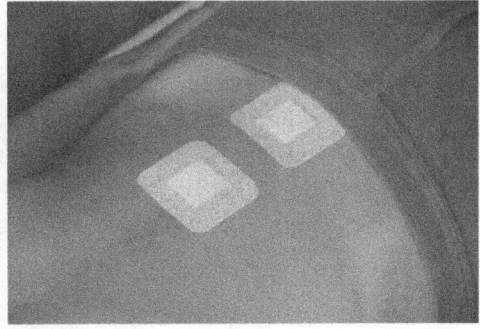

Figure 6.32.5 Zhu Shui San Application at Guan Yuan (RN-4)

33. Seminal Emission

Seminal emission refers to abnormally frequent or excessive emissions of semen without sexual contact. There are two types of seminal emission; dream emission and seminal efflux. Dream emission refers to emission of semen while dreaming; seminal efflux describes emission of semen when the patient is awake. It is often accompanied by dizziness, a fatigued spirit and lack of strength, devitalized essence-spirit and dull aching lumbar region and knees. This pattern usually has the following causes: effulgent sovereign and ministerial fire causing non-interaction of the heart and kidney; damp-heat and phlegm-fire pouring downward to harass essence chamber; taxation damageing the heart and spleen causing a failure of qi to contain essence; kidney deficiency, uncontrollable loss of semen and unconsciousness, resulting in insecurity of the essence gate. This pattern is often found in male sexual dysfunction, prostatitis, neurosism, cystospermitis and orchiditis.

Main Symptoms: Frequent involuntary emissions of semen, more than twice a week.

Acupoints:

- *Primary points:* Shen Shu (BL-23), Ming Men (DU-4), Zhong Ji (RN-3), Gao Huang (BL-43), Shen Men (HT-7).

- *Symptomatic points:* Dream emission: Xin Shu (BL-15), Guan Yuan (RN-4), Tai Chong (LR-3); Seminal efflux: Qi Hai (RN-6), San Yin Jiao (SP-6), Zhi Shi (BL-52).

Moxibustion Method:

- Gentle Moxa: Apply moxa for 6–20 minutes per acupoint, once daily, each treatment repeated 10 times. (Figure 6.33.1)

- Moxa on Ginger: Apply 5–10 cones per acupoint, once or twice a day, 10 days for a course of treatment. (Figure 6.33.2)

- Moxa on Fu Zi Cake: Apply 2–3 cones per acupoint, once daily, 10 days for a course of treatment. (Figure 6.33.3)

- Hua Jing Gao Application: Grind 10g each of Liu Huang (Sulfur) and Mu Ding Xiang (Caryophylli Fructus) into a fine powder, then pound two pieces of garlic into a pulp, mix them with a little She Xiang (Moschus), and make into pills as large as black soya beans, then cover with Zhu Sha (Cinnabaris). Deep-fry 50g of Chuan Jiao (Zanthoxyli Pericarpium), 20g each of Rou Gui (Cinnamomi Cortex), Fu Pian (Aconiti Radix Lateralis Praeparata Secta), Jiu Cai Zi (Allii Tuberosi Semen) and She Chuang Zi (Cnidii Fructus), and 300g of garlic with 500ml of Ma You (Sesami Oleum). Filter residue and continue to decoct until it shapes up. Then add some 250g of Guang Dan (Minium) and mix well into black plaster. Apply the black plaster to acupoints with the pill inside. Change the plaster after 3 days. (Figure 6.33.4)

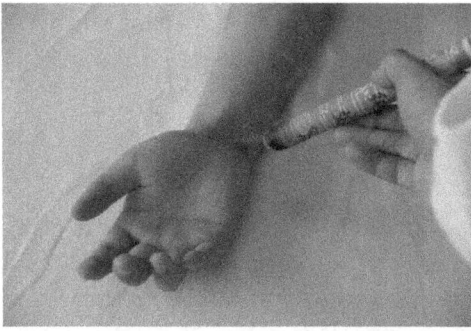

Figure 6.33.1 Gentle Moxa at Shen Men (HT-7)

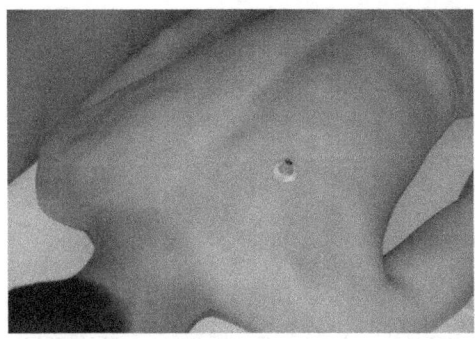

Figure 6.33.2 Moxa on Ginger at Gao Huang (BL-43)

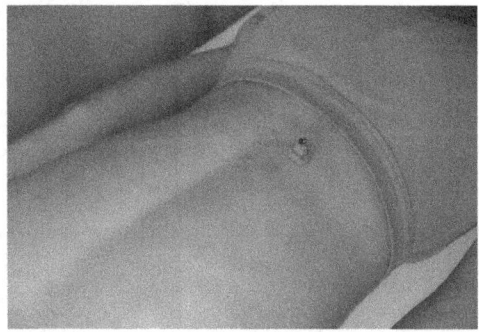

Figure 6.33.3 Moxa on Fu Zi Cake at Shen Shu (BL-23)

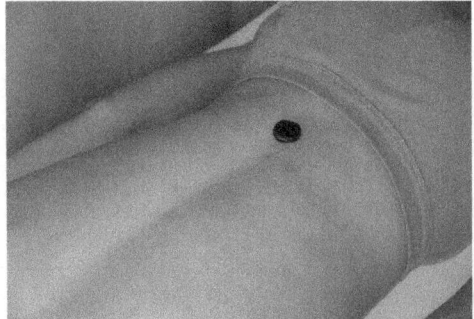

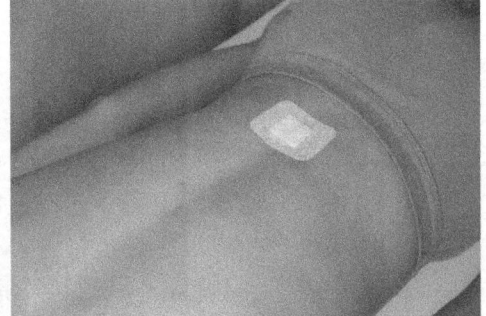

Figure 6.33.4 Hua Jing Gao Application at Ming Men (DU-4)

34. Impotence

Impotence is an abnormal physical or psychological state of males characterized by the inability to engage in sexual intercourse due to the failure to achieve or maintain an erection. It is often caused by debilitation of the life gate fire, damage to the heart and spleen, fright and fear damageing the kidney or liver depression. The pattern is often seen in male sexual dysfunction and some chronic deficiency conditions.

Main Symptoms: The penis cannot achieve or maintain erection, often accompanied by premature ejaculation.

Acupoints: Yang Jiao (GB-35), Ming Men (DU-4), Shen Shu (BL-23), Qi Hai (RN-6), Guan Yuan (RN-4), San Yin Jiao (SP-6).

Moxibustion Method:

- Gentle Moxa: Apply moxa for 20–30 minutes per acupoint, once daily; each treatment is repeated 10 times. Repeat after 3–5 days rest. (Figure 6.34.1)

- Moxa on Fu Zi Cake: Apply 3–5 cones per acupoint, 10 days for a course of treatment. (Figure 6.34.2)

- Warm Needle Moxa: Apply 6–20 minutes per acupoint every other day, 10 days for a course of treatment. Repeat after 10 days. (Figure 6.34.3)

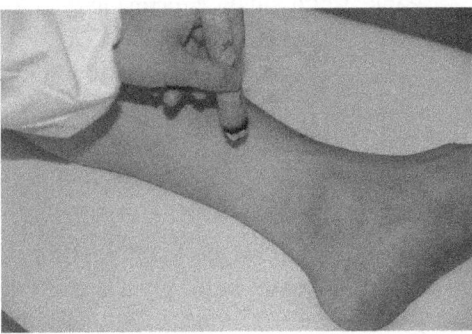

Figure 6.34.1 Gentle Moxa at San Yin Jiao (SP-6)

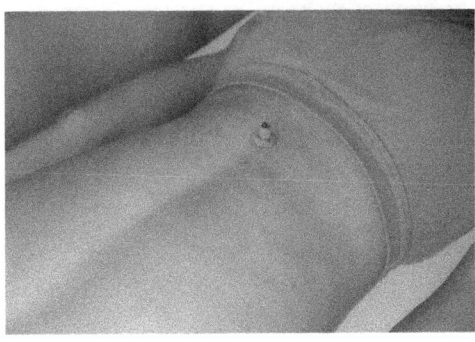

Figure 6.34.2 Moxa on Fu Zi Cake at Ming Men (DU-4)

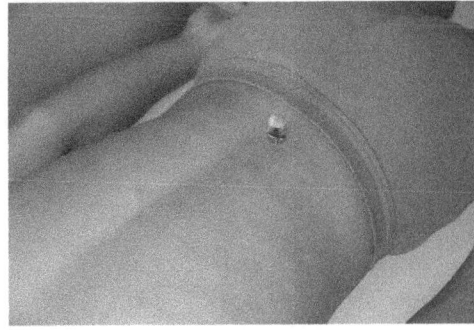

Figure 6.34.3 Warm Needle Moxa at Shen Shu (BL-23)

35. Leukaemia

Leukaemia is a malignant disease originating from the hematopoietic tissues or lymphocytes, manifesting as a proliferation of leukaemia cells in the bone marrow, peripheral blood, and other organs and tissues. Leukaemia, known as blood cancer in TCM, has the following causes: brewing toxic heat harassing essence-marrow, insufficiency of healthy qi, turbid pathogens binding internally, and internal static blood obstruction. The disease is directly bound up with the kidney, liver and spleen.

Main Symptoms: Infective fever, blood depletion, bleeding, bone pain, tenderness of the sternum, aggregative accumulation.

Acupoints: Da Zhui (DU-14), Zhong Wan (RN-12), Zu San Li (ST-36), Xin Shu (BL-15), Xue Hai (SP-10), Jue Gu (GB-39).

Moxibustion Method:

- Moxa on Ginger: Apply 5–7 cones the size of jujube seeds per acupoint, once daily or once every other day, 10 days for a course of treatment. Repeat after 5 days. (Figure 6.35.1)

- Scarring Moxa:* Apply 4–5 cones per acupoint. (Figure 6.35.2)

- Xiao Pi San Application: Grind the following herbs into fine powder: 30g each of Shui Hong Hua Zi (Polygoni Orientalis Fructus) and Pi Xiao (Natrii Sulfas Non-Purus), 12g each of Zhang Nao (Camphora), Tao Ren (Persicae Semen) and Tu Bie Chong (Eupolyphaga seu Steleophaga), 15g each of Sheng Nan Xing (Arisaematis Rhizoma Crudum) and Chuan Shan Jia (Manis Squama), 16g of Wang Bu Liu Xing (Vaccariae Semen), 15g each of Bai Jie Zi (Sinapis Albae Semen), Sheng Chuan Wu (Aconiti Radix Cruda) and Sheng Cao Wu (Aconiti Kusnezoffii Radix Cruda), 9g each of Sheng Bai Fu Zi (Typhonii Rhizoma Crudum) and Yuan Hu (Corydalis Rhizoma). Add 1.2g She Xiang (Moschus) and 3g Bing Pian (Borneolum), then mix well and store in a sealed container. Apply the above herb powder with some honey and vinegar on the area of splenomegaly, cover with oilpaper, bind up with gauze, and compress with a hot-water bottle. Perform once daily. (Figure 6.35.3)

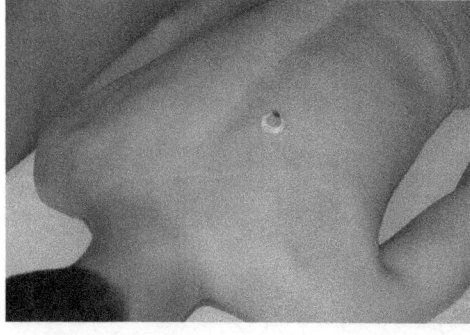
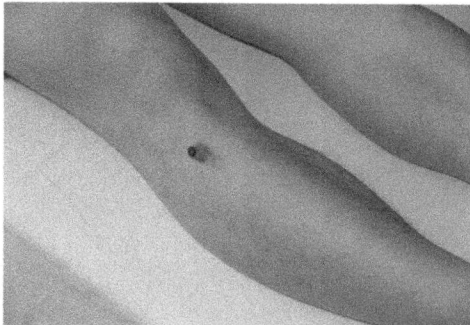

Figure 6.35.1 Moxa on Ginger at Xin Shu (BL-15)   *Figure 6.35.2 Scarring Moxa at Zu San Li (ST-36)*

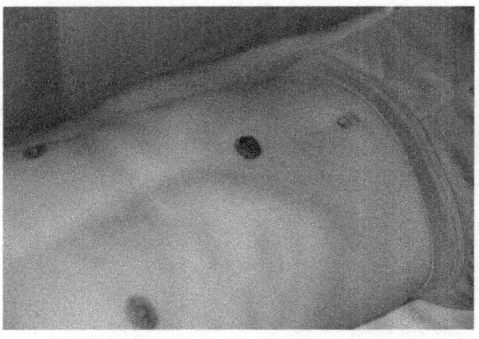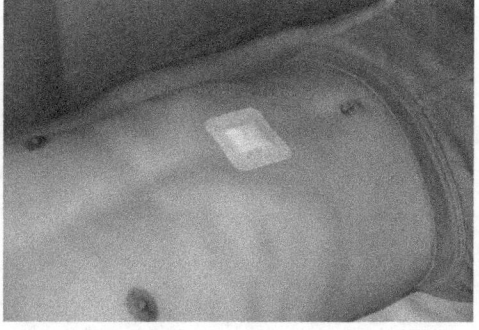

Figure 6.35.3 Xiao Pi San Application at Zhong Wan (RN-12)

36. Anaemia

Anaemia is a condition in which the blood is deficient of red blood cells, haemoglobin, or in total volume. It falls within the categories of blood deficiency, vacuity-taxation and sallow disease in TCM, and is characterized by chronic vacuity patterns. It is often caused by an innate deficiency or acquired loss of nourishment.

Main Symptoms: Dizziness, palpitations, shortness of breath, fatigue and a lack of strength, a poor appetite, abdominal distension, nausea and pale skin and mucosa.

Acupoints: Zu San Li (ST-36), Pi Shu (BL-20), Ge Shu (BL-17), Da Zhui (DU-14), Jue Gu (GB-39), Gan Shu (BL-18).

Moxibustion Method:

- Gentle Moxa: Apply moxa for 5–10 minutes per acupoint, once daily, and repeat 10 times for a course of treatment. (Figure 6.36.1)

- Moxa on Ginger: Apply 5–7 cones per acupoint, once daily, and repeat 10 times for a course of treatment. Repeat the course of treatment after 3 days. (Figure 6.36.2)

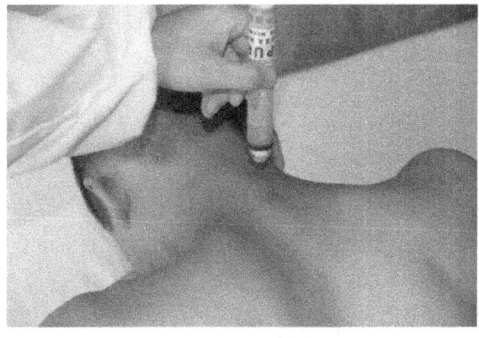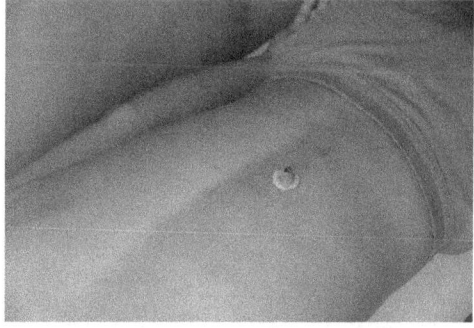

Figure 6.36.1 Gentle Moxa at Da Zhui (DU-14)   *Figure 6.36.2 Moxa on Ginger at Pi Shu (BL-20)*

- Non-scarring Moxa: Apply 3–5 cones per acupoint, once daily, and repeat 10 times for a course of treatment. Repeat the course of treatment after 3–5 days. (Figure 6.36.3)

- Warm Needle Moxa: Apply moxa for 5–10 minutes per acupoint, once daily, and repeat 10 times for a course of treatment. (Figure 6.36.4)

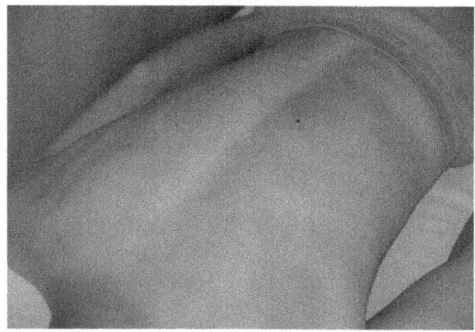
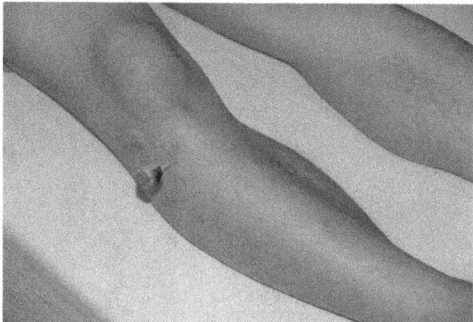

Figure 6.36.3 Non-scarring Moxa at Gan Shu (BL-18)

Figure 6.36.4 Warm Needle Moxa at Zu San Li (ST-36)

37. Hyperthyroidism

Hyperthyroidism is a condition in which the thyroid gland produces too much thyroid hormone. The condition is characterized by enlargement of the thyroid gland, increased metabolic rate, protruding eyes, pretibial myxoedema and acropachy. It falls within the category of goitre in TCM. The disease usually has the following causes: qi stagnation, congealing and binding of phlegm and yin damage induced by affect-mind internal damage or physical factors.

Main Symptoms: An enlarged thyroid gland, protruding eyes, restlessness, an increased appetite, weight loss and fatigue.

Acupoints: Fee Shu (BL-13), Xin Shu (BL-15), Zu San Li (ST-36), Feng Chi (GB-20), Yin Ling Quan (SP-9), San Yin Jiao (SP-6).

Moxibustion Method:

- Gentle Moxa: Apply moxa for 5–15 minutes per acupoint, once daily, each treatment repeated 10 times. (Figure 6.37.1)

- Moxa on Ginger: Apply 3–5 cones per acupoint, once daily, each treatment repeated 10 times. Repeat the treatment course after 3–5 days rest. (Figure 6.37.2)

- Moxa on Garlic: Apply 5–10 cones per acupoint, once daily, each treatment repeated 10 times. (Figure 6.37.3)

- Non-scarring Moxa: Apply 3–5 cones the size of broad beans per acupoint, once daily or every other day, each treatment repeated 10 times. (Figure 6.37.4)

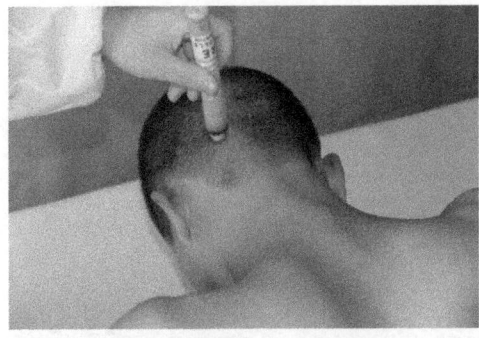

Figure 6.37.1 Gentle Moxa at Feng Chi (GB-20)

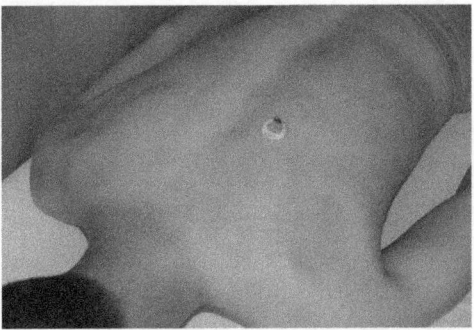

Figure 6.37.2 Moxa on Ginger at Xin Shu (BL-15)

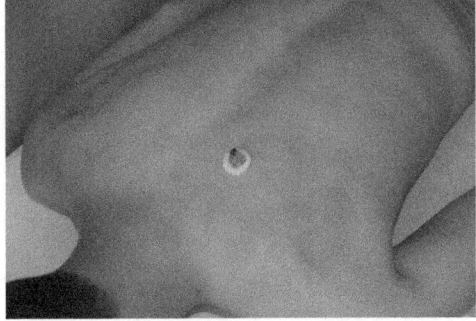

Figure 6.37.3 Moxa on Garlic at Fei Shu (BL-13)

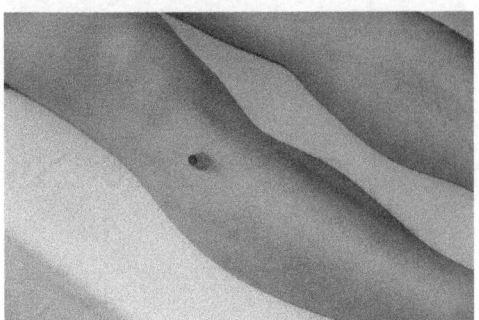

*Figure 6.37.4 Non-scarring Moxa at Zu San Li
(ST-36)*

38. Diabetes

Diabetes is a metabolic disorder and known as dispersion-thirst in TCM. It is characterized by polydipsia, polyphagia, polyuria and emaciation. The disease usually has the following causes: dietary irregularities damageing the spleen and stomach; emotional depression obstructing qi dynamics; overwork causing internal rise of deficient fire; or an innate deficiency resulting in static blood.

Main Symptoms: Polydipsia, polyphagia, polyuria, emaciation.

Acupoints:

- *Primary points:* Guan Yuan (RN-4), Yi Shu (between BL-17 and BL-18), Yang Chi (SJ-4), San Yin Jiao (SP-6), Qi Hai (RN-6).

- *Symptomatic points:* Polydipsia: Fei Shu (BL-13), Chi Ze (LU-5), Zhong Fu (LU-1); Polyphagia: Zhong Wan (RN-12), Zu San Li (ST-36), Pi Shu (BL-20); Polyuria: Ming Men (DU-4), Shen Shu (BL-23), Zhong Ji (RN-3).

Moxibustion Method:

- Gentle Moxa: Apply moxa for 15–20 minutes per acupoint, once daily or every other day, and repeat 10 times for a course of treatment. (Figure 6.38.1)

- Cone Moxa: Apply 3–5 wheat-sized cones per acupoint, once daily and repeat 10 times for a course of treatment. Repeat the treatment course after 20 days rest. (Figure 6.38.2)

- Moxa on Ginger: Apply 6–30 cones per acupoint, once every other day, and repeat 10 times for a course of treatment. (Figure 6.38.3)

- Warm Needle Moxa: Apply moxa for 5–10 minutes per acupoint, once every other day, and repeat 10 times for a course of treatment. (Figure 6.38.4)

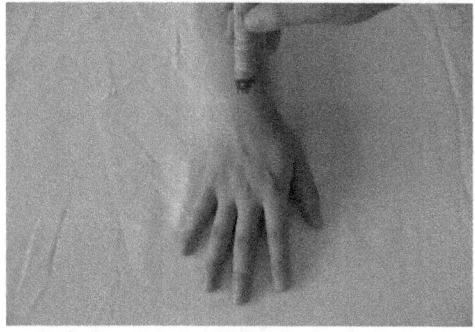 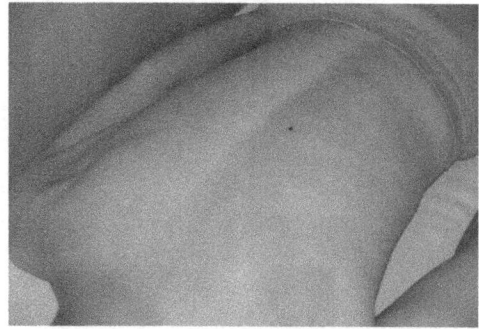

Figure 6.38.1 Gentle Moxa at Yang Chi (SJ-4)   Figure 6.38.2 Cone Moxa at Yi Shu (between BL-17 and BL-18)

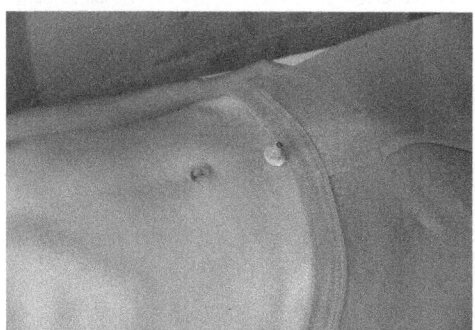 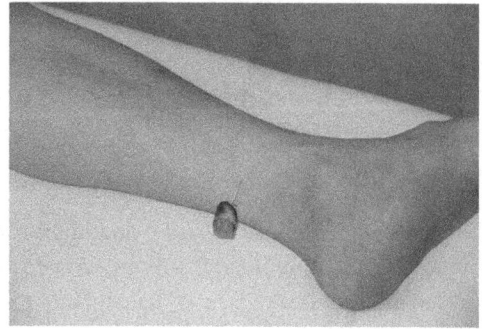

Figure 6.38.3 Moxa on Ginger at Guan Yuan (RN-4)   Figure 6.38.4 Warm Needle Moxa at San Yin Jiao (SP-6)

39. Obesity

Obesity is a nutritional disorder manifesting as a far higher amount of body fat than is healthy or desirable. The key symptoms are a body weight of more than 120% of standard weight, which is accompanied by dizziness, a fatigued spirit, no strength to speak and a shortness of breath. The disease has the following causes: innate factors, debility in old age, excessive consumption of fatty and sweet foods, extended periods of lying or sitting, a lack of exercise, right vacuity or affect-mind ill-being.

Main Symptoms: The weight is 20% more than standard body weight.

Acupoints: Zu San Li (ST-36), Pi Shu (BL-20), Qu Chi (LI-11), Feng Long (ST-40), Yin Ling Quan (SP-9), San Yin Jiao (SP-6).

Moxibustion Method:

- Gentle Moxa: Apply moxa for 6–15 minutes per acupoint, once daily or every other day, each treatment repeated 10 times. Repeat the treatment course after 3 days. (Figure 6.39.1)

- Moxa on Ginger: Apply 3–5 cones per acupoint, once or twice a day, each treatment repeated 20 times. Repeat the treatment course after 3 days. (Figure 6.39.2)

- Non-scarring Moxa: Apply 5–7 cones per acupoint, once every other day. Continue for 2–3 months. (Figure 6.39.3)

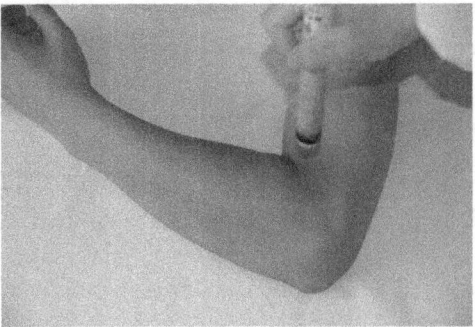

Figure 6.39.1 Gentle Moxa at Qu Chi (LI-11)

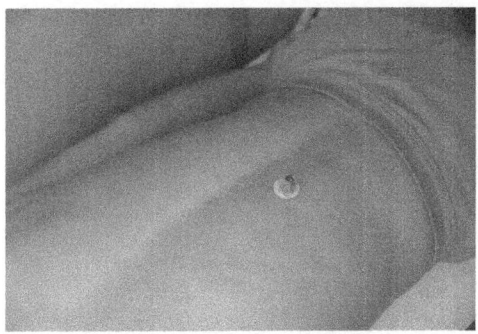
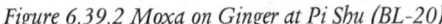
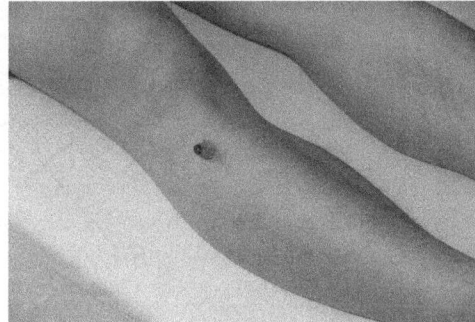

Figure 6.39.2 Moxa on Ginger at Pi Shu (BL-20)   *Figure 6.39.3 Non-scarring Moxa at Zu San Li (ST-36)*

40. Rheumatic Arthritis

Rheumatic arthritis is a kind of acute or chronic inflammation of connective tissue that is common and recurrent. The key symptoms are wandering aching pain and heaviness or soreness in the joints and muscles. It is an allergic disease beginning with an acute onset of fever and joint pain. The disease falls in the category of impediment pattern in TCM, and is usually caused by external pathogens exploiting vacuity or accumulated phlegm and stasis.

Main Symptoms: Wandering aching pain, heaviness or soreness in the joints and muscles.

Acupoints:

- *Primary points:* Qu Quan (LR-8), Da Zhui (DU-14), Zu San Li (ST-36), Yin Ling Quan (SP-9), Ashi points.

- *Symptomatic points:* Shoulder: Jian Yu (LI-15), Jian Liao (SJ-14), Jian Qian (EX-UE-12); Elbow: Qu Chi (LI-11), Shou San Li (LI-10), Chi Ze (LU-5); Wrist: Wai Guan (SJ-5), Yang Chi (SJ-4), He Gu (L-4); Hip: Huan Tiao (GB-30), Feng Shi (GB-31), Bi Guan (ST-31); Knee: Xi Yan (EX-LE-5), Liang Qiu (ST-34), Xue Hai (SP-10); Ankle: Jie Xi (ST-41), Qiu Xu (GB-40), Zhao Hai (KI-6).

Moxibustion Method:

- Gentle Moxa: Apply moxa for 15–20 minutes per acupoint, once daily, each treatment repeated 10 times. (Figure 6.40.1)

- Moxa on Ginger: Apply 3–5 cones per acupoint, once daily, each treatment repeated 10 times. (Figure 6.40.2)

- Direct Moxa: Dip a piece of Tao Zhi (Persicae Ramulus) approximately 17–20cm long and as thick as a thumb in sesame oil, then ignite it. Blow it out and press it on the acupoints or affected parts that have been covered with 3–5 layers of cotton paper, until the skin reddens. Apply moxa once daily. (Figure 6.40.3)

- Medicinal Scarring Cone Moxa:* Grind the following herbs into a fine powder: 1000g Chen Ai Rong (aged Artemisiae Argyi Folium Tritum), 50g each of Liu Huang (Sulfur), Fang Feng (Saposhnikoviae Radix), Cang Zhu (Atractylodis Rhizoma), Shi Cang Pu (Acori Tatarinowii Rhizoma), Xiao Hui Xiang (Foeniculi Fructus), Huo Xiang (Agastaches Herba), Feng Qiu (Liquidambaris Fructus) and Chen Pi (Citri Reticulatae Pericarpium), and 1g of She Xiang (Moschus). Make the herb powder into cones the size of a mung bean. Choose 2–4 acupoints each time and inject 0.5–1ml of 2% ethocaine intracutaneously, and then apply moxa. Apply 6–100 cones according to the acupoints and the patient's condition, until eschar appears. Finally cover the eschar with a sterile gauze. (Figure 6.40.4)

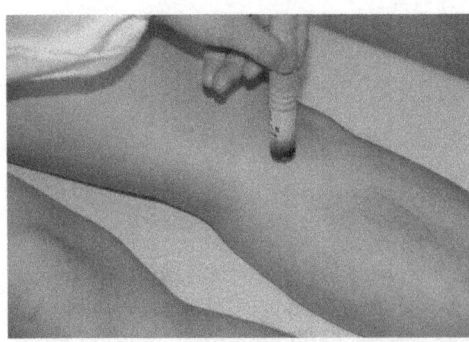

Figure 6.40.1 Gentle Moxa at Yin Ling Quan (SP-9)

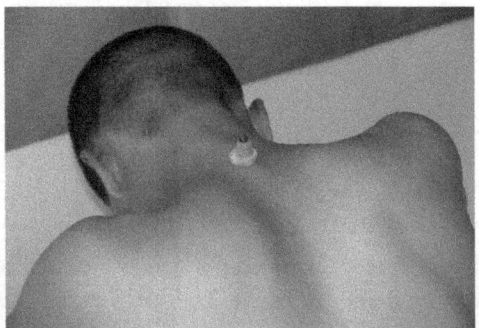

Figure 6.40.2 Moxa on Ginger at Da Zhui (DU-14)

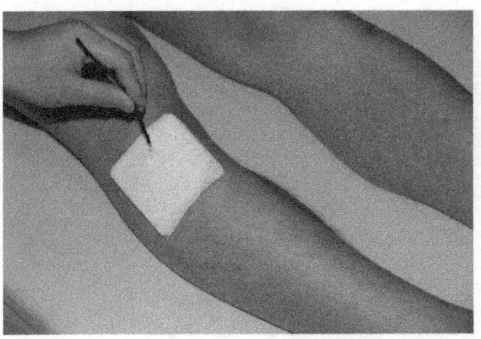 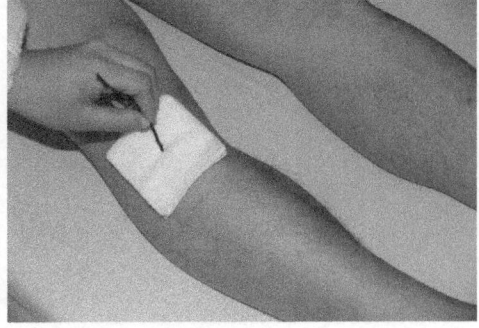

Figure 6.40.3 Direct Moxa at Zu San Li (ST-36)

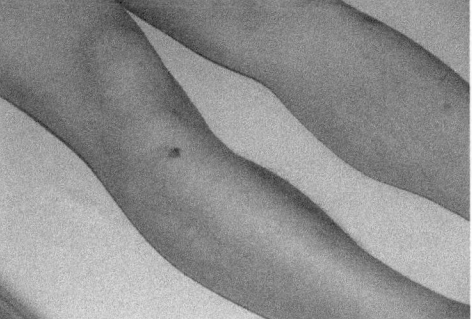

Figure 6.40.4 Medicinal Scarring Cone Moxa at Zu San Li (ST-36)

- Wu Zhu Yu Application: Mix an appropriate amount of Wu Zhu Yu (Evodiae Fructus) powder with yellow wine, and fry into a paste. Cover the acupoints with some pieces of cloth, then put on the warm herb paste. Change the paste when it becomes cool. Apply moxa on 2–4 acupoints each time, once or twice daily, and repeat 5 times for a course of treatment. (Figure 6.40.5)

- Jin Fang Steam Treatment: Jin Jie (Schizonepeta), Fang Feng (Radix Sileris), Ai Ye (Folium Artemisiae Argyi) and shelled Da Suan (Garlic). Add 30g each of the above ingredients and some water into a basin and bring to the boil. Treat the affected parts with the herb steam for 1–2 hours each time. Wipe the skin after treatment to protect against cold invasion. Apply the steam moxa once daily, and repeat 5 times for a course of treatment. Repeat after 3 days. (Figure 6.40.6)

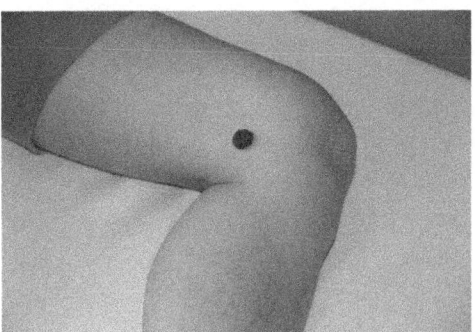 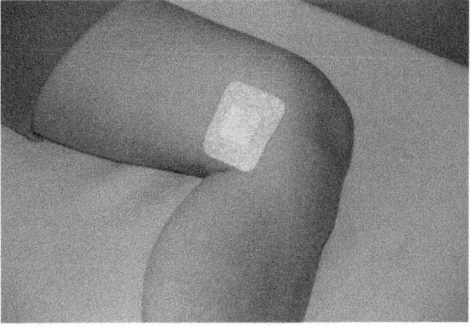

Figure 6.40.5 Wu Zhu Yu Application at Qu Quan (LR-8)

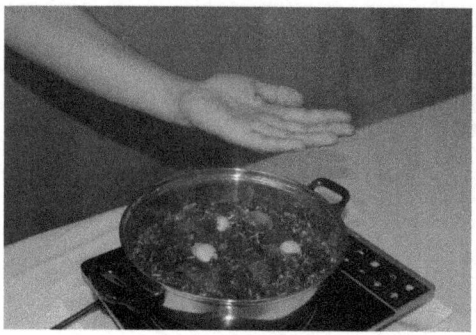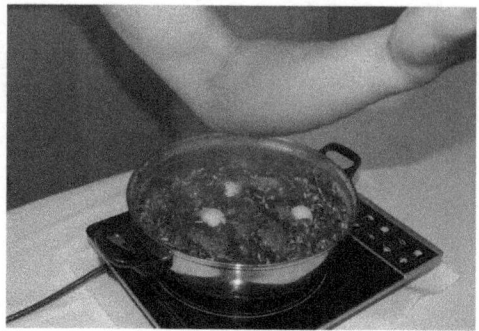

Figure 6.40.6 Jin Fang Steam Treatment at Ashi Points

41. Rheumatoid Arthritis

Rheumatoid arthritis (RA) is a kind of commonly seen systemic autoimmune disease manifesting as chronic infection of the joints. The features of this disease are constant, repetitive, progressive articulatory synovitis, drainage, cell proliferation and pannus formation. Symmetrical pathological changes of the facet joints of the hands, wrist and feet are commonly seen. RA is equivalent to the TCM disease known as lame impediment. It can occur due to external contraction of wind, cold and damp pathogens; contraction of heat pathogens or formation of pathogenic heat. These exhaust qi and damage the blood and viscera.

Main Symptoms: Stiffness in the morning, symmetrical multiple swelling of the facet joints, restricted joint movement, and even rigidity and deformation.

Acupoints: Da Zhu (BL-11), Qu Chi (LI-11), Zu San Li (ST-36), Da Zhui (DU-14), Yang Ling Quan (GB-34), Ashi points.

Moxibustion Method:

- Moxa on Ginger: Apply 5–7 moxa cones to each acupoint. Perform once every other day. One treatment course consists of 10 treatments. (Figure 6.41.1)

- Gentle Moxa: Apply moxa to each acupoint for 15–20 minutes. Perform once daily. One treatment course consists of 10 treatments. (Figure 6.41.2)

- Scarring Moxa:* Apply 6–20 moxa cones to each acupoint, using cones approximately the size of a soybean or wheat kernel. Perform once every 2–4 weeks. (Figure 6.41.3)

- Fumigation Moxa: Ignite a moxa cone, put it in a fumigation device and fix it at the point. Apply 1 cone each time. Perform once every morning and evening, and continue for 5 days. Perform once daily after symptomatic relief. (Figure 6.41.4)

- Wei Ling Xian Application: Take fresh Wei Ling Xian (Clematidis Radix Folium), mash into a paste, add brown sugar, mash and melt down. Apply the paste, approximately 1–1.5cm in diameter, to each point. When sensations of wind blowing and ants crawling occur, wait for 2–3 minutes, then remove the medicine and flush the local area with clean water. If blisters appear, let them subside naturally; to prevent infection, don't puncture blisters. (Figure 6.41.5)

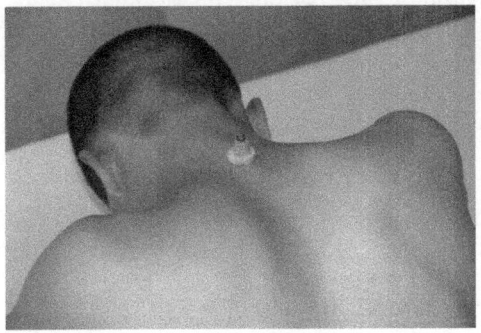

Figure 6.41.1 Moxa on Ginger at Da Zhui (DU-14)

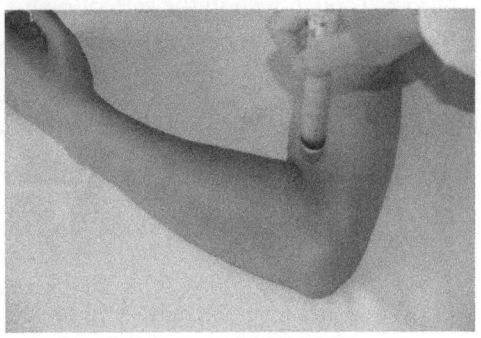

Figure 6.41.2 Gentle Moxa at Qu Chi (LI-11)

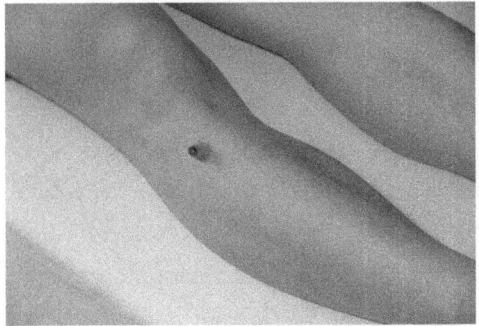

Figure 6.41.3 Scarring Moxa at Zu San Li (ST-36)

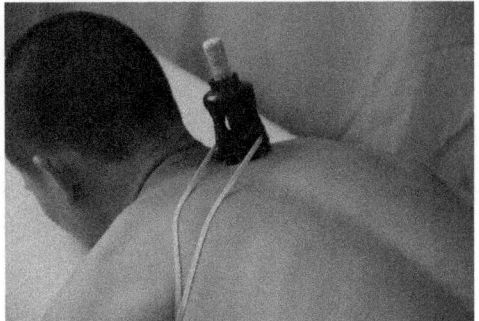

Figure 6.41.4 Fumigation Moxa at Da Zhu (BL-11)

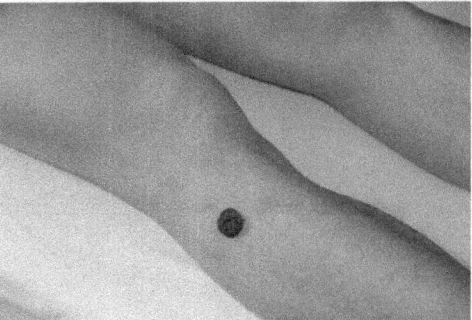

Figure 6.41.5 Wei Ling Xian Application at Yang Ling Quan (GB-34)

42. Atrophy Syndrome

Atrophy syndrome refers to slack, weak and chronically disabled tendons, and in extreme cases muscle atrophy and paralysation. The most common clinical manifestation is weakness of the legs. The most common causes include lung heat damageing the fluids and failing to distribute fluids; spreading damp-heat causing disharmony of qi and blood; deficiency of spleen and stomach causing dysfunction of transportation of food essences;

liver and kidney depletion causing marrow exhaustion, sinew atrophy or phlegm and blood stasis obstructing the collaterals, as well as tendon and vessel malnutrition. This syndrome is often seen in the case of motor neuron disease, peripheral nerve injury, acute infectious polyradiculoneuritis, brain paralysis and external injuring paraplegia in Western medicine.

Main Symptoms: Weak and feeble limbs, slack tendons, muscle atrophy and paralysation.

Acupoints:

- *Primary points:* Zu San Li (ST-36), San Yin Jiao (SP-6), Bi Guan (ST-31), Yang Gu (SI-5).

- *Symptomatic points:* Body fluid impairment due to lung heat: Qu Chi (LI-11), Tai Yuan (LU-9), Xia Ju Xu (ST-39); Spreading damp-heat: Zhong Wan (RN-12), Yin Ling Quan (SP9), Qu Chi (LI-11); Spleen and stomach deficiency: Pi Shu (BL-20), Qi Hai Shu (BL-24), Jie Xi (ST-41); Liver-kidney depletion: Gan Shu (BL-18), Shen Shu (BL-23), Yang Ling Quan (GB-34), Xuan Zhong (GB-39); Phlegm and blood stasis obstructing the collaterals: Shen Shu (BL-23), Qu Chi (LI-11), Xue Hai (SP10), Liang Qiu (ST-34).

Moxibustion Method:

- Cone Moxa: Apply 3–5 moxa cones to each acupoint. Perform once daily. One treatment course consists of 15 treatments. (Figure 6.42.1)

- Gentle Moxa: Apply moxa to each acupoint for 6–20 minutes. Perform once daily. One treatment course consists of 10 treatments. (Figure 6.42.2)

- Moxa on Shan Yao: Take fresh Shan Yao and soak it in diluted saline solution, cut into 0.2cm pieces and apply to each point, apply 4–8 cones on each piece. Perform once daily. One treatment course consists of 10 treatments. (Figure 6.42.3)

- Pressing Moxa: Apply pressing moxa to each point 5–10 times. Perform once daily. One treatment course consists of 10 treatments. (Figure 6.42.4)

- Warm Needle Moxa: Apply moxa to each acupoint for 6–15 minutes. Perform once daily. One treatment course consists of 10 treatments. (Figure 6.42.5)

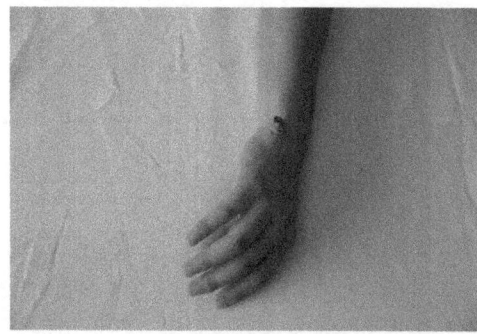

Figure 6.42.1 Cone Moxa at Yang Gu (SI-5)

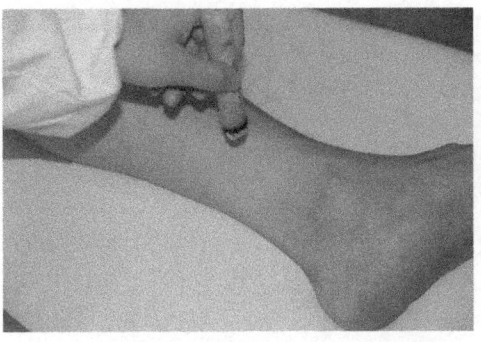

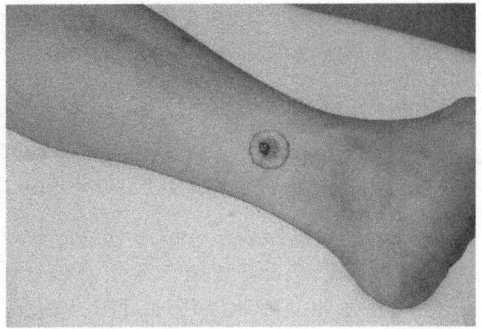

Figure 6.42.2 Gentle Moxa at San Yin Jiao (SP-6)   *Figure 6.42.3 Moxa on Shan Yao at San Yin Jiao (SP-6)*

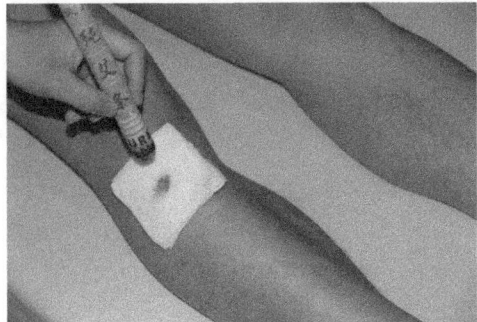

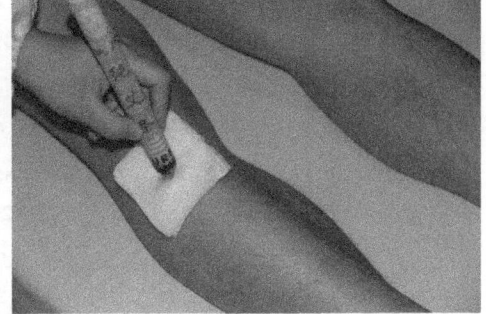

Figure 6.42.4 Pressing Moxa at Zu San Li (ST-36)

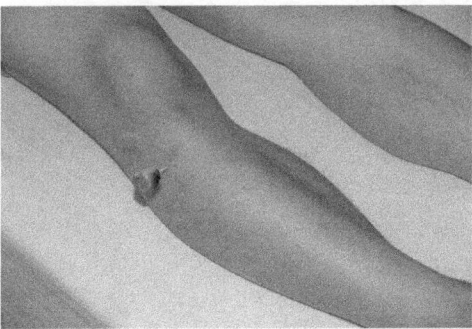

Figure 6.42.5 Warm Needle Moxa at Zu San Li (ST-36)

43. Epilepsy

Epilepsy is a set of clinical syndromes featuring paroxysmal malfunction of the central nervous system resulting from excessive discharge of cerebral neurons. It manifests as recurrent dysfunction of the movement, sense, behaviour and vegetative nervous systems. It is equivalent to epilepsy in TCM. It can occur due to a congenital predisposition, excessive fear and exhaustion, sequelae of other diseases, head injuries, as well as dysfunction of the zang-fu organs, wind phlegm or blood stasis clouding the clear orifices and causing mental confusion.

Main Symptoms: Sudden loss of consciousness, foaming at the mouth, convulsions and becoming conscious when moved. These epileptic events occur repeatedly.

Acupoints:

- *Primary points:* Bai Hui (DU-20), Tai Chong (LR-3), Feng Long (ST-40), Shen Zhu (DU-12), Jiu Wei (RN-15), Xin Shu (BL-15).

- *Symptomatic points:* Attack period: Feng Fu (DU-16), Nei Guan (PC-6), Shen Men (HT-7), Zhong Wan (RN-12); Rest period: Shen Shu (BL-23), San Yin Jiao (SP-6), Shen Que (RN-8), Qi Hai (RN-6).

Moxibustion Method:

- Moxa on Ginger: Apply 6–30 moxa cones to each acupoint, using cones approximately the size of a soybean. Perform once daily. One course of treatment consists of 7–10 treatments. (Figure 6.43.1)

- Gentle Moxa: Apply moxa to each acupoint for 6–15 minutes. Perform once daily. One course of treatment consists of 10 treatments. (Figure 6.43.2)

- Scarring Cone Moxa:* Apply 3–5 moxa cones to each acupoint. Perform once monthly for 4 months altogether. (Figure 6.43.3)

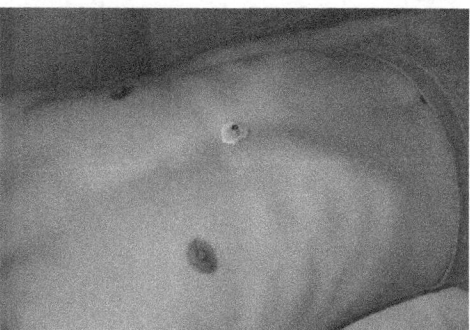

Figure 6.43.1 Moxa on Ginger Jiu Wei (RN-15)

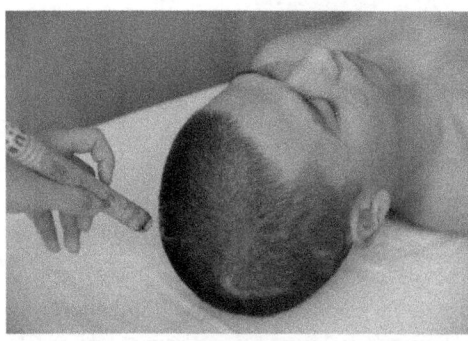

Figure 6.43.2 Gentle Moxa at Bai Hui (DU-20)

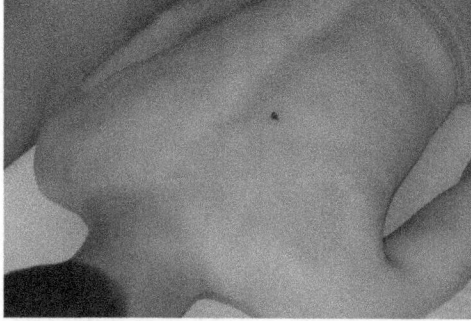

Figure 6.43.3 Scarring Cone Moxa at Xin Shu (BL-15)

- Juncibustion:* Apply juncibustion once to each acupoint. Perform twice per month. (Figure 6.43.4)

- Moxa on Yang Sui Ding:* Take 500g of Ai Ye (Artemisiae Argyi Folium), 120g of Liu Huang (Sulfur), 6g of She Xiang (Moschus) and 0.9g of both Xi Niu Huang (Bovis Bezoar Occidentale) and Zhen Zhu Fen (Margarita Pulverata). First put the Ai Ye into a pan and add 1000ml water, decoct them until there is only 120ml of water left, then make Yang Sui Ding (lozenges) according to the instructions. Choose 1 point for each treatment, put a thin round sheet of paper on it, then apply a wheat kernel-sized piece of Yang Sui Ding to the point and ignite it. Burn 1 cone at a time until blisters appear, bind and fix with a surgical dressing; let the blisters be absorbed naturally. Perform once monthly. (Figure 6.43.5)

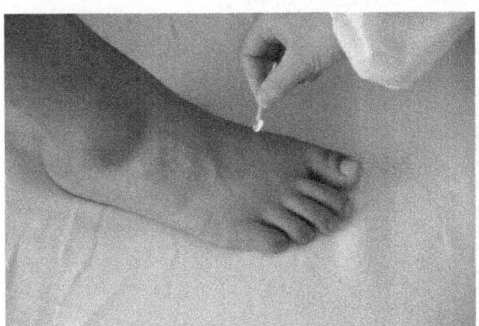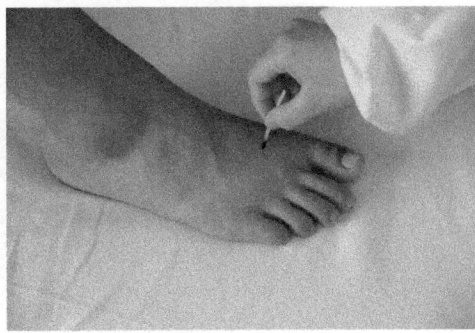

Figure 6.43.4 Juncibustion at Tai Chong (LR-3)

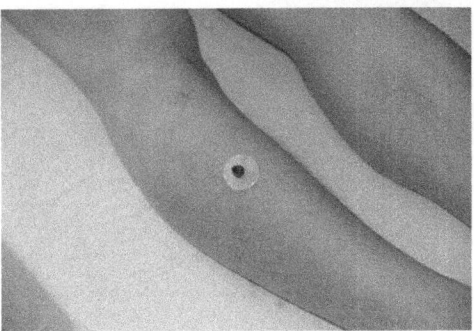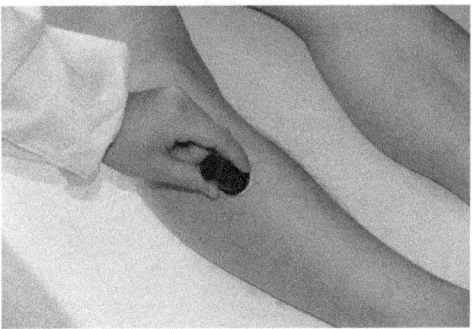

Figure 6.43.5 Moxa on Yan Sui Ding at Feng Long (ST-40)

44. Panasthenia

Panasthenia refers to the weakening of mental abilities resulting from long-term emotional tension and mental stress. It manifests clinically as mental excitability and exhaustion. It is often accompanied by headache, dyssomnia, dysphoria, emotional irritability and other disorders of the body. It is associated with the mind depletion category of disease-patterns in TCM. It usually occurs due to liver qi depression; phlegm-fire harassing the heart; liver depression and spleen deficiency; yin deficiency with effulgent fire; dual deficiency of the heart and spleen; heart deficiency with timidity; non-interaction between the heart and kidney.

Main Symptoms: Fatigue, insomnia, forgetfulness, dizziness and headache.

Acupoints: Xin Shu (BL15), Bai Hui (DU-20), Zu San Li (ST-36), Nei Guan (PC-6), Shen Men (HT-7).

Moxibustion Method:

- Gentle Moxa: Apply moxa to each acupoint for 6–20 minutes. Perform once daily. One treatment course consists of 10 treatments. (Figure 6.44.1)

- Non-scarring Moxa: Apply 3–7 moxa cones to each acupoint. Perform once daily. One treatment course consists of 10 treatments. (Figure 6.44.2)

- Warm Needle Moxa: Apply moxa to each acupoint for 6–15 minutes. Perform once every other day. One treatment course consists of 10 treatments. (Figure 6.44.3)

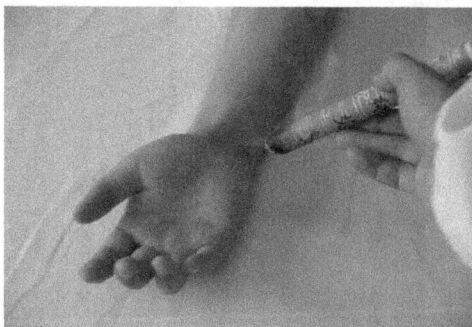

Figure 6.44.1 Gentle Moxa at Shen Men (HT-7)

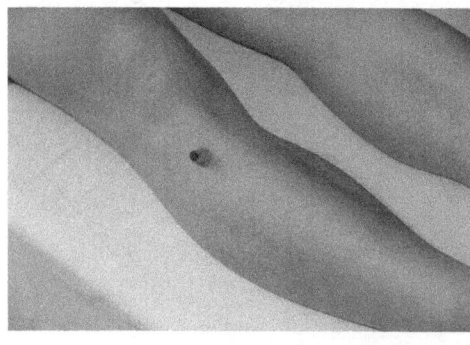

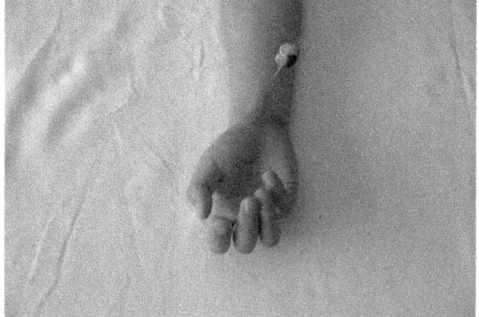

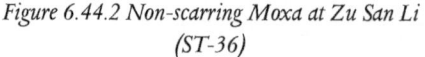

Figure 6.44.2 Non-scarring Moxa at Zu San Li (ST-36)   *Figure 6.44.3 Warm Needle Moxa at Nei Guan (PC-6)*

45. Insomnia

Insomnia, also called sleeplessness, is a condition manifesting as difficulty sleeping. Mild cases present as a difficulty falling asleep, being able to fall sleep but being easily woken up, not being able to fall asleep again after waking up, or sleeping in fits and starts. In severe cases patients cannot fall sleep throughout the night. It is often accompanied by headache, dizziness, palpitations, forgetfulness, excessive dreaming and other symptoms. It usually occurs due to deficiency causing a lack of spirit preservation; yin deficiency with effulgent fire causing a failure of yin to constrain yang; heart vacuity and gallbladder timidity causing agitation of heart spirit; phlegm-heat or repletion fire harassing the heart spirit. This pattern is often seen in neurasthenia, neurosis and anaemia.

Main Symptoms: Difficulty sleeping.

Acupoints: San Yin Jiao (SP-6), Shen Men (HT-7), Xin Shu (BL15), Bai Hui (DU-20), Nei Guan (PC-6), Zu San Li (ST-36).

Moxibustion Method:

- Moxa on Ginger: Apply 5–10 moxa cones to each acupoint, using cones approximately the size of a soybean. Perform once every evening. One treatment course consists of 5 treatments. (Figure 6.45.1)

- Gentle Moxa: Apply moxa to each acupoint for 6–15 minutes. Perform once every evening. One treatment course consists of 7 treatments. (Figure 6.45.2)

- Moxa on Celery Root: Take celery root, cut it into 0.2cm pieces and apply to each point. Apply 3–5 cones of moxa on each piece. Perform once every evening. (Figure 6.45.3)

- Zhen Zhu San Application: Take equivalent amounts of Zhen Zhu powder, Dan Shen powder, Liu Huang powder and Bing Pian, and mix them and apply to Yong Quan (KI-1). Perform once every evening. One treatment course consists of 7 treatments. (Figure 6.45.4)

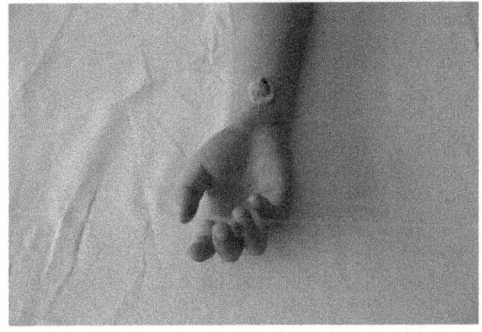
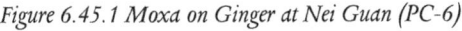
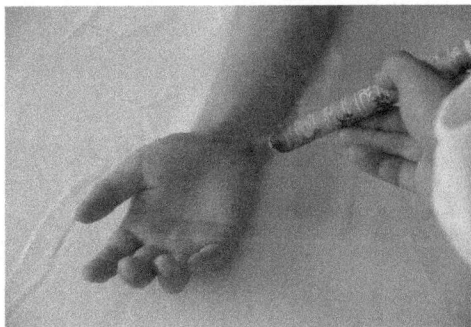

Figure 6.45.1 Moxa on Ginger at Nei Guan (PC-6)   *Figure 6.45.2 Gentle Moxa at Shen Men (HT-7)*

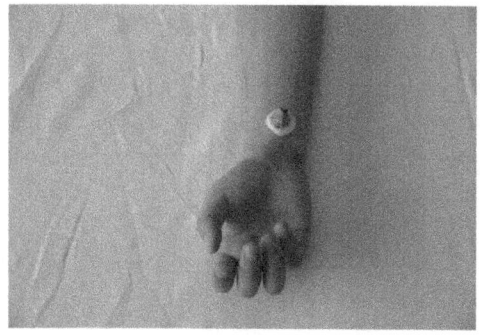

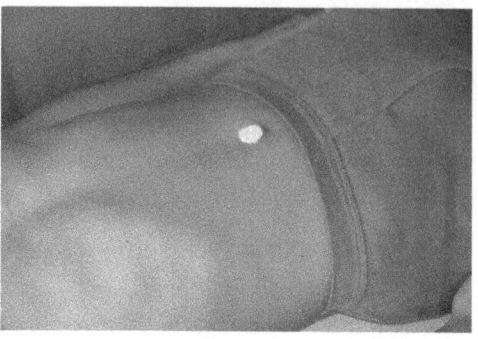

Figure 6.45.3 Moxa on Celery Root at Nei Guan (PC-6)

Figure 6.45.4 Zhen Zhu San Application at Shen Que (RN-8)

46. Facial Paralysis

Facial paralysis refers to a disease involving facial drooping of the mouth and eye to one side. The onset is often sudden and the patient often wakes up with one side of the face numb or even paralyzed. The wrinkles on the forehead either become shallow or disappear, the palpebral fissure becomes larger, the naso-labial groove becomes shallow, and the corner of the mouth droops and is deviated to the healthy side. It often occurs due to contraction of external pathogens causing blockage of qi and blood or insufficient anti-pathogenic energy causing vacuity of the meridians and insecurity of exterior's defensive capabilities. It is equivalent to peripheral facial paralysis in Western medicine.

Main Symptoms: Dry mouth and eyes.

Acupoints:

- *Local points:* Di Cang (ST-4), Jia Che (ST-6), Xia Guan (ST-7), Yi Feng (SJ-17), Yang Bai (GB-14), Qian Zheng (on the cheek, 0.5 *cun* in front of the earlobe).

- *Distant points:* He Gu (LI-4), Zu San Li (ST-36).

Moxibustion Method:

- Moxa on Ginger or Garlic: Apply 5–7 moxa cones to each acupoint. Perform once every evening. One treatment course consists of 7 treatments. (Figure 6.46.1)

- Gentle Moxa: Apply moxa to each acupoint for 6–15 minutes. Perform once every evening. One treatment course consists of 7 treatments. (Figure 6.46.2)

- Heavenly Moxa (Blistering Moxibustion):* Grind 3 Ban Mao (Mylabris) and 3 grains of Ba Dou (Crotonis Fructus) into a powder, and mix with sesame oil to make a paste. Spread the paste on sterilized gauze and apply to Di Cang (ST-4), Jia Che (ST-6), and Xia Guan (ST-7). Perform for 5 hours in summer and 8 hours in winter. Apply to 2 points each time and repeat once every 7 days. One course of treatment consists of 4 treatments. If blisters occur on local skin, bind with a surgical dressing and keep clean; let the blisters be absorbed naturally. (Figure 6.46.3)

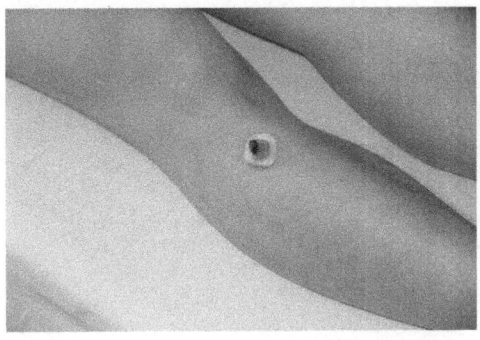

Figure 6.46.1 Moxa on Ginger or Garlic at Zu San Li (ST-36)

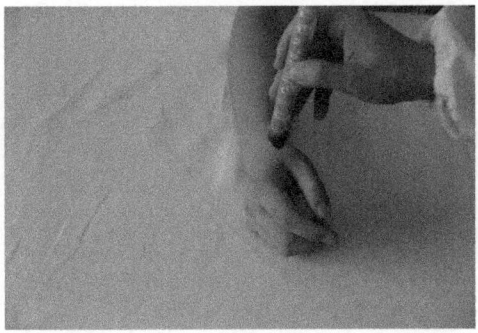

Figure 6.46.2 Gentle Moxa at He Gu (LI-4)

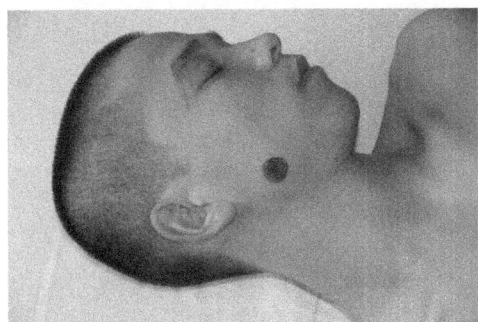

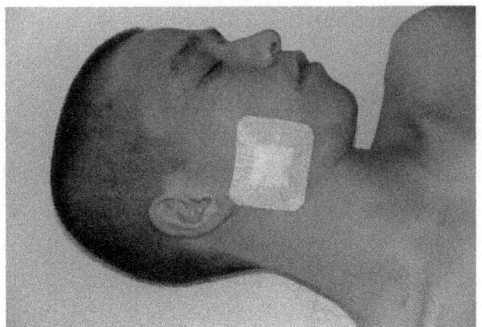

Figure 6.46.3 Heavenly Moxa at Jia Che (ST-6)

- Xian E Bu Shi Cao Application: Take adequate fresh E Bu Shi Cao (Centipedae Herba), mash and apply to the affected cheek, change every other day. (Figure 6.46.4)

- Qian Zheng Gao Application: Take 10g of Bi Ma Ren (Ricini Semen) and 30g of Song Xiang (Pini Resina), and grind them into a powder for further use. Take 1 litre of water and bring to the boil, add Bi Ma Ren powder and boil for a further 5 minutes. Then add Song Xiang, simmer on a low heat for 3–4 minutes, pour into a basin with cold water (approximately 1 kg of water) and make into a paste. Cut the paste into 3g pieces for further use. Take one piece of paste, soften it with boiled water and spread it on a piece of round cloth. Apply the cloth to Xia Guan (ST-7) or Jia Che (ST-6), fix it with tape and change every 5 days. (Figure 6.46.5)

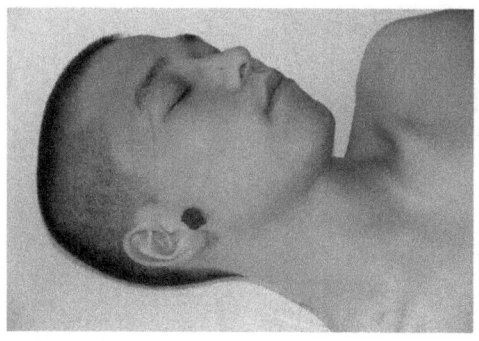

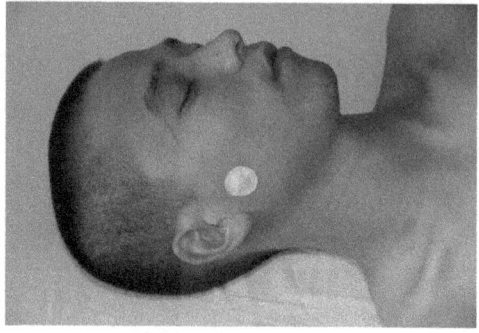

Figure 6.46.4 Xian E Bu Shi Cao Application at Qian Zheng

Figure 6.46.5 Qian Zheng Gao Application at Xia Guan (ST-7)

47. Sciatica

Sciatica refers to a syndrome manifesting as radiating pain along the path of the sciatic nerve. It is often classified into root sciatica and trunk sciatica. It usually occurs due to contraction of external pathogens or injury causing qi stagnation and blood stasis. Root sciatica is often secondary to lumbar spinal stenosis, lumbar intervertebral disc protrusion, rachitis and spina bifida. Trunk sciatica is often secondary to arthritis of the hip, sacroiliitis, hip injury, pelvic inflammatory disease, tumour and piriformis syndrome.

Main Symptoms: Radiating, burning, shock-like pain in the waist, hip, posterior side of the thigh, lateral side of the crus and foot.

Acupoints:

- *Primary points:* Waist Jia Ji points (EX-B2), Ju Liao (GB-29), Huan Tiao (GB-30), Zhi Bian (BL-54), Wei Zhong (BL-40).

- *Symptomatic points:* Lumbago: Shen Shu (BL-23), Guan Yuan Shu (BL-26); Hip pain: Ci Liao (BL-32); Pain in the posterior thigh: Cheng Fu (BL36), Yin Men (BL-37); Pain below the knee: Zu San Li (ST-36), Da Zhui (DU-14), Yang Ling Quan (GB-34), Cheng Shan (BL-57), Xuan Zhong (GB-39), Kun Lun (BL-60).

Moxibustion Method:

- Non-scarring Moxa: Apply 3–7 moxa cones to each acupoint. Perform once daily during the acute period and once every other day during the chronic period. One treatment course consists of 6 treatments. (Figure 6.47.1)

- Moxa on Ginger: Apply 5–7 moxa cones to each acupoint, using cones approximately the size of a date pit or horsebean. Perform once daily. One treatment course consists of 7–10 treatments. There should be a 3–5 day interval between 2 courses. (Figure 6.47.2)

- Gentle Moxa: Apply moxa to each acupoint for 6–20 minutes. Perform 1–2 times daily. One treatment course consists of 7–10 treatments. There should be a 3–5 day interval between 2 courses. (Figure 6.47.3)

- Juncibustion:* Perform once daily. One treatment course consists of 10 treatments. (Figure 6.47.4)

- Wu Zhu Yu Application: Mash Wu Zhu Yu (Evodiae Fructus) into a powder, stored in a bottle for further use. Take some powder, mix it with yellow wine, fry in a pan, and then make it into paste. Spread the paste on several pieces of cyan cloth and apply them to different points. Change the cloth when it becomes cold. Choose 2–4 points each time and perform 1–2 times daily. One treatment course consists of 5 treatments. (Figure 6.47.5)

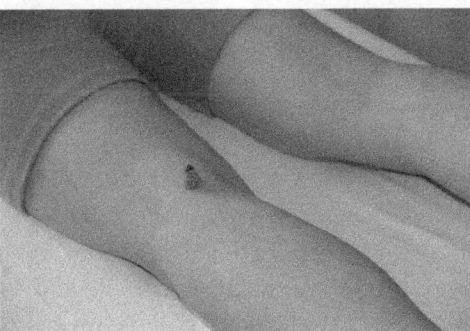

Figure 6.47.1 Non-scarring Moxa at Wei Zhong (BL-40)

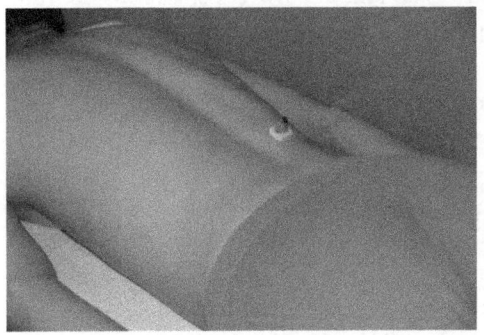
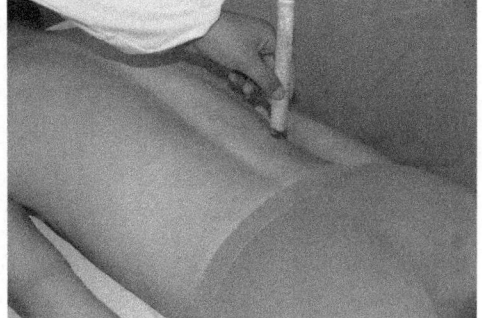

Figure 6.47.2 Moxa on Ginger at Shen Shu (BL-23)   *Figure 6.47.3 Gentle Moxa at Shen Shu (BL-23)*

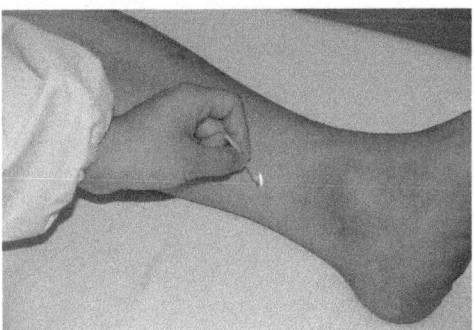
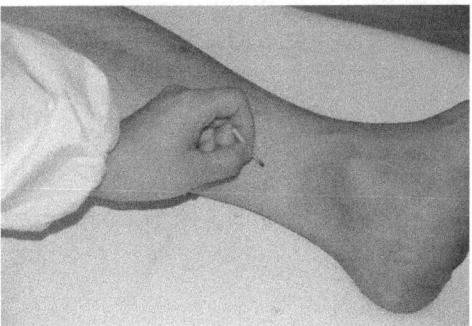

Figure 6.47.4 Juncibustion at San Yin Jiao (SP-6)

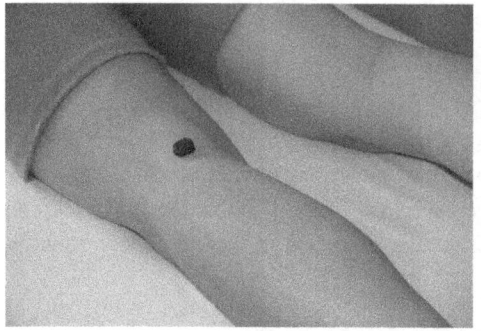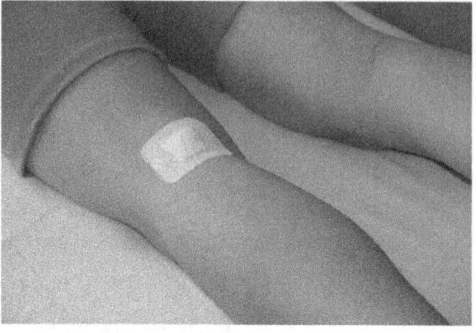

Figure 6.47.5 Wu Zhu Yu Application at Wei Zhong (BL-40)

48. Spontaneous Sweating and Night Sweats

Spontaneous sweating and night sweats are conditions in which the disordered discharge of sweat results from yin-yang disharmony and insecurity of interstices. Spontaneous sweating refers to sweating occurring constantly during daytime, especially when moving, that is not due to external environment factors. Night sweats refer to sweating when sleeping that ceases upon waking up. It usually occurs due to deficiency of lung qi causing exterior deficiency and insecurity; nutritional and defensive disharmony causing dysfunction of the exterior's defensive capabilities; deficiency of heart blood preventing heart liquid from being stored; yin deficiency with effulgent fire forcing fluids to escape. It is often seen in cases of hyperthyroidism, autonomic nerve dysfunction, rheumatic fever and tuberculosis in Western medicine.

Main Symptoms: Spontaneous sweating: sweating constantly during daytime, especially when moving; Night sweats: sweating when sleeping, which ceases upon waking up.

Acupoints: Night sweats: Yin Xi (HT-6), Gan Shu (BL-18), Chi Ze (LU5), Fei Shu (BL-13), Zhong Ji (RN-3), Hou Xi (SI-3); Spontaneous sweating: Yang Ling Quan (GB-34), Da Zhui (DU-14), He Gu (LI-4), Fu Liu (KI-7), Yu Ji (LU-10), Zhao Hai (KI-6).

Moxibustion Method:

- Non-scarring Moxa: Apply 3–5 moxa cones to each acupoint. Perform 1–2 times daily until sweating ceases. (Figure 6.48.1)

- Gentle Moxa: Apply moxa to each acupoint for 15 minutes. Perform once daily. One treatment course consists of 10 treatments. (Figure 6.48.2)

- Juncibustion:* Apply juncibustion to Yin Xi (HT-6) once. (Figure 6.48.3)

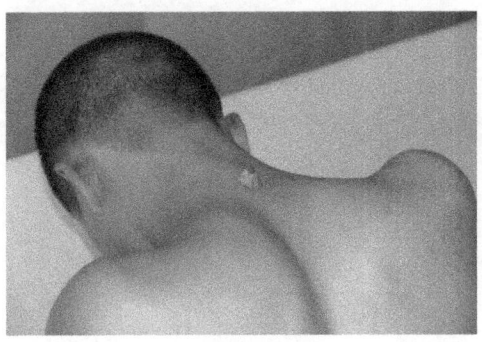

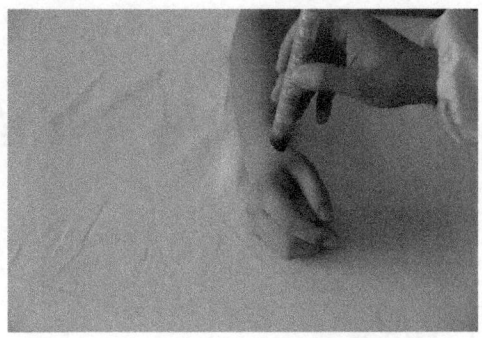

Figure 6.48.1 Non-scarring Moxa at Da Zhui (DU-14)

Figure 6.48.2 Gentle Moxa at He Gu (LI-4)

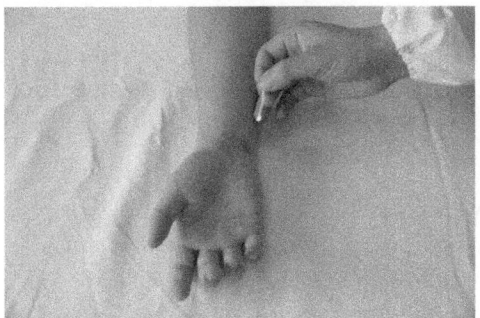

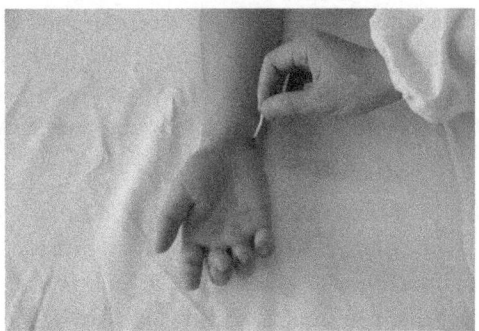

Figure 6.48.3 Juncibustion at Yin Xi (HT-6)

CHAPTER 7

Musculoskeletal Diseases

1. Stiff Neck

Stiff neck refers to a type of condition that involves acute simple rigidity, pain in the neck and nape, and limitation of movement. Stiff neck is usually caused by one of the following: an inappropriate sleeping posture; an inappropriate pillow height; invasion of wind and cold into the neck causing tension of the sinews. This disease is often seen in cases of neck muscle strain and contusion, neck rheumatism and degenerative changes of the cervical vertebra. It can also be caused by synovial incarceration or partial dislocation of the cervical facet joints.

Main Symptoms: One side of the neck experiences sudden rigidity and pain upon waking in the morning. In extreme cases the rigidity and pain spreads to the shoulder or upper arm of the same side. The patient's head often slants towards the affected side, movement is limited and there is obvious tenderness under pressure without redness or swelling.

Acupoints: Luo Zhen (M-UE-24), Hou Xi (SI-3), Xuan Zhong (GB-39), Ashi points.

Moxibustion Method:

- Gentle Pole Moxa: Apply moxa to each point for 15–20 minutes. Perform treatment once per day. Three treatments comprise one course of treatment. (Figure 7.1.1)

- Moxa on Ginger: Using moxa cones the size of a grain of wheat; apply moxa to each point for 15–20 minutes. Perform treatment once per day. Three treatments comprise one course of treatment. (Figure 7.1.2)

- Warm Needle Moxa: Apply moxa to each point for 15–20 minutes. Perform treatment once per day. Three treatments comprise one course of treatment. (Figure 7.1.3)

- Zhuang-style Medicated Thread Moxa: Using medicated thread that has undergone the herbal medicine soaking process, light the thread, shake the wrist to extinguish the flame, and quickly tap the glowing tip of the thread on the area or acupoint, like a sparrow pecking. One peck is the equivalent of one cone. Apply 3 cones to each acupoint. Perform once per day. Three treatments comprise one course of treatment (Figure 7.1.4)

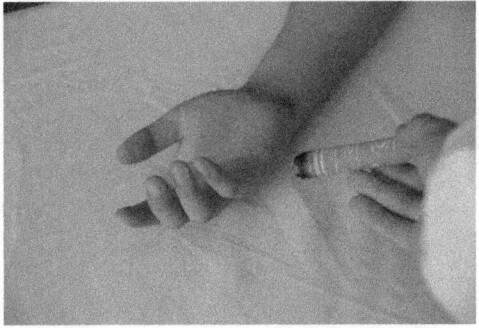

Figure 7.1.1 Gentle Pole Moxa at Hou Xi (SI-3)

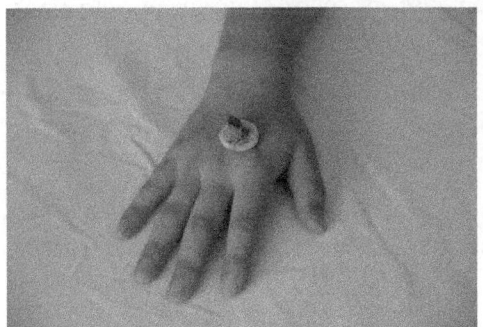

Figure 7.1.2 Moxa on Ginger at Luo Zhen (M-UE-24)

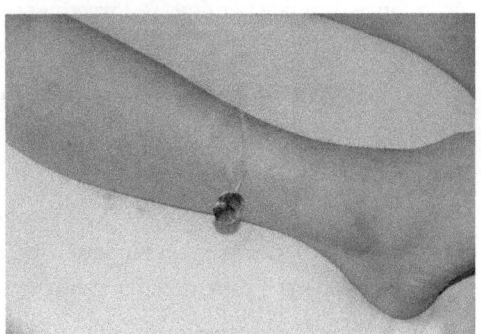

Figure 7.1.3 Warm Needle Moxa at Xuan Zhong (GB-39)

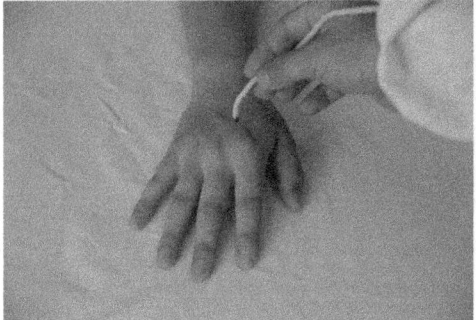

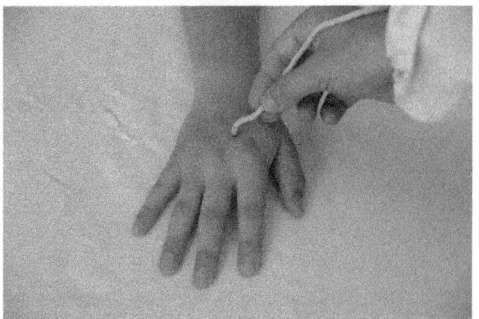

Figure 7.1.4 Zhuang-style Medicated Thread Moxa at Luo Zhen (M-UE-24)

2. Cervical Spondylopathy

Cervical spondylopathy, also called cervical syndrome, refers to a group of clinical symptoms that stimulate and compress cervical nerve roots, the spinal cord, vertebral arteries and cervical sympathetic nerves. This may be caused by hyperplastic inflammation of the cervical spine, cervical intervertebral disc extrusion and degenerative changes of the cervical zygapophyseal joints or ligaments. Cervical spondylopathy is usually caused by one of the following: debility in old age, deficiency of the liver and kidney, depriving sinews and bones of nourishment; or sedentary behaviour causing wearing of qi, taxation causing injury of the sinews and flesh; or contraction of external pathogens or strain and contusion bringing about meridian vessel obstruction.

Main Symptoms: The major features of cervical spondylopathy are local pain involving the occiput, neck, nape, shoulder, back and upper limbs; progressive disorder of sensation and movement. Mild cases experience dizziness, headache, pain and numbness of upper limbs, while severe cases can cause paralysis and even be life-threatening.

Acupoints: Da Zhui (DU-14), Tian Zhu (BL-10), Hou Xi (SI-3), Cervical Jia Ji points.

Moxibustion Method:

- Gentle Pole Moxa: Apply moxa to each point for 5–10 minutes. Perform treatment once or twice per day. Ten treatments comprise one course of treatment, with a 3–5 day interval between each treatment course. (Figure 7.2.1)

- Moxa on Ginger: Use moxa cones the size of a jujube seed. Apply 3–6 cones per acupoint, once per day, 7–10 treatments comprise one course of treatment. (Figure 7.2.2)

- Warm Needle Moxa: Apply 2–3 cones per acupoint, once per day or every other day, 7–10 treatments comprise one course of treatment, with a 3–5 day interval between each treatment course. (Figure 7.2.3)

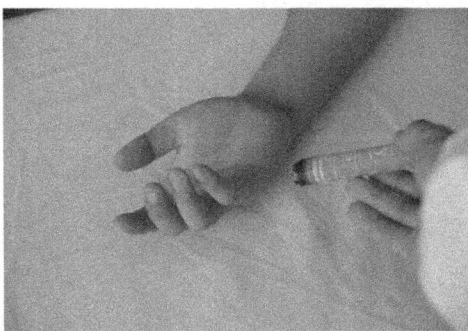

Figure 7.2.1 Gentle Pole Moxa at Hou Xi (SI-3)

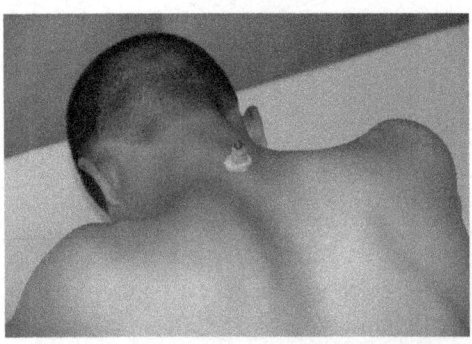
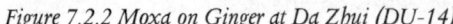

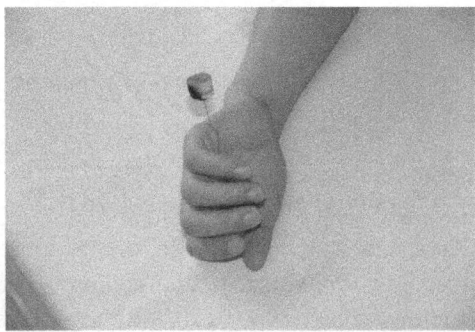

Figure 7.2.2 Moxa on Ginger at Da Zhui (DU-14)   *Figure 7.2.3 Warm Needle Moxa at Hou Xi (SI-3)*

3. Soft Tissue Injury

Soft tissue injury mainly refers to injury of various soft tissues without bone fracture, dislocation or injured skin; especially tendon and ligament injury. Soft tissue injury most often occurs around the joints and is usually caused by one of the following: strong trauma, torsion, traction and compression. It can also be caused by a weak constitution, excessive taxation and invasion of wind-cold-damp pathogens.

Main Symptoms: Local swelling and pain, ecchymosed skin, limitation of joint movement, even immobility of the joint.

Acupoints:

- *Primary points:* Local Ashi points.

- *Symptomatic points:* Elbow: Shou San Li (LI-10), Qu Chi (LI-11), Zhou Liao (LI-12), Chi Ze (LU-5); Wrist: Yang Xi (LI-5), Yang Chi (SJ-4), Yang Gu (SI-5), Wai Guan (SJ-5), Da Ling (PC-7), Zhi Gou (SJ-6), Tai Yuan (LU-9); Lumbar region: Shen Shu (BL-23), Wei Zhong (BL-40), Kun Lun (BL-60), Yao Yang Guan (DU-3), Zhi Bian (BL-54), Yin Men (BL-37), Ming Men (DU-4); Knee: Yang Ling Quan (GB-34), Yin Ling Quan (SP-9), Zu San Li (ST-36), Liang Qiu (ST-34), Xue Hai (SP-10), Cheng Shan (BL-57), Wei Zhong (BL-40); Ankle: Kun Lun (BL-60), Tai Xi (KI-3), Shen Mai (BL-62), Jie Xi (ST-41), Xuan Zhong (GB-39), Qiu Xu (GB-40), Zhong Feng (LR-4).

Moxibustion Method:

- Gentle Pole Moxa: Apply moxa to each point for 6–15 minutes. Perform treatment once or twice per day. Three treatments comprise one course of treatment. (Figure 7.3.1)

- Moxa on Ginger: Use moxa cones the size of a soybean. Apply 4–6 cones per acupoint, once or twice per day. Three treatments comprise one course of treatment. (Figure 7.3.2)

- Warm Moxa Device: Perform treatment for 30–40 minutes. Ten treatments comprise one course of treatment, altogether 3–4 courses, with a 2–4 day interval between each treatment course. (Figure 7.3.3)

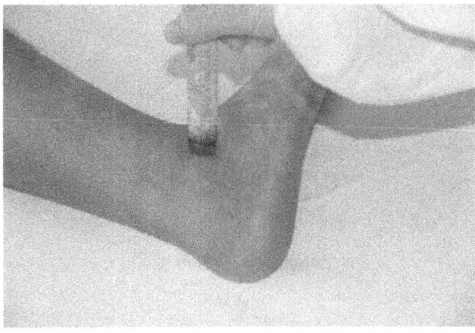

Figure 7.3.1 Gentle Pole Moxa at Kun Lun (BL-60)

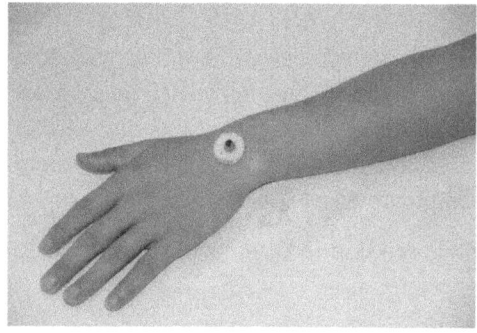

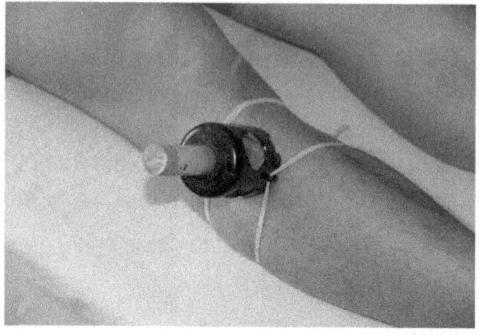

Figure 7.3.2 Moxa on Ginger at Yang Chi (SJ-4)   *Figure 7.3.3 Warm Moxa Device at Zu San Li (ST-36)*

- Medicinal Pen Moxa: Tap medicinal moxa on points. Perform treatment twice per day. Three treatments comprise one course of treatment. (Figure 7.3.4)

- Lightning-Fire Needle: Apply to the local skin repeatedly (approximately 7–10 times) until the skin reddens. Perform treatment once per day. Seven treatments comprise one course of treatment. (Figure 7.3.5)

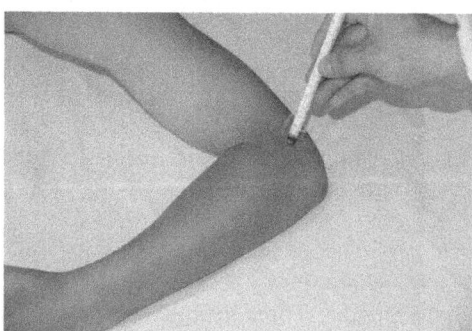

Figure 7.3.4 Medicinal Pen Moxa at Qu Chi (LI-11)

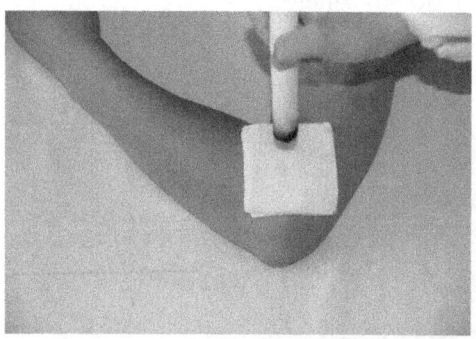

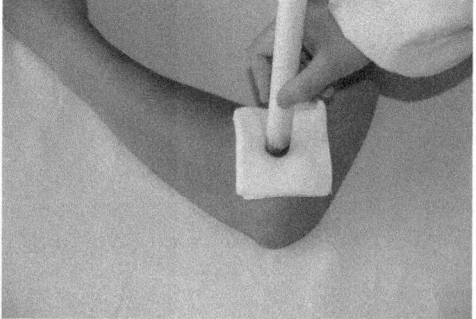

Figure 7.3.5 Lightning-Fire Needle at Qu Chi (LI-11)

4. Lumbar Pain

Lumbar pain refers to pain experienced in the unilateral or bilateral lumbar region, or middle of the spine. Lumbar pain is usually caused by one of the following: injury of lumbar region and disturbance of qi-blood circulation causing tension of vessels and networks; contraction of external pathogens; or kidney deficiency causing a lack of nourishment to the lumbar region. In modern medicine, lumbar pain is attributed to diseases of the spine, adjacent tissues or internal organs, and can achieve significant relief from moxibustion.

Main Symptoms: Clinically, the main symptom is pain of the lumbar region, such as mild and intermittent pain, pain in a fixed location, distending and uncomfortable pain, or stabbing pain which becomes even more acute under pressure.

Acupoints: Shen Shu (BL-23), Yao Yang Guan (DU-3), Yang Ling Quan (GB-34), Wei Zhong (BL-40), Ming Men (DU-4).

Moxibustion Method:

- Gentle Pole Moxa: Apply moxa to each point for 6–15 minutes. Perform treatment once per day, 3–5 treatments comprise one course of treatment. (Figure 7.4.1)

- Cone Moxa: Apply 3–5 cones per acupoint, with 10 cones used at Shen Shu (BL-23), once per day, 3–5 treatments comprise one course of treatment. (Figure 7.4.2)

- Moxa on Fu Zi Cake: Apply 3–5 cones per acupoint, with 6–15 cones used at Shen Shu (BL-23) and Yao Yang Guan (DU-3), once per day, 3–5 treatments comprise one course of treatment. (Figure 7.4.3)

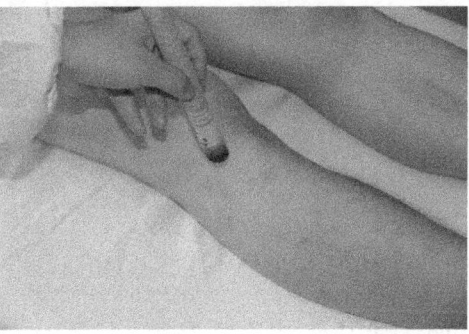

Figure 7.4.1 Gentle Pole Moxa at Yang Ling Quan (GB-34)

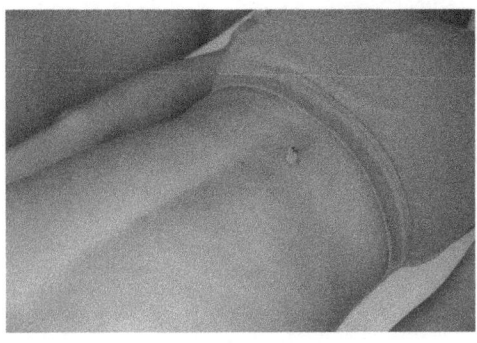

Figure 7.4.2 Cone Moxa at Shen Shu (BL-23)

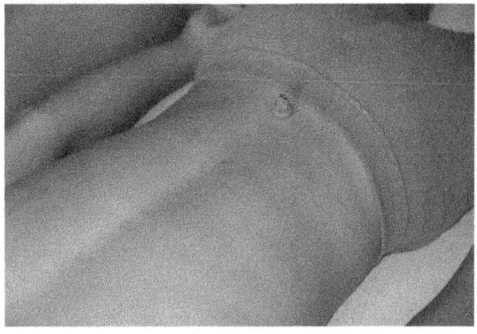

Figure 7.4.3 Moxa on Fu Zi Cake at Yao Yang Guan (DU-3)

5. Tennis Elbow

Tennis elbow refers to a common condition, the main symptoms of which are elbow pain and disturbance of elbow joint movement. Tennis elbow is usually caused by one of the following: cold-dampness invading the channels and collaterals of the elbow, or engageing in long-term vigorous exercise involving pronation and wrist extension. In modern medicine, it is equivalent to external humeral epicondylitis.

Main Symptoms: The lateral side of elbow joint experiences pain, a weak grip and pain aggravated by forearm rotation. In extreme cases the pain spreads to the forearm, upper arm or shoulder.

Acupoints: Zhou Liao (LI-12), Shou San Li (LI-10), Shou Wu Li (LI-13), Ashi points.

Moxibustion Method:

- Moxa on Ginger: Apply 5–7 cones per acupoint, once per day. Seven treatments comprise one course of treatment. (Figure 7.5.1)

- Warm Needle Moxa: Perform treatment for 15–20 minutes, once per day. Six treatments comprise one course of treatment. (Figure 7.5.2)

- Cone Moxa: Use moxa cones the size of a wheat-grain. Apply 7 cones per acupoint, once per day. Sterilize the moxa-area with 75% alcohol after treatment, without bandageing. The area should heal after one week. If there is still pain at that time, continue with moxibustion. (Figure 7.5.3)

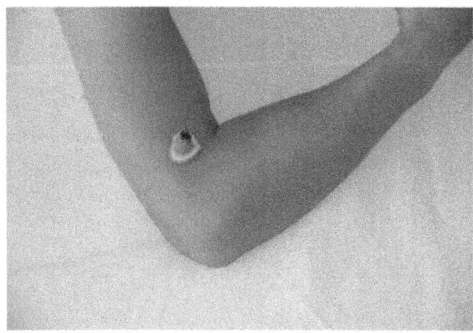

Figure 7.5.1 Moxa on Ginger at Zhou Liao (LI-12)

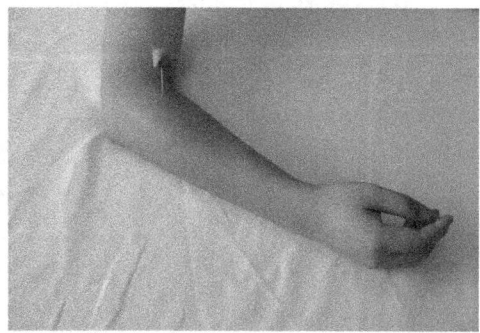

Figure 7.5.2 Warm Needle Moxa at Shou San Li (LI-10)

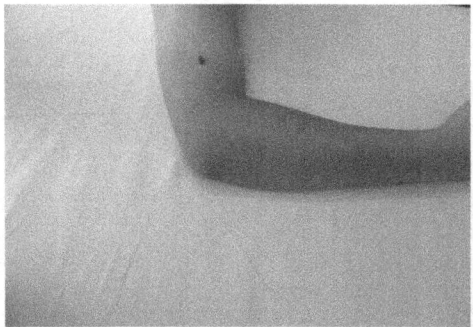

Figure 7.5.3 Cone Moxa at Shou Wu Li (LI-13)

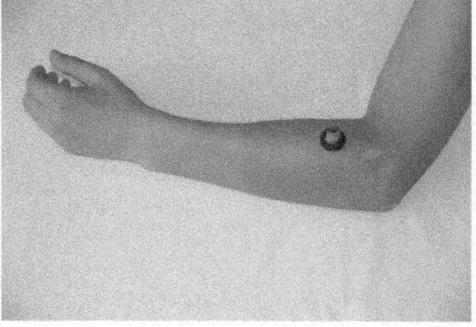

Figure 7.5.4 Moxa on Medicinal Cake at Shou San Li (LI-10)

- Moxa on Medicinal Cake: Apply 2–3 cones per acupoint, once per day (or every other day). Five treatments comprise one course of treatment. (Figure 7.5.4)

- Zhuang-style Medicated Thread Moxa: Apply 1–2 cones per acupoint, once per day. Ten treatments comprise one course of treatment, with a 3–4 day interval between each treatment course. (Figure 7.5.5)

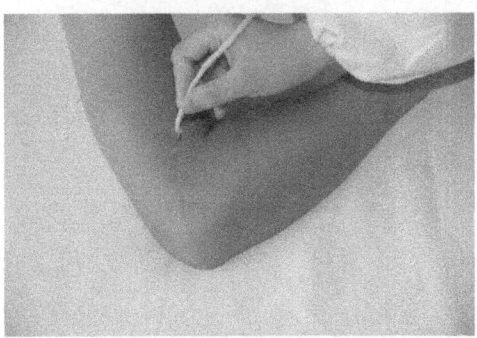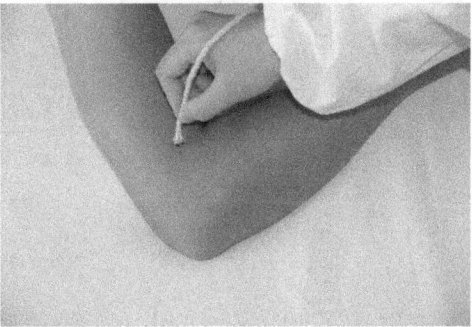

Figure 7.5.5 Zhuang-style Medicated Thread Moxa at Zhou Liao (LI-12)

6. Heel Pain

Heel pain refers to pain in the heel area caused by acute or chronic injury. Heel pain is usually caused by the following: liver-kidney depletion causing sinews and vessels to be deprived of nourishment, further contraction of wind-cold-dampness pathogen or external injury, or taxation detriment causing qi stagnation and blood stasis.

Main Symptoms: Heel and sole pain when standing or walking, a desire to avoid touching the ground, and obvious tenderness when pressed. The pain can spread forward to the forefoot and is aggravated by moving and walking and is alleviated by resting.

Acupoints: Zhao Hai (KI-6), Kun Lun (BL-60), Shen Mai (BL-62), Xuan Zhong (GB-39), Ashi points.

Moxibustion Method:

- Pecking Sparrow Moxa: Apply moxa to each point for 5–15 minutes. Perform treatment once every other day. Fourteen treatments comprise one course of treatment. (Figure 7.6.1)

- Warm Needle Moxa: Apply moxa to each point for 5–15 minutes, once per day. Six treatments comprise one course of treatment. (Figure 7.6.2)

- Moxa on Ginger: Apply 3–5 cones per acupoint, once per day or twice per day (AM and PM). Seven treatments comprise one course of treatment. (Figure 7.6.3)

- Moxa on Medicinal Cake: Apply moxa to each point for 6–15 minutes. Perform treatment once per day. Ten treatments comprise one course of treatment, with a 7-day interval between each treatment courses. (Figure 7.6.4)

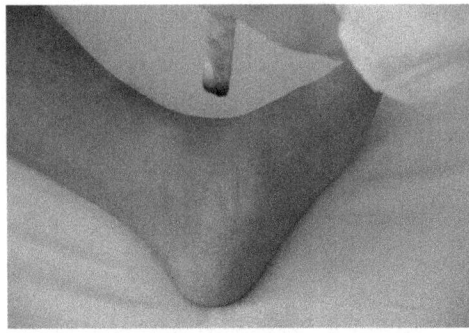 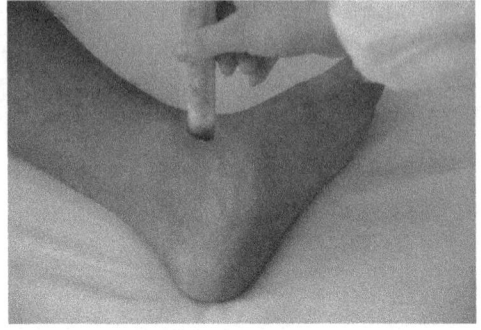

Figure 7.6.1 Pecking Sparrow Moxa at Zhao Hai (KI-6)

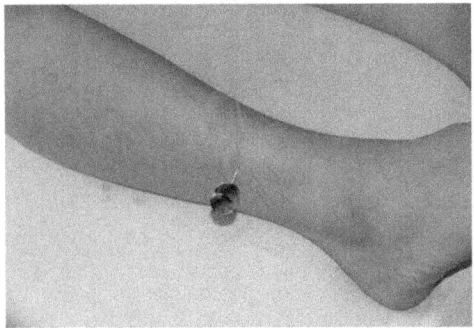

Figure 7.6.2 Warm Needle Moxa at Xuan Zhong (GB-39)

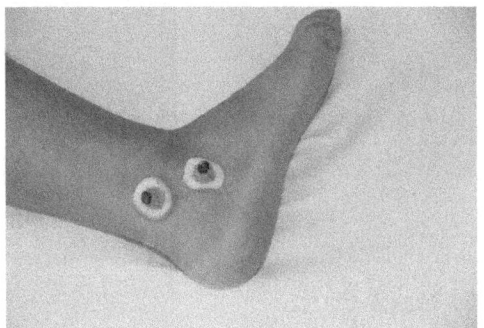

Figure 7.6.3 Moxa on Ginger at Kun Lun (BL-60)

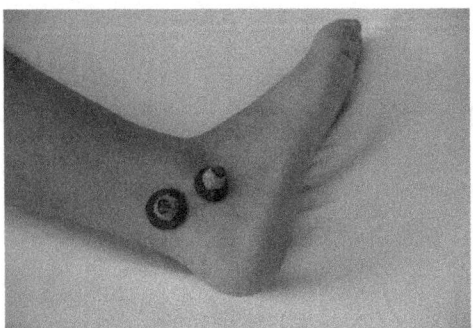

Figure 7.6.4 Moxa on Medicinal Cake at Kun Lun (BL-60) and Shen Mai (BL-62)

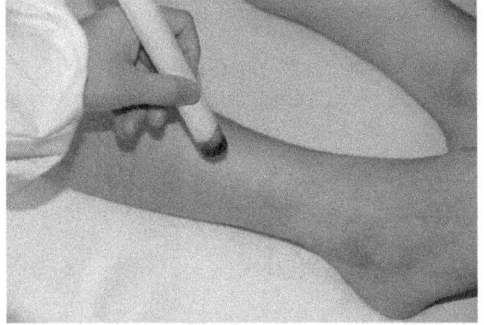

Figure 7.6.5 Medicinal Moxa at Xuan Zhong (GB-39)

- Medicinal Moxa: Using herbal drugs that have undergone the desiccative process, grind 80g of Shen Jin Cao (Lycopodii Herba), 60g of Hong Hua (Carthami Flos), 50g of Zhi Ma Qian Zi (mix-fried Strychni Semen), 100g of Chuan Xiong (Chuanxiong Rhizoma), 100g of Dan Shen (Salviae Miltiorrhizae Radix) and 60g of Gui Zhi (Cinnamomi Ramulus) into a fine powder and blend for treatment. Take 30g of the powder and mix it with moxa floss and wrap tightly with three pieces of thick cotton paper to make a medicinal pole 20cm long and 1.5cm in diameter.

Apply moxa to each point for 1–2 minutes. Perform treatment once every other day. Three treatments comprise one course of treatment, with an interval of 2 days between each course. (Figure 7.6.5)

7. Scapulohumeral Periarthritis

Scapulohumeral periarthritis refers to a disease in which the soft tissue surrounding the shoulder joint suffers from chronic aseptic inflammation. In Chinese medicine, it is called frozen shoulder or shoulder impediment. The main symptoms are pain of the shoulder joint, difficulty lifting and raising the shoulder and coldness of the shoulder. It is usually caused by one of the following: contraction of wind-cold, overwork, sudden sprain and contusion, or habitual lying in a lateral position causing chronic compression of sinews and vessels.

Main Symptoms: In the early stage, the pain is severe but the patient can remain active; in the later stage, the main symptoms are functional disturbance of the shoulder with less pain than before.

Acupoints: Jian Zhen (SI-9), Jian Qian (M-UE-48), Jian Yu (LI-15), Zhong Ping (extra point; 1 *cun* below Zu San Li), Yang Ling Quan (GB-34), Ashi points.

Moxibustion Method:

- Moxa on Medicinal Cake: Apply moxa to each point for 20–30 minutes. Perform treatment once per day. Ten treatments comprise one course of treatment. (Figure 7.7.1)

- Moxa on Ginger: Apply 5–7 cones per acupoint, once per day. Seven treatments comprise one course of treatment. (Figure 7.7.2)

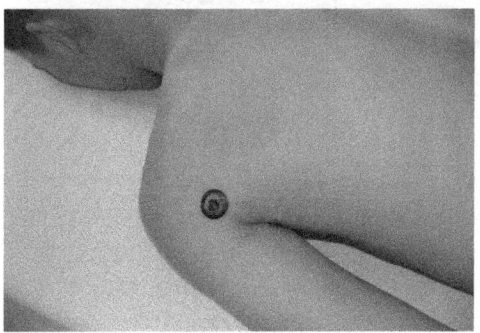 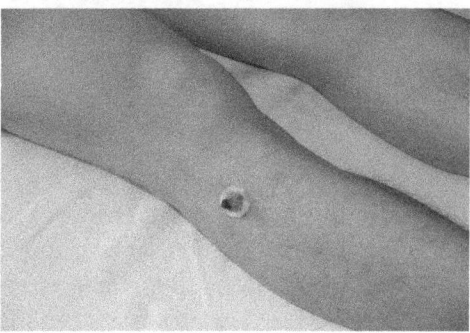

Figure 7.7.1 Moxa on Medicinal Cake at Jian Zhen (SI-9)   *Figure 7.7.2 Moxa on Ginger at Yang Ling Quan (GB-34)*

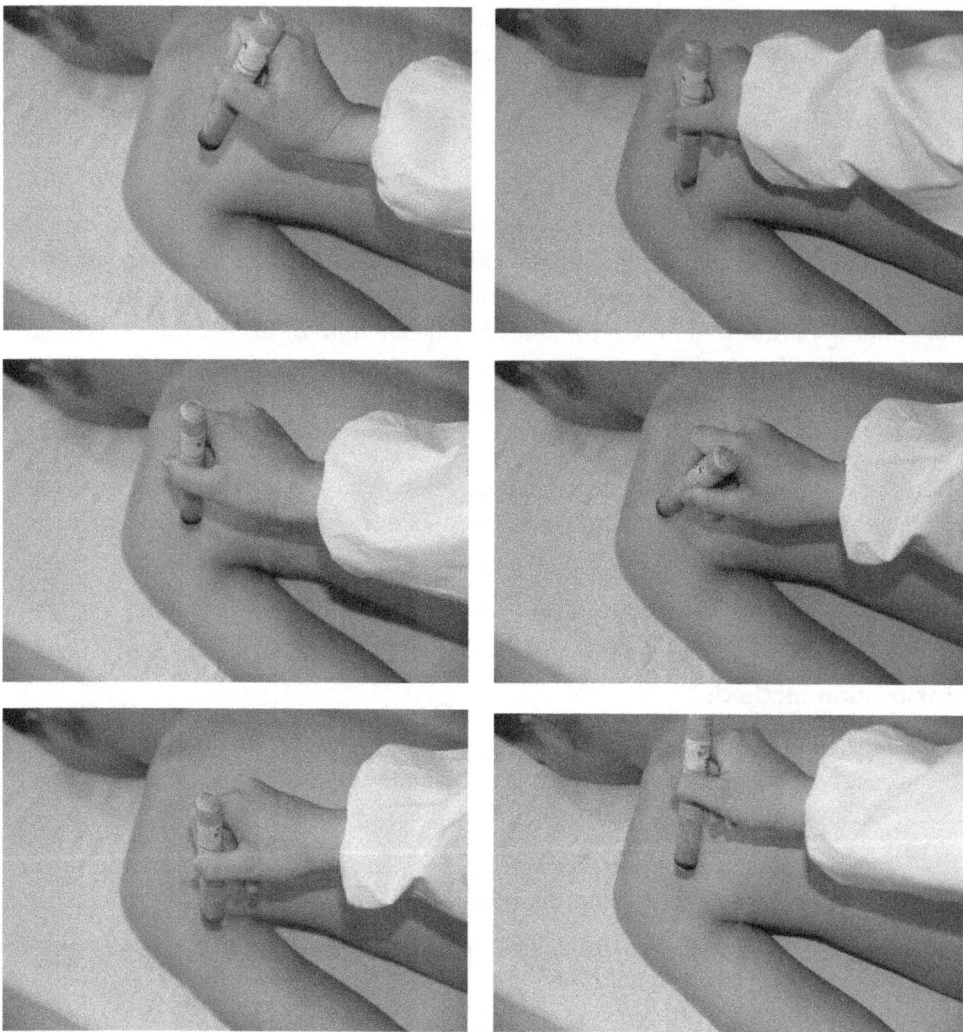

Figure 7.7.3 Heat Sensitivity Moxa at Jian Zhen (SI-9)

- Heat Sensitivity Moxa: There are four steps: circling; pecking; to and fro; gentle moxa. First, perform circling moxibustion for 2 minutes to warm up local qi and blood; then use pecking sparrow moxibustion for 2 minutes to reinforce sensitization; next, perform to and fro moxibustion along the channels in order to inspire meridian qi; finally, use gentle moxa to encourage transmission of sensation and open the channels and collaterals. Perform treatment once per day, for 14 days consecutively. (Figure 7.7.3)

- Gentle Moxa: Apply moxa to each point for 15–20 minutes. Perform treatment once per day. Ten treatments comprise one course of treatment, with an interval of 3–4 days between each course. (Figure 7.7.4)

- Cone Moxa: Apply 3–5 cones per acupoint. Perform treatment once every other day. Twenty days comprise one course of treatment. (Figure 7.7.5)

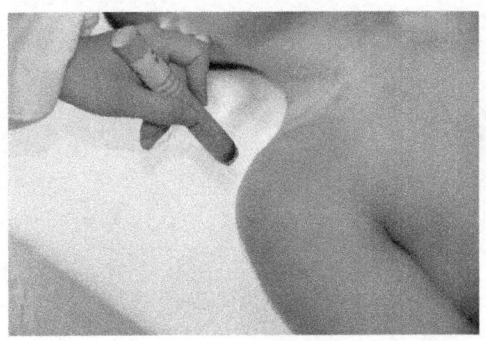

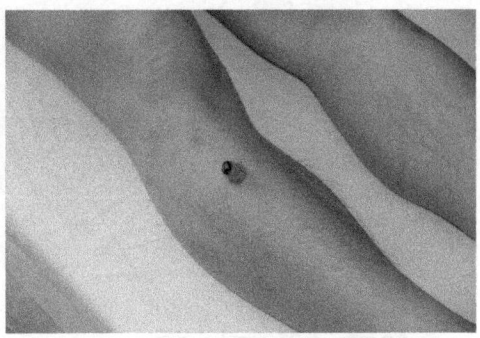

Figure 7.7.4 Gentle Moxa at Jian Yu (LI-15)   *Figure 7.7.5 Cone Moxa at Zhong Ping*

CHAPTER 8

Paediatric Conditions

1. Infantile Vomiting

Infantile vomiting is a disease in which food or sputum rises adversely from the stomach to the mouth. It is usually caused by the following: external pathogens invading the stomach, internal food damage, roundworms, external injury or a severe fright causing stomach qi to rise upward. It is commonly seen in infants and is equivalent to infantile vomiting in Western medicine.

Main Symptoms: Vomiting.

Acupoints:

- *Primary points:* Pi Shu (BL-20), Wei Shu (BL-21), Zu San Li (ST-36), Nei Guan (PC-6).

- *Supporting points:* Xia Wan (RN-10), Tian Shu (ST-25), Zhong Wan (RN-12).

Moxibustion Method:

- Gentle Moxa: Choose 4–6 points. Apply moxa to each acupoint for 5–10 minutes. Perform once daily. One treatment course consists of 10 treatments. (Figure 8.1.1)

- Moxa on Ginger: Choose 4–6 points. Apply 5–7 moxa cones to each acupoint. Perform once daily. One treatment course consists of 10 treatments. (Figure 8.1.2)

- Moxa on Fu Zi Cake: Take an appropriate amount of Fu Zi (Aconiti Radix Lateralis Praeparata), grind it into a powder and mix with an appropriate amount of flour and water to made a cake. Choose 2–3 points. Apply 3–5 moxa cones to each acupoint. Perform once daily. One treatment course consists of 10 treatments. (Figure 8.1.3)

- Non-scarring Moxa: Choose 3–5 points. Apply 3–5 moxa cones to each acupoint. Perform directly on the skin once every other day. One treatment course consists of 10 treatments. (Figure 8.1.4)

- Pecking Sparrow Moxa: Choose 5–6 points. Apply moxa to each acupoint for 5–10 minutes. Perform once or twice daily. One treatment course consists of 10 treatments. (Figure 8.1.5)

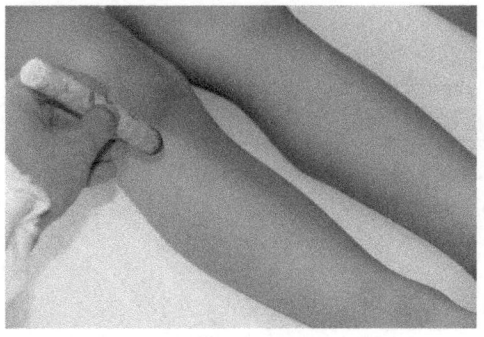

Figure 8.1.1 Gentle Moxa at Zu San Li (ST-36)

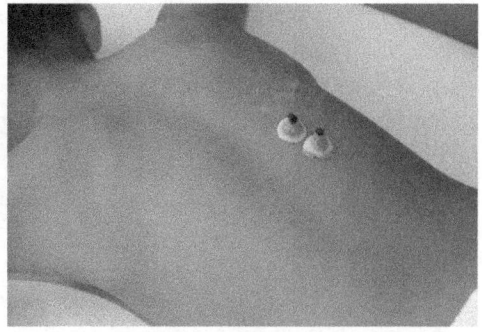

Figure 8.1.2 Moxa on Ginger at Pi Shu (BL-20) and Wei Shu (BL-21)

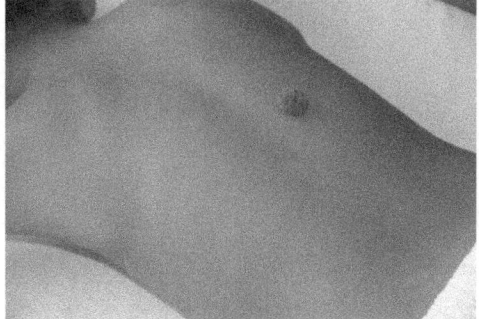

Figure 8.1.3 Moxa on Fu Zi Cake at Pi Shu (BL-20)

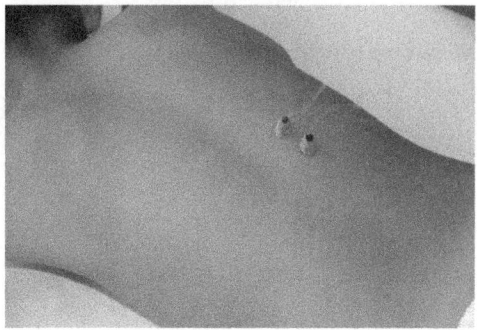

Figure 8.1.4 Non-scarring Moxa at Pi Shu (BL-20) and Wei Shu (BL-21)

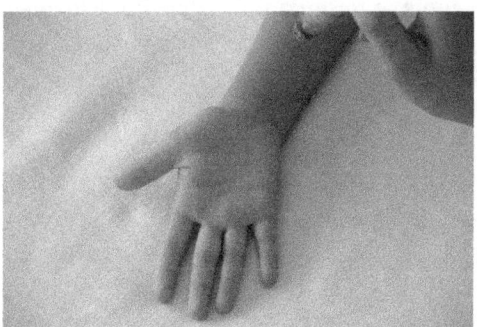

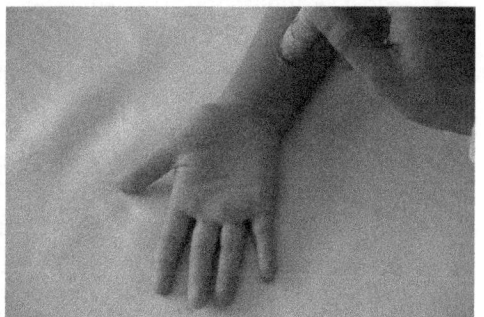

Figure 8.1.5 Pecking Sparrow Moxa at Nei Guan (PC-6)

2. Infantile Malnutrition with Accumulation

Infantile malnutrition with accumulation is a chronic disease that causes damage to the spleen and stomach and influences the growth and development of children. The condition results from a deficiency of innate natural endowment or acquired deficiency of breast milk; premature weaning; inappropriate feeding; chronic eating disorder; worm accumulation and a misuse of medication. Injury to the spleen and stomach with the subsequent disorder of transportation and transformation causes a functional disorder of digestion and absorption. This leads to a deficiency of qi and blood production so that viscera and muscles cannot be nourished and malnutrition with accumulation results. It is equivalent to infantile malnutrition or some parasitic disease in Western medicine and is commonly seen in infants less than 5 years old.

Main Symptoms: Emaciation with a sallow complexion, dry and thin hair, enlarged head and thin neck, swollen abdomen, exposed blue veins and irregular bowel movements.

Acupoints:

- *Primary points:* Si Feng (EX-UE-10), Zu San Li (ST-36), Zhong Wan (RN-12), Pi Shu (BL-20).

- *Supporting points:* Zhang Men (LR-13), Wei Shu (BL-21), Jian Li (RN-11), Tian Shu (ST-25), San Yin Jiao (SP-6).

Moxibustion Method:

- Gentle Moxa: Choose 2–3 points. Apply 3–5 moxa cones to each acupoint. Perform once daily. One treatment course consists of 7 treatments. (Figure 8.2.1)

- Bai Fan Application: Take 30g of Bai Fan (Alumen) powder, mix with mature vinegar and apply to Yong Quan (KI-1). Perform once every night. (Figure 8.2.2)

- E Wei Application: Take 10g of E Wei (Ferulae Resina), 7 grains of Xing Ren (Armeniacae Semen), 1 Wu Gong (Scolopendra) (remove the head and legs), and 3 pieces of scallion white with tassels, mash and apply to the umbilical region. Perform once daily. (Figure 8.2.3)

- Ban Xia Application: Take equivalent weights of fresh Ban Xia (Pinelliae Rhizoma Crudum) and Xiang Fu (Cyperi Rhizoma), grind them into a powder, mix with egg white, apply to Yong Quan (KI1), bind and fix. Perform once every night. (Figure 8.2.4)

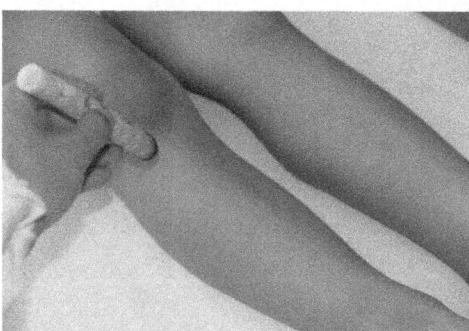

Figure 8.2.1 Gentle Moxa at Zu San Li (ST-36)

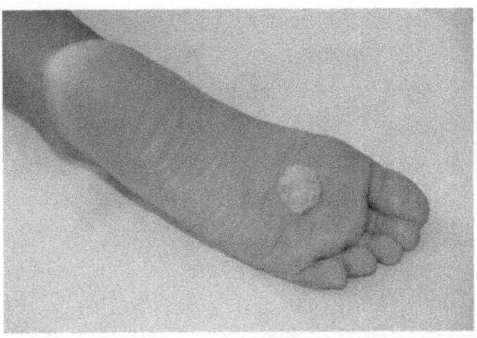 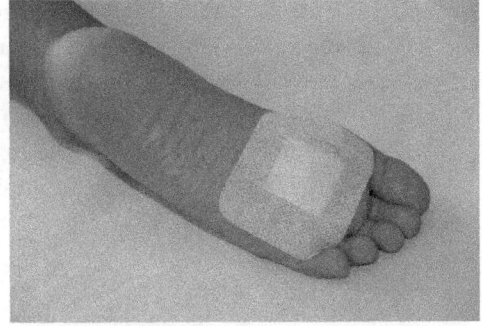

Figure 8.2.2 Bai Fan Application at Yong Quan (KI-1)

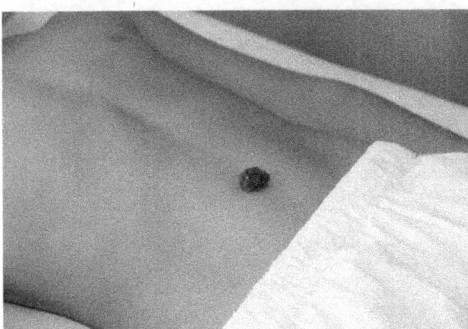 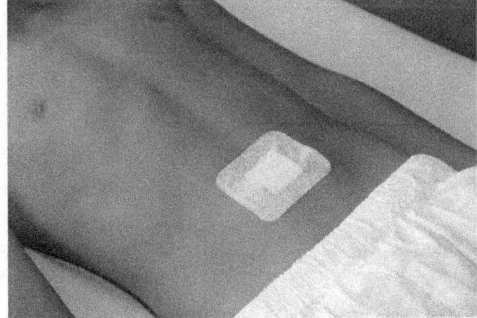

Figure 8.2.3 E Wei Application at Shen Que (RN-8)

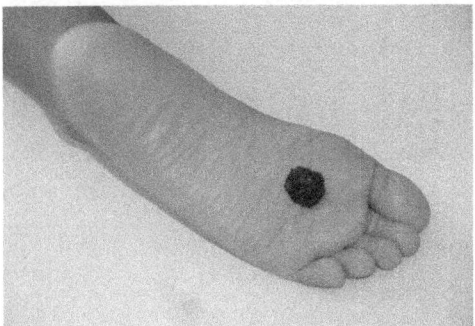 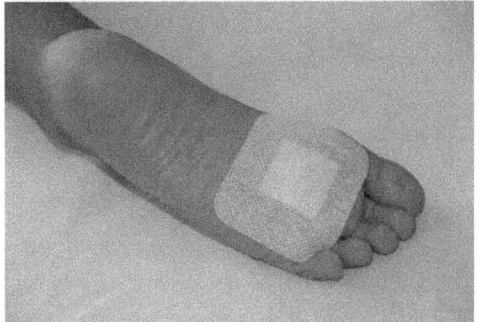

Figure 8.2.4 Ban Xia Application at Yong Quan (KI-1)

- Mu Xiang Compound Application: Take 12g each of Mu Xiang (Aucklandiae Radix), Chen Pi (Citri Reticulatae Pericarpium) and Lai Fu Zi (Raphani Semen), 10g each of San Leng (Sparganii Rhizoma), E Zhu (Curcumae Rhizoma) and Bin Lang (Arecae Semen), and 3g of Jiang Huang (Curcumae Longae Rhizoma), grind into a powder, mix with sesame oil into a paste and apply to Zhong Wan (RN-12). Perform once daily. (Figure 8.2.5)

- Shi Jun Zi Compound Application: For worm accumulation syndrome, take 10g each of Shi Gao (Gypsum Fibrosum), Dang Shen (Codonopsis Radix) and Bai Zhu (Atractylodis Macrocephalae Rhizoma), 9g each of Dang Gui (Angelicae Sinensis Radix), San Leng (Sparganii Rhizoma), E Zhu (Curcumae Rhizoma), Shan

Zhi (Gardeniae Fructus), Hei Bai Chou (Pharbitidis Semen) and Long Dan Cao (Gentianae Radix), 6g each of Hu Huang Lian (Picrorhizae Rhizoma), Da Huang (Rhei Radix et Rhizoma), Bin Lang (Arecae Semen), Mu Xiang (Aucklandiae Radix) and Chen Pi (Citri Reticulatae Pericarpium), 3g each of Ba Dou (Citri Reticulatae Pericarpium) and Xiong Huang (Realgar), grind into a powder, mix with honey into a paste and apply to the umbilical region. Perform once daily. (Figure 8.2.6)

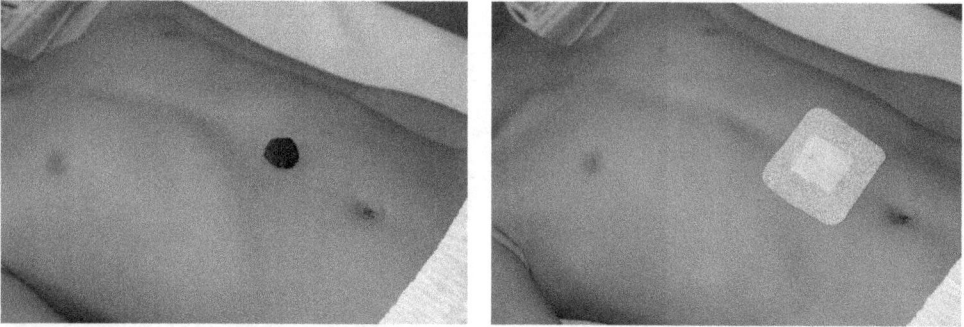

Figure 8.2.5 Mu Xiang Compound Application at Zhong Wan (RN-12)

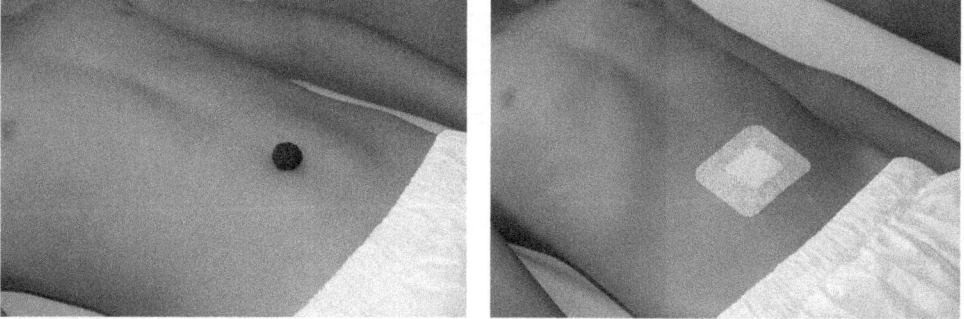

Figure 8.2.6 Shi Jun Zi Compound Application at Shen Que (RN-8)

3. Infantile Enuresis

Children's enuresis is a disease in which a child over 3 years old has urinary incontinence when sleeping and is aware of what happened only after waking up. It usually occurs due to the following: deficiency of kidney qi; depletion of original qi of the lower energizer; spleen-lung deficiency; lower energizer damp-heat causing bladder retention failure. In Western medicine it is considered to be caused by a functional disorder of the cerebral cortex or subcortical nerve centre. If a child occasionally suffers from nocturnal bedwetting due to excessive playing, a lack of sleep, exhaustion or drinking too much before going to bed, then it is not considered to be infantile enuresis.

Main Symptoms: Enuresis while sleeping, usually at midnight or at dawn, once a night for several nights or several times in one night.

Acupoints:

- *Primary points:* Zhong Ji (RN-3), Pang Guang Shu (BL28), San Yin Jiao (SP-6), Qi Hai (RN-6), Guan Yuan (RN-4), Ming Men (DU-4).

- *Supporting points:* Ci Liao (BL-32) (clinical experience point for enuresis), Shen Que (RN-8).

Moxibustion Method:

- Gentle Moxa: Choose 2–3 points. Apply moxa to each acupoint for 5–10 minutes. Perform once daily. One course of treatment consists of 7 treatments. (Figure 8.3.1)

- Moxa on Ginger: Choose 3–5 points, and apply 5–7 cones approximately the size of a grain of wheat to each point. Perform once daily. One course of treatment consists of 7 treatments. (Figure 8.3.2)

- Pecking Sparrow Moxa: Apply moxa to Ming Men (DU-4) and Guan Yuan (RN-4) respectively for 6–15 minutes. Perform once daily. (Figure 8.3.3)

- Hair Dryer Treatment: Direct the hair dryer towards Guan Yuan (RN-4), Zhong Ji (RN-3), San Yin Jiao (SP-6) for 10 minutes each. Perform once daily. (Figure 8.3.4)

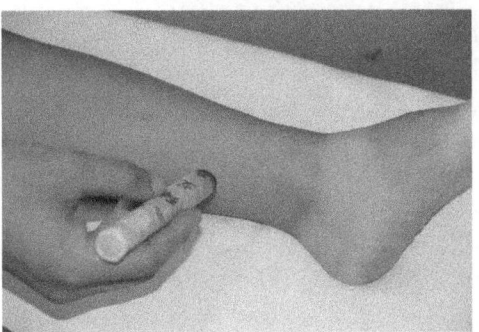
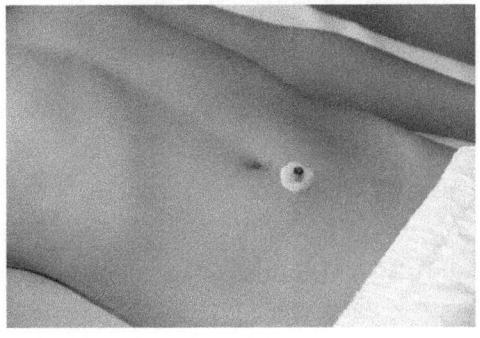

Figure 8.3.1 Gentle Moxa at San Yin Jiao (SP-6)   *Figure 8.3.2 Moxa on Ginger at Qi Hai (RN-6)*

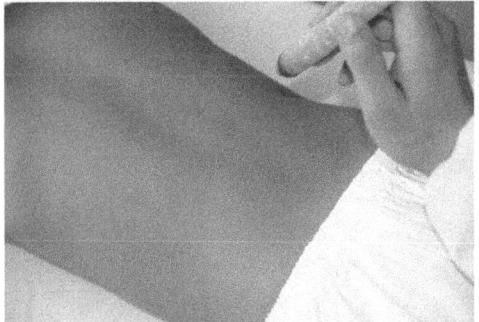
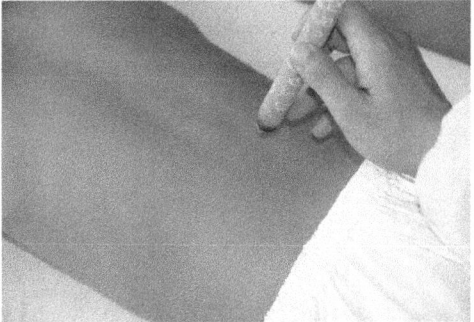

Figure 8.3.3 Pecking Sparrow Moxa at Ming Men (DU-4)

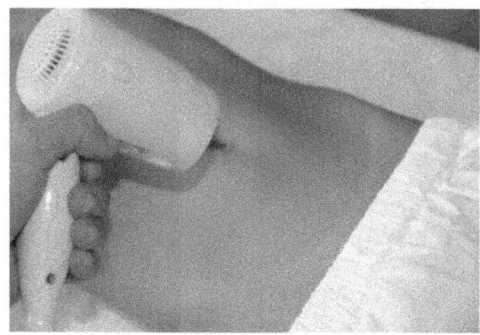

Figure 8.3.4 Hair Dryer Treatment at Guan Yuan (RN-4)

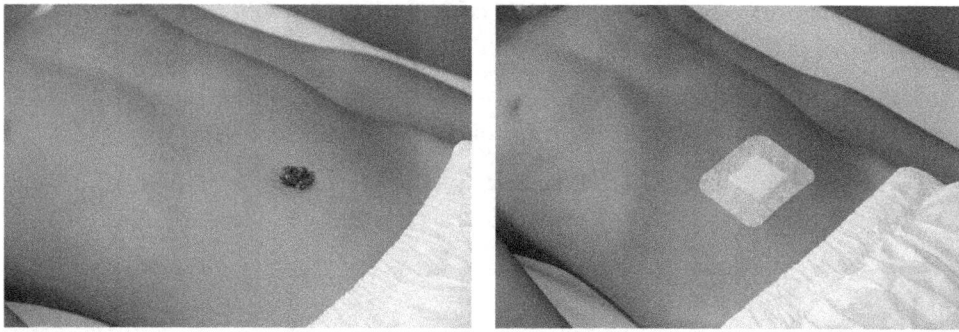

Figure 8.3.5 Bu Gu Zhi Application at Shen Que (RN-8)

- Bu Gu Zhi Application: Apply 0.3g of Bu Gu Zhi (Psoraleae Fructus) to the umbilical region, bind and fix. Change once every two days. (Figure 8.3.5)

- Xiong Huang Application: Mash 30g of Xiong Huang (Realgar) with 2 pieces of scallion and apply to Shen Que (RN-8) every night; remove the next day. (Figure 8.3.6)

- Ding Xiang Application: Take 3 grains of Ding Xiang (Caryophylli Flos), grind them into a powder, mix with cooked rice to make a cake and apply to the umbilical region. Perform once every night. (Figure 8.3.7)

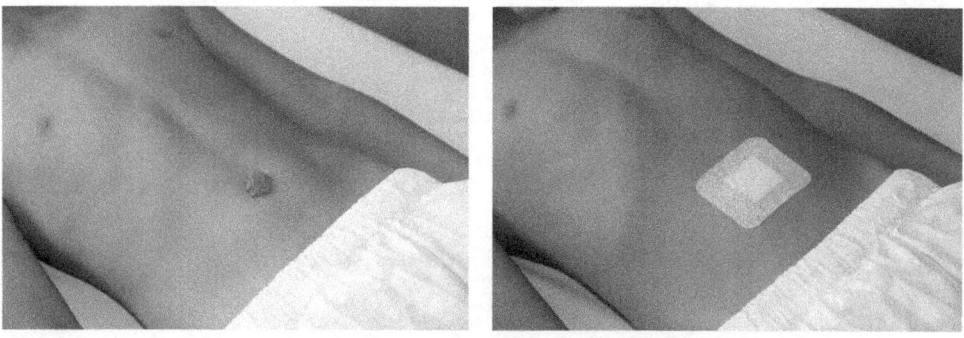

Figure 8.3.6 Xiong Huang Application at Shen Que (RN-8)

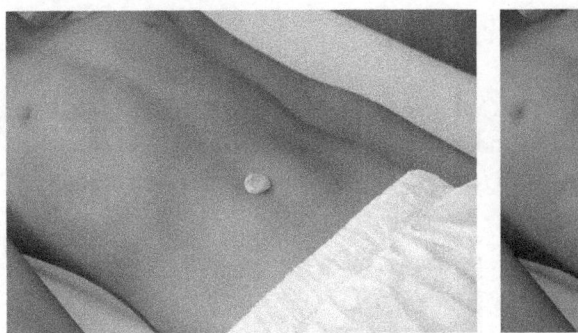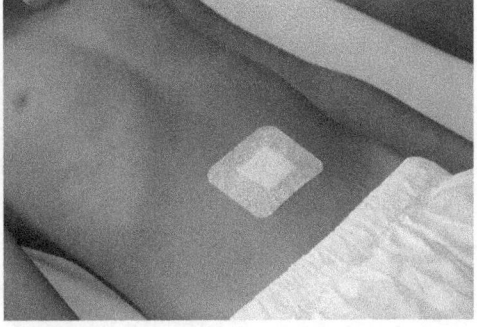

Figure 8.3.7 Ding Xiang Application at Shen Que (RN-8)

4. Infantile Whooping Cough

Whooping cough is a disease in which a paroxysmal spasmodic cough occurs with a whooping inhalation; known as a cock-crowing echo. It usually occurs as a result of the following: external contraction causing retention of turbid phlegm that obstructs the respiratory tract and causes lung qi to rise to the throat rather than diffuse. It is commonly seen in winter and spring and lasts for 2–3 months. It can be divided into three periods: first cough, spasmodic cough and recovery. The younger the infant, the more severe the condition. Western medicine considers it to be an infectious respiratory disease caused by bordetella pertussis.

Main Symptoms: Paroxysmal spasmodic cough occuring with a whooping inhalation, known as cock-crowing echo. First cough is similar to cold symptoms and mainly manifests as a cough, running nose, a slight chill and fever. In the spasmodic cough period there is severe coughing that is not relieved until a large amount of phlegm is coughed up or stomach content is vomited; the spasmodic cough can occur over 10 times or tens of times in one attack. In the recovery period the cough is relieved and the coughing sound is weak. Chronic illness can lead to deficiency of lung yin and spleen-stomach vacuity.

Acupoints:

- *Primary points:* Lie Que (LU-7), Fei Shu (BL-13), Feng Men (BL-12), Feng Long (ST-40).

- *Symptomatic points:* First cough: He Gu (LI-4), Wai Guan (SJ-5); Spasmodic cough period: Tian Tu (RN-22), Kong Zui (LU-6); Recovery period: Tai Yuan (LU-9), Tai Bai (SP-3), Pi Shu (BL-20), Zu San Li (ST-36).

Moxibustion Method:

- Gentle Moxa: Apply moxa to each acupoint for 6–20 minutes. Perform once daily. One course of treatment consists of 5 treatments. (Figure 8.4.1)

- Moxa on Ginger: Apply 1–3 moxa cones to each acupoint, using cones approximately the size of a grain of wheat. Perform the procedure 1–2 times daily. It is better to apply moxa on garlic after blood-letting. One course of treatment consists of 5 treatments. (Figure 8.4.2)

- Medicinal Moxa: Take 60g of Yi Mu Cao (Leonuri Herba) and 30g of Xia Ku Cao (Prunellae Spica), fry them until hot and grind them into a powder. Mix the powder with yellow wine and apply to Qi Hai (RN-6). Change once daily and continue for a week. (Figure 8.4.3)

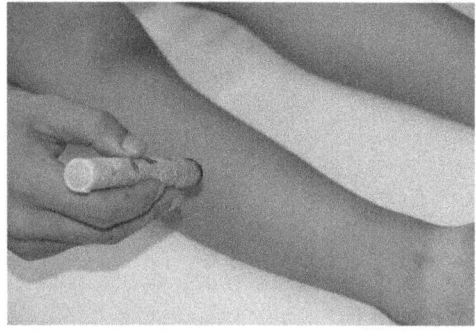

Figure 8.4.1 Gentle Moxa at Zu San Li (ST-36)

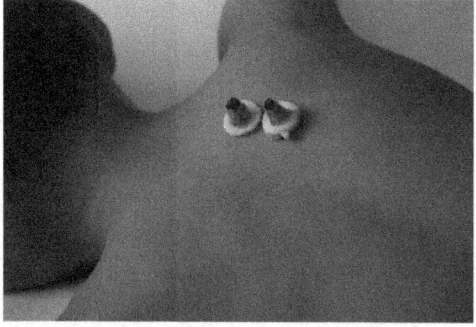

Figure 8.4.2 Moxa on Ginger at Fei Shu (BL-13) and Feng Men (BL-12)

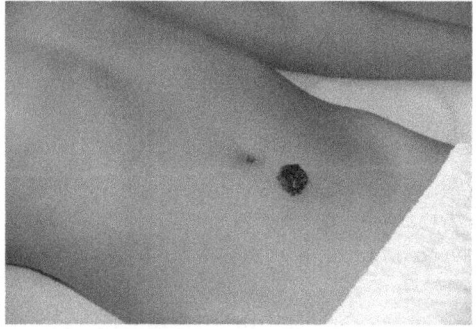

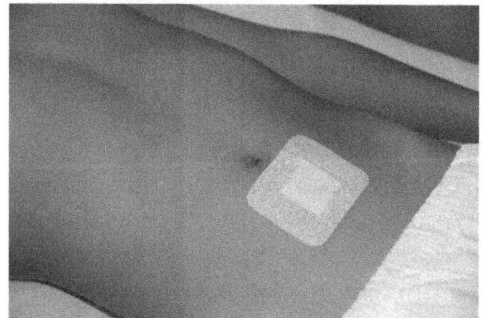

Figure 8.4.3 Medicinal Moxa at Qi Hai (RN-6)

5. Infantile Diarrhoea

Infantile diarrhoea is a stomach and intestinal tract condition in which the frequency of bowel movements increases, the faeces are thin or water-like and contain some undigested food. It usually occurs due to the following factors: contraction of external pathogens; internal injury of food combined with a predisposing weakness of spleen and stomach causing injury to spleen and stomach; this results in a disorder of transportation and transformation. It frequently occurs in summer and autumn, and is commonly seen in infants between 6 months and 2 years old. It is one of the main causes that leads to malnutrition, poor growth, underdevelopment and, even, death. It is equivalent to dyspepsia and acute and chronic enteritidis.

Main Symptoms: The frequency of bowel movements increases; the faeces are thin or water-like and contain undigested food.

Acupoints:

- *Primary points:* Da Chang Shu (BL-25), Zu San Li (ST-36), Zhong Wan (RN-12), Shen Que (RN-8).

- *Supporting points:* Tian Shu (ST-25), Shang Ju Xu (ST-37).

Moxibustion Method:

- Moxa on Ginger: Choose 3–4 points. Apply 3–5 moxa cones to each acupoint. Perform once daily. One course of treatment consists of 7 treatments. (Figure 8.5.1)

- Moxa on Salt: Fill the umbilical fossa with salt; apply moxa on Shen Que (RN-8). Perform once daily. (Figure 8.5.2)

- Circling Moxa: Choose 3–4 points. Apply moxa cones to each acupoint for 5 minutes. Perform once daily until the local skin reddens. (Figure 8.5.3)

- Medicinal Application: Choose 3–5 points each time, take equivalent amounts of Wu Zhu Yu (Evodiae Fructus), Ding Xiang (Caryophylli Flos) and Bai Jie Zi (Sinapis Albae Semen), and mix with a small amount of She Xiang (Moschus) and Bing Pian (Borneolum). Steam the herbs and make them into pills approximately the size of mung beans. Apply to the points and fix with a plaster. Change once daily. (Figure 8.5.4)

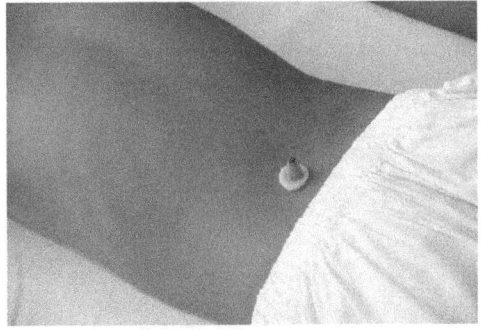 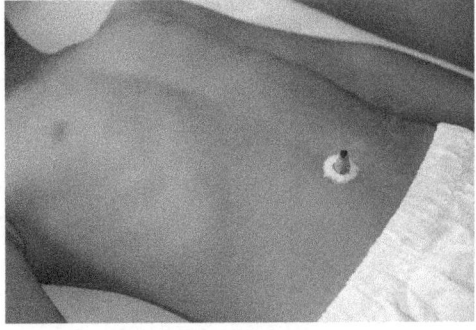

Figure 8.5.1 Moxa on Ginger at Da Chang Shu (BL-25) *Figure 8.5.2 Moxa on Salt at Shen Que (RN-8)*

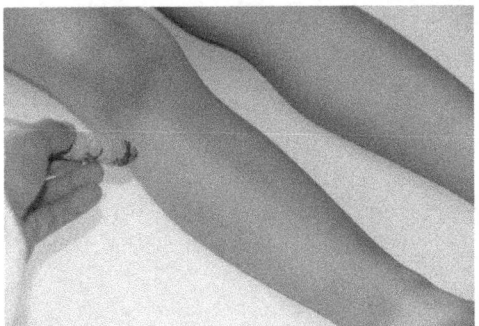 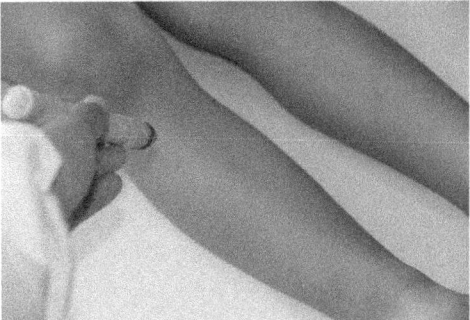

Figure 8.5.3 Circling Moxa at Zu San Li (ST-36)

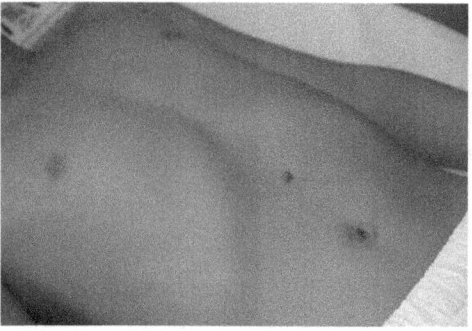
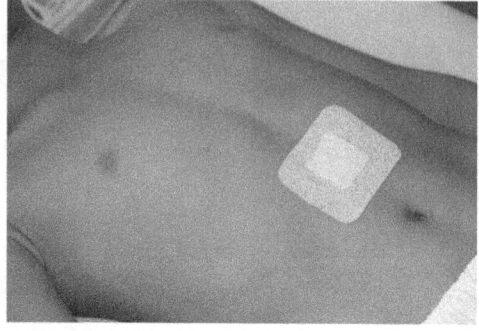

Figure 8.5.4 Medicinal Application at Zhong Wan (RN-12)

- Ding Gui San Application: Take equivalent amounts of Ding Xiang (Caryophylli Flos) and Rou Gui (Cinnamomi Cortex), grind them into a powder, apply to the umbilical fossa, and fix with a plaster. Change every 2–3 days. (Figure 8.5.5)

- Fu Zi Application: To treat vacuity-cold diarrhoea, grind 15g of Fu Zi (Aconiti Radix Lateralis Praeparata) and 30g of Pao Jiang (Zingiberis Rhizoma Praeparatum) into a powder. Using 2g each time, apply to the umbilical fossa. Next take an appropriate amount of salt and scallions, fry them until they become hot and wrap them in a piece of cloth and gently rub it on the navel and belly. Perform once daily. To treat chronic diarrhoea, take an appropriate amount of Fu Zi, mash and mix with some Rou Gui, apply to the palms and the bottom of the foot, bind and fix until a warm sensation arrives at the extremities. Perform once daily. (Figure 8.5.6)

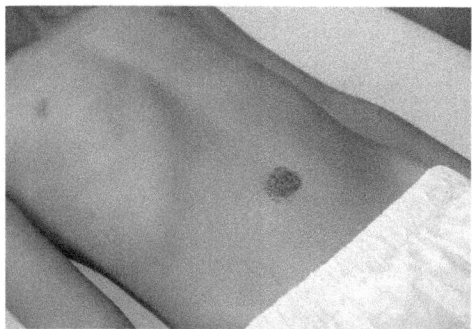
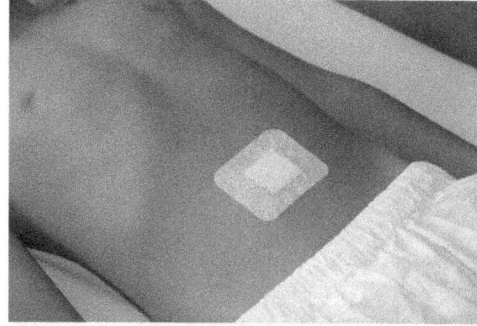

Figure 8.5.5 Ding Gui San Application at Shen Que (RN-8)

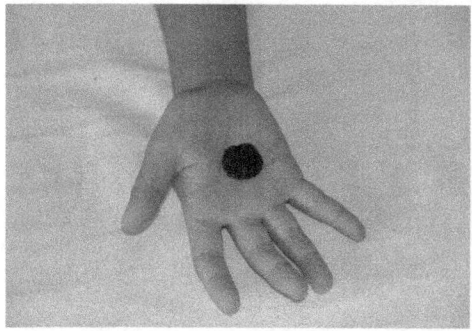
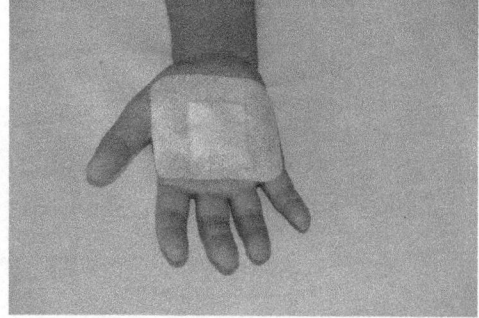

Figure 8.5.6 Fu Zi Application on the Palm

6. Infantile Convulsions

Convulsions are commonly referred to as spasms, and mainly manifest as convulsions of the limbs, a stiff neck, lockjaw, upward looking eyes, and even coma. Clinically, it can be classified into acute convulsions and chronic convulsions depending on whether there is a high fever induced by external contraction or a history of severe or chronic disease. Acute convulsions are usually due to contraction of external pathogens causing retaining of internal phlegm-heat; it is related to heart, pericardium, liver and kidney. Chronic convulsions are caused by chronic vomiting and diarrhoea or delayed acute convulsions; it is related to liver, spleen and kidney. In Western medicine it is also referred to as infantile convulsions and is seen in a plethora of conditions such as high grade fever, Japanese encephalitis, epidemic meningitis and primary epilepsy. It is more prevalent in children between the ages of 1 and 5.

Main Symptoms: It mainly manifests as convulsions of the limbs, a stiff neck, lockjaw, and even coma. It is occasionally accompanied by foaming at the mouth and incontinence. In severe cases, there may be dysfunction of breathing and circulation as well as shallow breathing and purple lips; it can also lead to choking and death.

Acupoints:

- *Primary points:* Shui Gou (DU-26), Zhong Chong (PC-9), He Gu (LI-4), Tai Chong (LR-3).

- *Symptomatic points:* Acute convulsions: add Shi Xuan (EX-UE11), Bai Hui (DU-20); Remission stage: add Da Zhui (DU-14), Feng Long (ST-40); Chronic convulsion: Gan Shu (BL-18), Pi Shu (BL-20), Wei Shu (BL-21), Shen Shu (BL-23), Ming Men (DU-4), Qi Hai (RN-6), Guan Yuan (RN-4), Zu San Li (ST-36), Shen Que (RN-8).

Moxibustion Method:

- *In an attack stage:* At first perform swift pricking bleeding at Shi Xuan (EX-UE-11), next apply 5 moxa cones respectively to Da Zhui (DU-14), Guan Yuan (RN-4), He Gu (LI-4) and Zu San Li (ST-36) until local skin reddens and the spasm ceases.

- *In remission stage:*

   ◦ Gentle Moxa: Choose 2–3 of the above points. Apply 1 moxa to each point. Perform once daily. (Figure 8.6.1)

   ◦ Earthworm Application: Clean 7 live earthworms and mash them up with honey. Apply to Xin Hui (DU-22) in acute convulsions; apply to the sole of the foot in chronic convulsions, and remove after 24 hours. (Figure 8.6.2)

   ◦ Zao Jiao Application: Take several pieces of Zao Jiao (Gleditsiae Fructus), soak them in children's urine, remove, dry, and grind into powder, then mix with breast milk and apply to Xin Hui (DU-22). (Figure 8.6.3)

   ◦ Wu Zhu Yu Application: Acute convulsions: take 10g of Wu Zhu Yu (Evodiae Fructus), 6g of Huang Lian (Coptidis Rhizoma), 3g of Fu Zi (Aconiti Radix Lateralis Praeparata), and grind into a powder. Mix with vinegar to make a paste; apply the paste to Yong Quan (KI-1) bilaterally (Figure 8.6.4). Chronic convulsions: take 3g each of Wu Zhu Yu, Quan Xie (Scorpio) and Bai Fan (Alumen), grind into a powder and place an appropriate amount on 1/4 piece of Fu Gui Zi Jin Gao; warm and apply to Yong Quan (KI-1) and Lao Gong (PC-8). Retain until a warm sensation arrives in the extremities. (Figure 8.6.5)

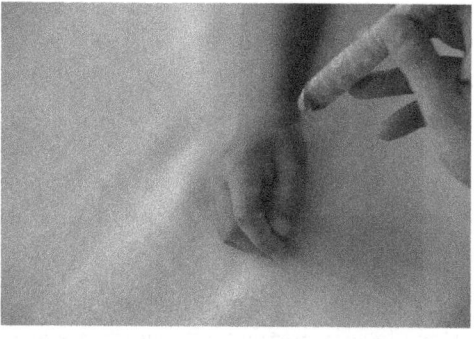

Figure 8.6.1 Gentle Moxa at He Gu (LI-4)

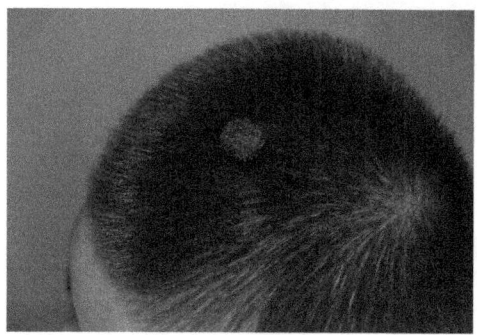

Figure 8.6.2 Earthworm Application at Xin Hui (DU-22)

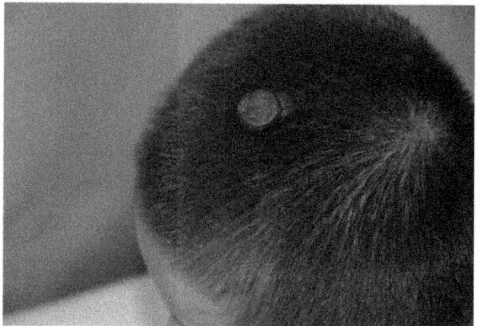

Figure 8.6.3 Zao Jiao Application at Xin Hui (DU-22)

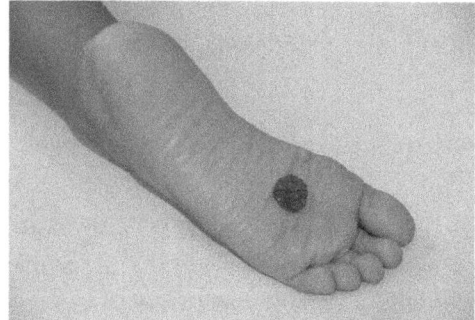

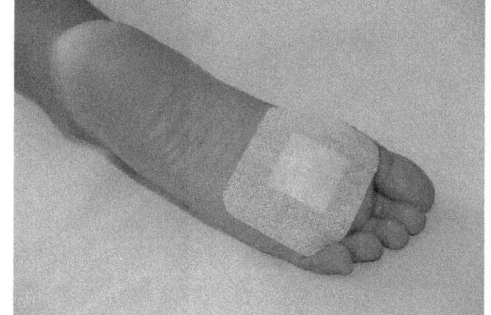

Figure 8.6.4 Wu Zhu Yu Application at Yong Quan (KI-1)

- ◦ Shi Chang Pu Hot Compress: Mix an appropriate amount of fresh Chang Pu (Acori Tatarinowii Rhizoma) and Ai Ye (Artemisiae Argyi Folium Crudum) with ginger juice, scallion juice, sesame oil and vinegar, fry until hot and wrap in a piece of cloth and gently rub it on the head, chest, back and extremities. (Figure 8.6.6)

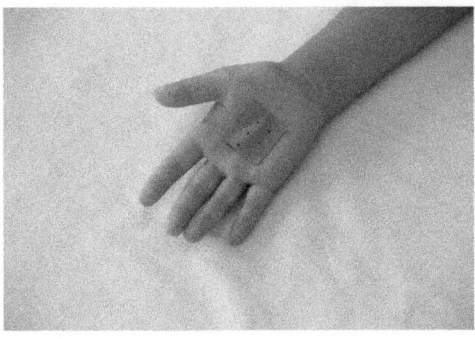

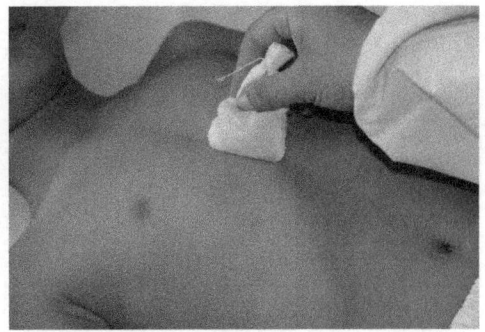

Figure 8.6.5 Wu Zhu Yu Application at Lao Gong (PC-8)

Figure 8.6.6 Shi Chang Pu Hot Compress at the Front of the Chest

7. Infantile Mumps

Infantile mumps is an acute infectious disease recognized by swollen cheeks with a fever and aches, or swelling without reddening. It is also called epidemic parotitis and, traditionally, toad plague. It is usually due to contraction of wind-heat mixed with epidemic pathogens that block the Shaoyang channel. It occurs after contraction of the mumps virus and transmitted via saliva. It is more prevalent in children between the ages of 5 and 10, and usually occurs in winter and spring. Children become immune after infection.

Main Symptoms: Unilateral or bilateral swollen cheeks with fever and aching.

Acupoints:

- *Primary points:* Jiao Sun (SJ-20), Er Gen (R-1, R-3), Lie Que (LU-7), Yi Feng (SJ-17), Jia Che (ST-6).

- *Supporting points:* Da Ying (ST-5), Wai Bian Tao (LO-7, 8, 9).

Moxibustion Method:

- Juncibustion:* Dip a piece of Juncus bufonius in oil and ignite. Quickly burn Jiao Sun (SJ-20), Er Gen (R-1, R-3) once. Treatment is effective when a clear pop or explosive sound is heard. If the patient is not cured, do it again 3 days later. (Figure 8.7.1)

- Pole Moxa: Choose 4–5 points each time. Perform once daily. (Figure 8.7.2)

- Circling Moxa: Choose 3–4 points. Apply moxa cones to each acupoint for 5 minutes. Perform once daily until the local skin reddens. (Figure 8.7.3)

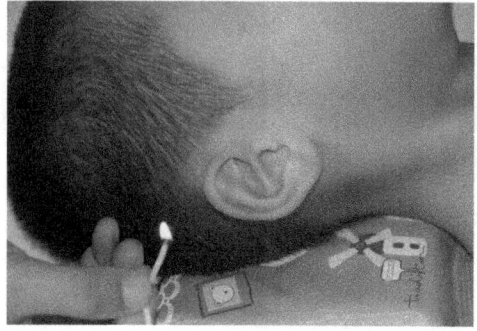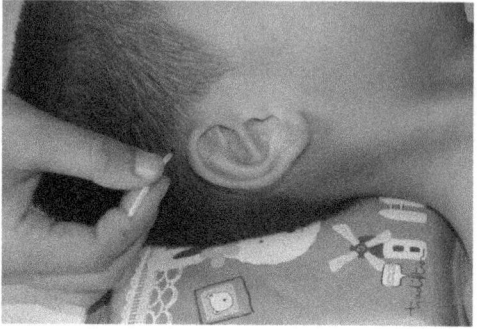

Figure 8.7.1 Juncibustion at Jiao Sun (SJ-20)

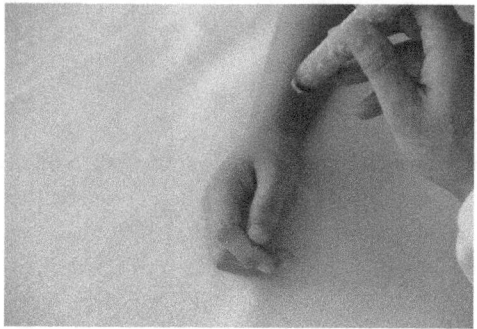

Figure 8.7.2 Pole Moxa at Lie Que (LU-7)

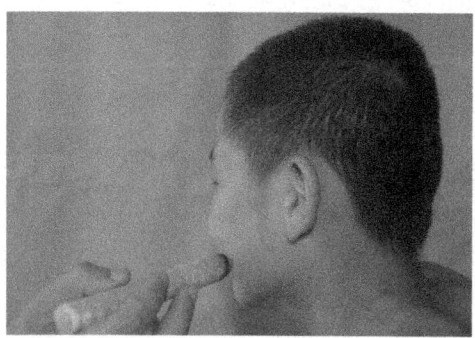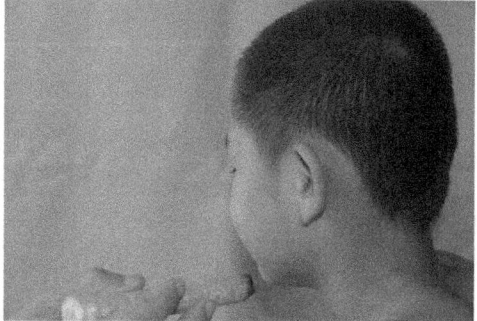

Figure 8.7.3 Circling Moxa at Jia Che (ST-6)

- Qing Dai San Application: Take some Qing Dai (Indigo Naturalis) powder, mix with rice vinegar and apply to the swollen areas. In addition perform to and fro moxa on Yi Feng (SJ-17) and Er Gen (R-1, R-3). Perform moxa once daily, apply powder 5–6 times daily and continue for 3–5 days. (Figure 8.7.4)

- Matchstick Moxa:* Choose Jiao Sun (SJ-20) of the affected side (unilateral or bilateral), and after disinfection ignite the match and press it on the acupoint. (Figure 8.7.5)

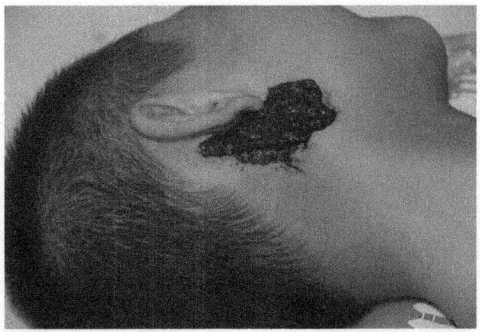

Figure 8.7.4 Qing Dai San Application at Yi Feng (SJ-17)

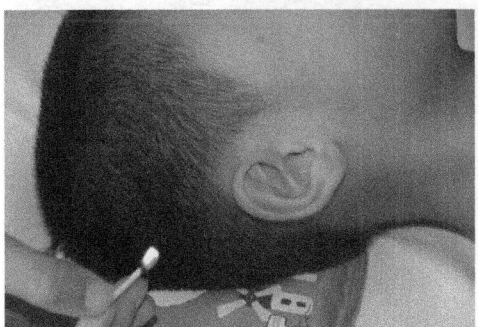 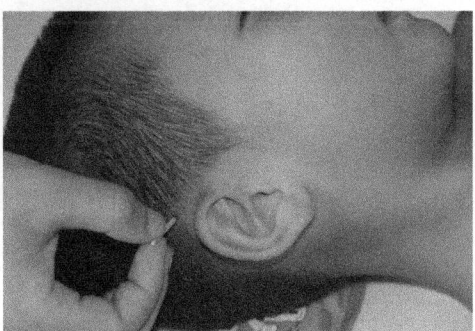

Figure 8.7.5 Matchstick Moxa at Jiao Sun (SJ-20)

8. Infantile Night Crying

Infantile night crying refers to a condition in which the infant continually or intermittently cries and can't sleep at night. It can be due to deficiency of qi and vitality, heart heat rising, food damage or fright. It is commonly seen in infants less than 1 year old, and also known as night crying in Western medicine.

Main Symptoms: The infant keeps crying and can't sleep at night, but is normal in the daytime.

Acupoints:

- *Primary points:* Shen Que (RN-8), Bai Hui (DU-20), Yong Quan (KI-1), Lao Gong (PC-8).

- *Supporting points:* Tong Li (HT-5), Zhong Chong (PC-9), Zhong Wan (RN-12).

Moxibustion Method:

- Gentle Moxa: Choose 3–5 points each time. Apply moxa to each acupoint for 3 minutes. Perform once daily. (Figure 8.8.1)

- Moxa on Ginger: Choose Bai Hui (DU-20) and 2–3 supporting points. Apply 1–3 moxa cones to each acupoint before going to bed. Perform once daily. (Figure 8.8.2)

- Pecking Sparrow Moxa: Choose 3–5 points. Apply moxa to each acupoint for 5–10 minutes. Perform once or twice daily before going to bed. (Figure 8.8.3)

- Moxa on Salt: Apply an appropriate amount of salt; apply 3 moxa cones on the salt each time. Perform once daily. (Figure 8.8.4)

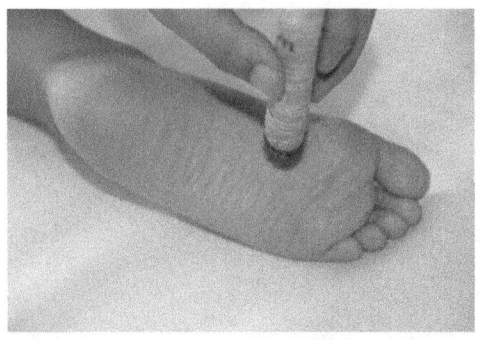

Figure 8.8.1 Gentle Moxa at Yong Quan (KI-1)

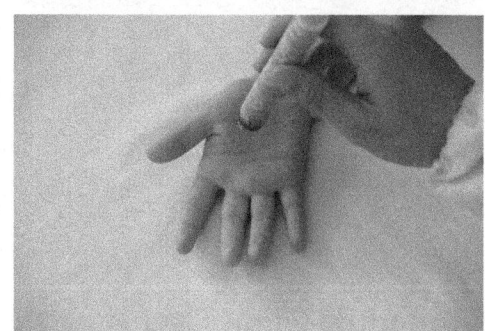

Figure 8.8.2 Moxa on Ginger at Bai Hui (DU-20)

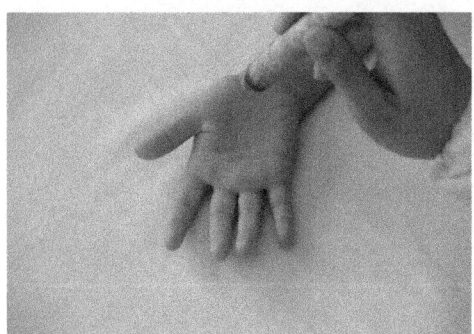

Figure 8.8.3 Pecking Sparrow Moxa at Lao Gong (PC-8)

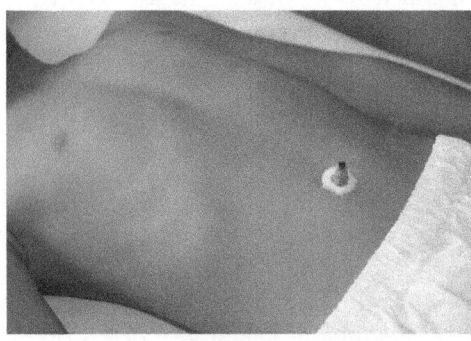

Figure 8.8.4 Moxa on Salt at Shen Que (RN-8)

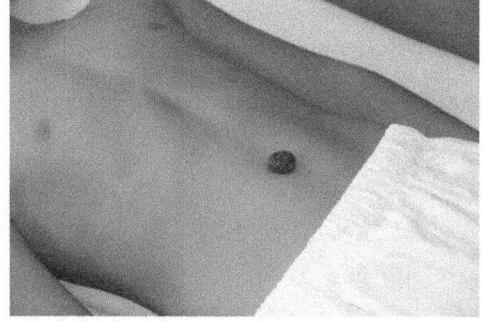

Figure 8.8.5 Moxa on Medicinal Cake at Shen Que (RN-8)

- Moxa on Medicinal Cake: Grind an appropriate amount of Wu Zhu Yu (Evodiae Fructus) and Rou Gui (Cinnamomi Cortex) into powder, mix with water to make a cake and apply on Zhong Wan (RN-12) or Shen Que (RN-8), in accordance with suspending moxa for 20 minutes. Perform once daily. (Figure 8.8.5)

- Hei Chou Application: Grind an appropriate amount of Hei Chou (Pharbitidis Semen Atrum) into powder; take 8–10g of the powder, mix with water to make plaster and apply to Shen Que (RN-8) before going to bed. Perform once daily. (Figure 8.8.6)

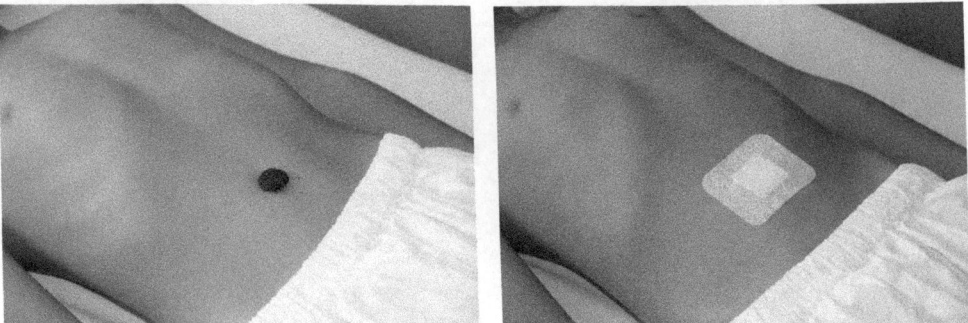

Figure 8.8.6 Hei Chou Application at Shen Que (RN-8)

9. Infantile Hernia

Infantile hernia is a condition that manifests as a feeling of heaviness in the testicle or umbilical region, and a bulge that can be palpated when coughing or standing but that decreases or disappears when laying in a horizontal position. It occurs due to cold congealing in the liver channel or a qi deficient constitution. It is also known as an inguinal hernia in Western medicine. It is more prevalent in infants less than 6 months old or between 1 and 2 years old.

Main Symptoms: A heavy feeling in the testicles or umbilical region, and a bulge that can be touched during coughing or crying but that decreases or disappears when laying in a horizontal position.

Acupoints:

- *Primary points:* Shen Que (RN-8), San Yin Jiao (SP-6), Tai Chong (LR-3), Qi Hai (RN-6), Guan Yuan (RN-4).

- *Supporting points:* Gui Lai (ST-29), Da Dun (LR-1), Da Ju (ST-27).

Moxibustion Method:

- Circling Moxa: Choose 3–4 points. Apply moxa cones to each acupoint for 5 minutes. Perform twice daily until the local skin reddens. (Figure 8.9.1)

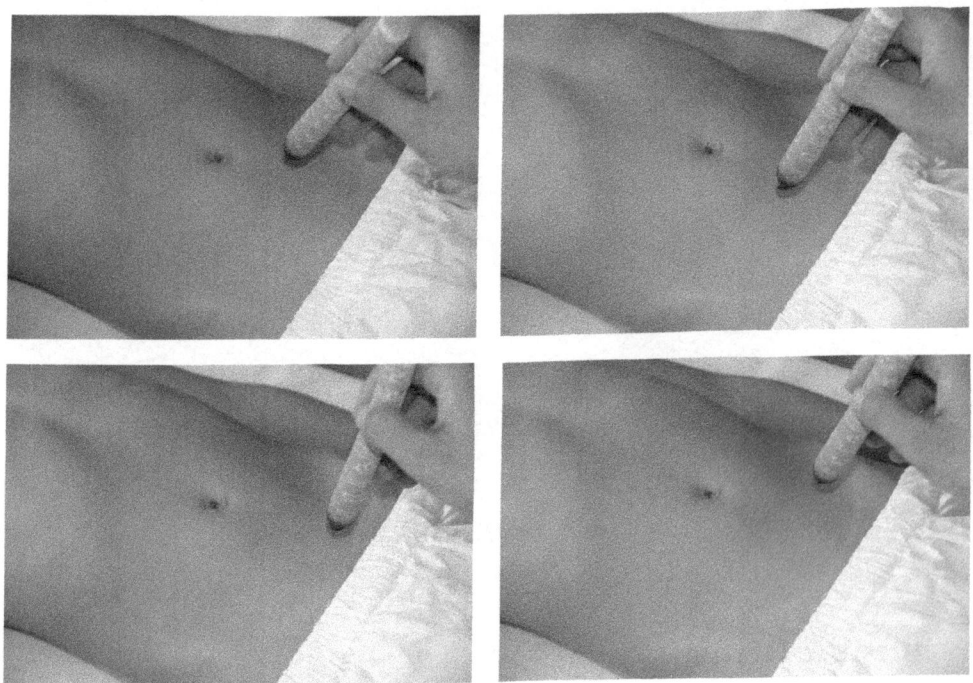

Figure 8.9.1 Circling Moxa at Qi Hai (RN-6)

10. Sequelae of Poliomyelitis

Sequelae of poliomyelitis refers to the late stage symptoms after the acute poliomyelitis, also known as infantile paralysis. It is usually due to epidemic pathogens invading the lung and stomach through the mouth and nose and harassing the channels. Western medicine considers it to be a disease caused by the polio virus invading the cells of the anterior angle of the spinal cord or motor neuron cells.

Main Symptoms: It manifests as paralysis of a unilateral arm or leg; ulcers of amyotrophy can be seen in chronic disease and accompanied by abnormality. Flaccid paralysis usually appears in the limbs, such as strephenopodia, strephexopodia and dropfoot.

Acupoints:

- *Primary points:* Pi Shu (BL-20), Wei Shu (BL-21), Zu San Li (ST-36), Shou San Li (LI-10), San Yin Jiao (SP-6), He Gu (LI-4).

- *Supporting points:* Wai Guan (SJ-5), Qu Chi (LI-11), Da Zhui (DU 14), Xuan Zhong (GB-39), Gan Shu (BL-18), Fu Tu (ST-32).

Moxibustion Method:

- Gentle Moxa: Choose 6–8 points each time. Apply moxa to each acupoint for 5–10 minutes. Perform once daily. One course of treatment consists of 15 treatments. (Figure 8.10.1)

- Non-scarring moxa: Choose 6–8 points each time. Apply 5–7 direct moxa cones to each acupoint. Perform once daily. One course of treatment consists of 10 treatments. (Figure 8.10.2)

- Gentle Moxa: Choose 3–4 points, first apply reinforcing manipulation until qi arrives, do not retain the needles; next apply gentle moxa to each acupoint for 5–10 minutes until the local skin becomes reddened with a little perspiration. Perform once every other day. One course of treatment consists of 1 month. (Figure 8.10.3)

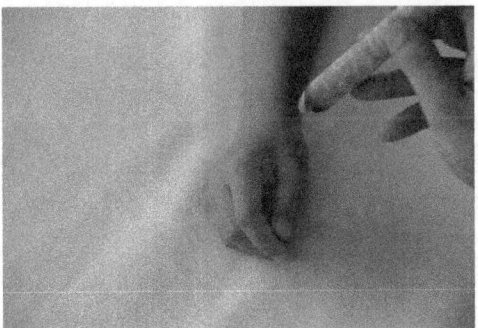

Figure 8.10.1 Gentle Moxa at He Gu (LI-4)

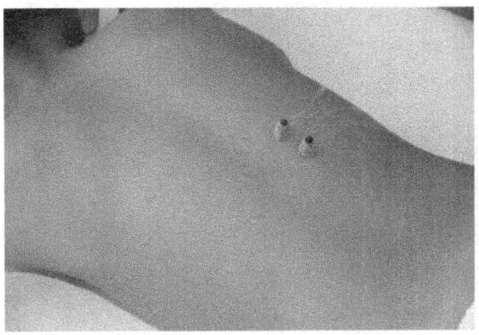
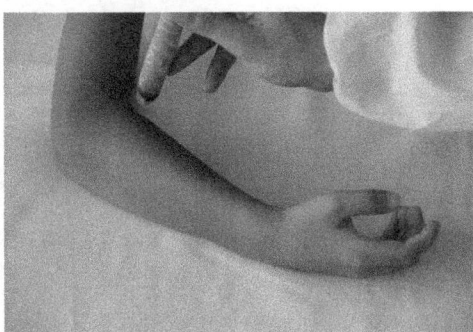

Figure 8.10.2 Non-scarring Moxa at Pi Shu (BL-20) and Wei Shu (BL-21)

Figure 8.10.3 Gentle Moxa at Shou San Li (LI-10)

11. Infantile Anorexia

Infantile anorexia is a disease that manifests as a chronic lack of appetite or anorexia, and in extreme cases even apastia. It is usually due to dietary inadequacy or long time dietary bias, as well as excessive snacking causing disharmony of spleen and stomach. A loss of nourishment after disease can also cause weakness of the spleen and stomach. It is commonly seen in preschool children and is equivalent to 'anorexia nervosa' in Western medicine.

Main Symptoms: Anorexia, severe food refusal, the child appears thin and lacks energy, a sallow complexion, anaemia, malnutrition, rickets, possible influences on growth and development.

Acupoints:

- *Primary points:* Pi Shu (BL-20), Wei Shu (BL-21), Zhong Wan (RN-12), Liang Men (ST-21), Zu San Li (ST-36), Gong Sun (SP-4).

- *Supporting points:* Shen Que (RN-8), Si Feng (EX-UE-10).

Moxibustion Method:

- Gentle Moxa: Apply moxa to each acupoint for 6–20 minutes. Perform once daily. One course of treatment consists of 10 treatments. (Figure 8.11.1)

- Jiao San Xian Compound Application: Grind equal amounts of scorch-fried Shan Cha (Crataegi Fructus Ustus), Shen Qu (Massa Medicata Fermentata Usta), Mai Ya (Hordei Fructus Germinatus Ustus), and fried Lai Fu Zi (Raphani Semen Frictum) into a powder. Mix with water to make a plaster and apply the plaster to Shen Que (RN-8) before going to bed. Remove the next day. One course of treatment consists of 10 treatments. (Figure 8.11.2)

- Pecking Sparrow Moxa: Choose 3–4 points. Apply moxa to each acupoint for 5–10 minutes. Perform once daily. One course of treatment consists of 10 treatments. (Figure 8.11.3)

- Moxa on Ginger: Apply 3–4 moxa cones to Zu San Li (ST-36). Perform once daily. One course of treatment consists of 3 treatments. Add needling of Si Feng (EX-UE-10); perform once every 3 days. (Figure 8.11.4)

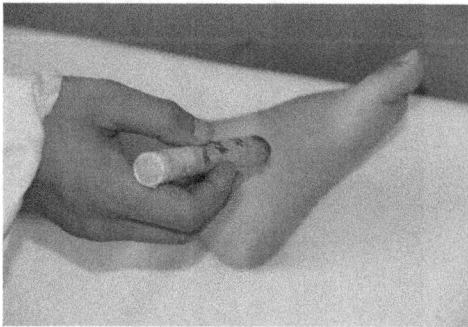

Figure 8.11.1 Gentle Moxa at Gong Sun (SP-4)

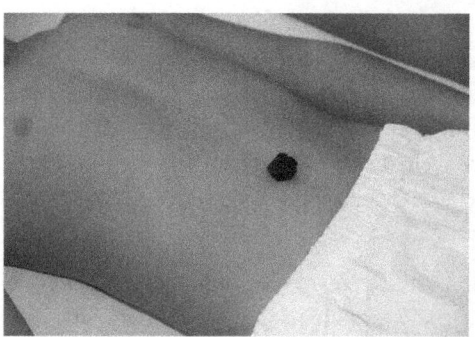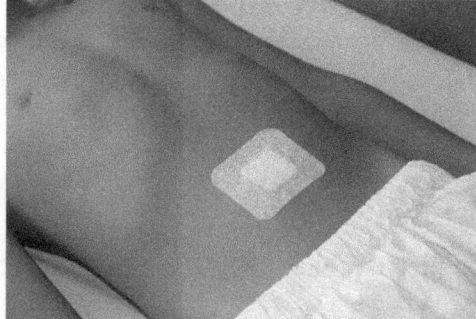

Figure 8.11.2 Jiao San Xian Compound Application at Shen Que (RN-8)

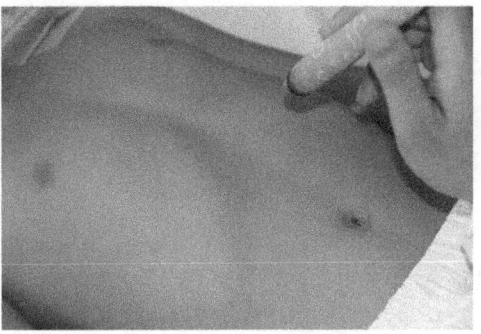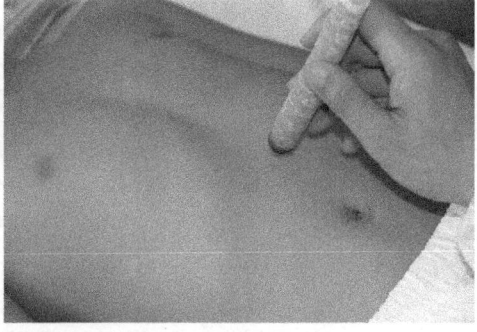

Figure 8.11.3 Pecking Sparrow Moxa at Zhong Wan (RN-12)

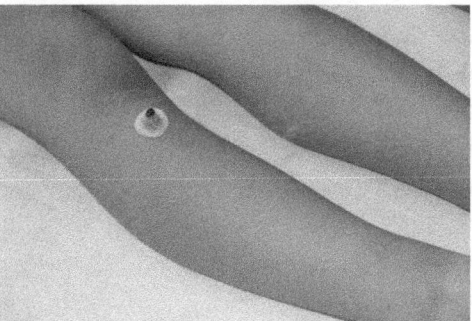

Figure 8.11.4 Moxa on Ginger at Zu San Li (ST-36)

12. Infantile Thrush

Infantile thrush manifests as ulcers of different sizes and at various positions in the oral mucosa such as the internal cheek, inner lip, gingiva, tongue and soft palate. Local aching, food refusal, salivating and dysphoria accompany it. It is usually due to the following: dietary inadequacy from eating too rich, greasy or hot food, causing heat toxins to be retained in the heart and spleen channel. It is equivalent to aphtha or aphthous stomatitis in Western medicine, which is caused by the herpes simplex virus or bacteria. It develops rapidly. If it invades the throat and oesophagus, it can easily influence breathing and suckling.

Main Symptoms: Ulcers occur in different sizes and at different positions in the oral mucosa such as the internal cheek, inner lip, gingiva, tongue and soft palate. Local aching, food refusal, salivating and dysphoria accompany it.

Acupoints:

- *Primary points:* Di Cang (ST-4), Zu San Li (ST-36), He Gu (LI-4), San Yin Jiao (SP-6).

- *Supporting points:* Yong Quan (KI-1), Lao Gong (PC-8), Shen Que (RN-8).

Moxibustion Method:

- Gentle Moxa: Choose 2–3 points. Apply moxa to each acupoint for 5–10 minutes. Perform 1–2 times daily. (Figure 8.12.1)

- Pecking Sparrow Moxa: Choose 2–3 points. Apply moxa to each acupoint for 5 minutes. Perform once daily. Apply moxa to Lao Gong (PC-8) and Yong Quan (KI-1) respectively for 10 minutes. (Figure 8.12.2)

- Wu Zhu Yu Application: Grind Wu Zhu Yu (Evodiae Fructus) into a powder and mix 10g of the powder with egg white to make a plaster; apply the plaster to Yong Quan (KI-1) bilaterally, bind and fix. Apply at night and remove the next morning. Perform once daily. (Figure 8.12.3)

- Xi Xin Application: Grind Xi Xin (Asari Herba) into a powder and mix 5g of the powder with vinegar to make a plaster; apply the plaster to Shen Que (RN-8). Perform once daily and take off the next morning. The treatment usually takes effect after 1–2 applications. (Figure 8.12.4)

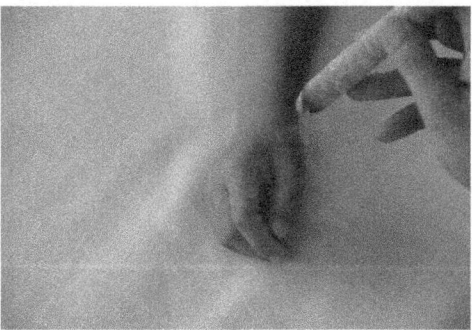

Figure 8.12.1 Gentle Moxa at He Gu (LI-4)

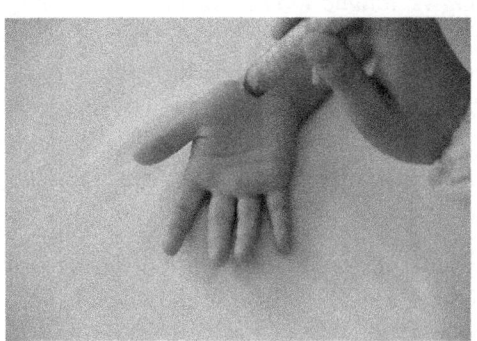
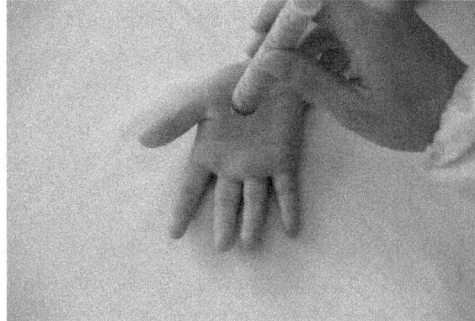

Figure 8.12.2 Pecking Sparrow Moxa at Lao Gong (PC-8)

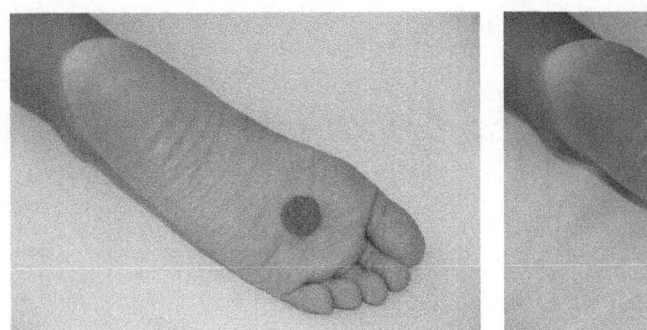
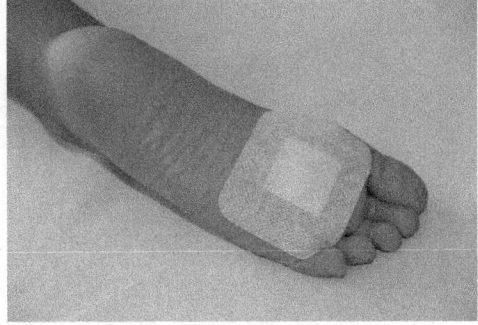

Figure 8.12.3 Wu Zhu Yu Application at Yong Quan (KI-1)

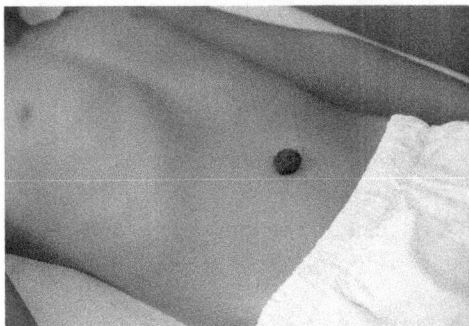
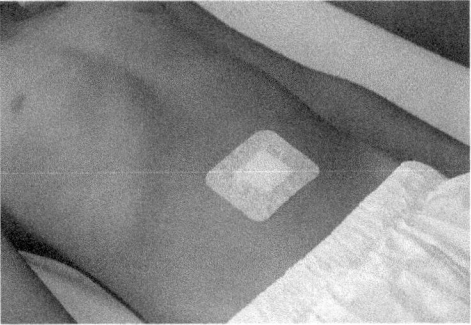

Figure 8.12.4 Xi Xin Application at Shen Que (RN-8)

CHAPTER 9

Gynaecological Conditions

1. Abnormal Menstruation

Abnormal menstruation refers to a condition in which the menstrual cycle and the colour, amount and quality of the menstrual blood all display abnormal changes, which are also accompanied by other symptoms. Abnormal changes in the menstrual cycle usually include advanced menstruation, delayed menstruation and an irregular menstrual cycle. This disease is closely related to the liver, spleen and kidney. The pathology can proceed in the following ways: liver depression transforming into fire and harassing the sea of blood; excessive thought and preoccupation injuring the spleen and leading to deficiency which results in a failure to contain blood; and kidney qi depletion resulting in a failure of the kidney to store. This disease is often seen in cases of dysfunctional uterine bleeding, as well as genital inflammation and tumours.

Main Symptoms: Advanced menstruation: menses occurring more than 7 days premature and, in severe cases, more than 10 days early. Delayed menstruation: menses delayed by more than 7 days, or even occurring once every 40 to 50 days. Irregular menstrual cycle: the cycle is advanced or delayed by 1 to 2 weeks, and continues for 2 menstrual cycles or more. At the same time abnormal changes in the colour, amount and quality of the menstrual blood occur.

Acupoints:

- *Primary points:* Guan Yuan (RN-4), Xue Hai (SP-10), San Yin Jiao (SP-6).

- *Symptomatic points:* Advanced menstruation: Gui Lai (ST-29), Zhong Ji (RN-3). Delayed menstruation: Qi Hai (RN-6), Zu San Li (ST-36). Irregular menstrual cycle: Xing Jian (LR-2), Gan Shu (BL-18).

Moxibustion Method:

- Gentle Moxa: Apply moxa to each acupoint for 6–20 minutes. Perform once daily. One treatment course consists of 5 treatments. (Figure 9.1.1)

- Moxa on Ginger: Apply 5–7 moxa cones to each acupoint, using cones approximately the size of a grain of wheat. Perform once daily. One treatment course consists of 5 treatments. (Figure 9.1.2)

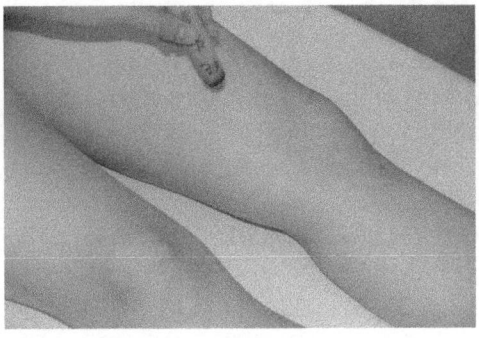

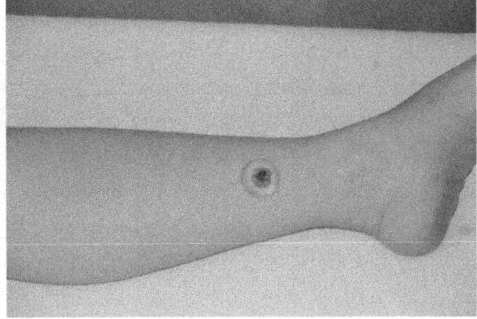

Figure 9.1.1 Gentle Moxa at Xue Hai (SP-10)   *Figure 9.1.2 Moxa on Ginger at San Yin Jiao (SP-6)*

- Medicinal Moxa: Fry 60g of Yi Mu Cao (Leonuri Herba) and 30g of Xia Ku Cao (Prunellae Spica), grind into a powder and mix with an appropriate amount of yellow wine (Vinum Aureum). Apply moxa to Qi Hai (RN-6). Change the herbs once daily and continue for one week. (Figure 9.1.3)

- Warm Needle Moxa: Apply standard needle moxa 3 to 5 days before menstruation is expected to occur. Each acupoint receives 3 to 5 cones of moxa (15 to 20 minutes of application). Perform once daily. One treatment course consists of 5 treatments. (Figure 9.1.4)

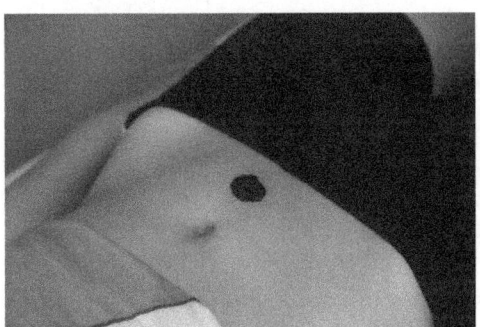

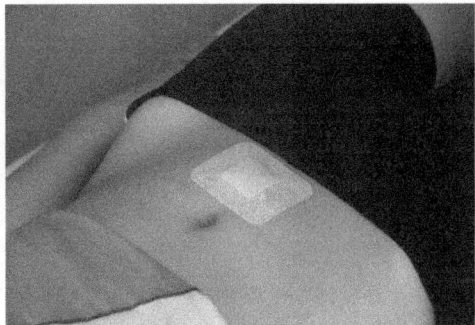

Figure 9.1.3 Medicinal Moxa at Qi Hai (RN-6)

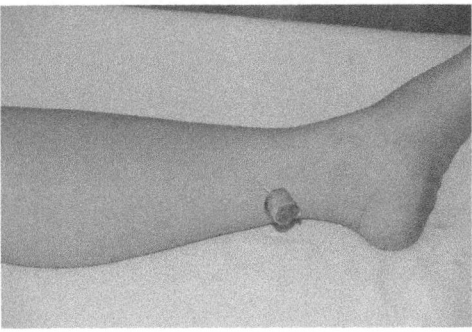

Figure 9.1.4 Warm Needle Moxa at San Yin Jiao (SP-6)

2. Dysmenorrhoea

Dysmenorrhoea refers to a condition in which cold pain, sometimes accompanied by nausea and vomiting, occurs in the lower abdomen before, during or after menstruation. It can radiate to the lumbosacral region, and can sometimes be too painful to endure. It is more prevalent in young unmarried women and usually occurs due to the following: contraction of external cold or drinking cold beverages causing cold pathogen to settle in the thoroughfare and controlling vessels; liver qi depression causing a blockage in the flow of blood; spleen and stomach deficiency causing deficiency of both qi and blood; insufficiency of liver and kidney causing deficiency of essence and blood. This condition is often seen in the case of endometriosis, acute or chronic pelvic inflammation, tumours, cervical stenosis or blockage. In Western medicine it is divided into primary dysmenorrhoea and secondary dysmenorrhoea.

Main Symptoms: Lower abdominal pain occurring before, during or after menstruation, which can be accompanied by pain and distension in the abdomen and breasts or the chest and rib cage. Pain occurring before menstruation is due to cold stagnation; pain occurring during menstruation is due to qi-stagnancy and blood stasis; pain occurring after menstruation is due to a deficiency of qi and blood.

Acupoints:

- *Primary points:* Di Ji (SP-8), Guan Yuan (RN-4), San Yin Jiao (SP-6).

- *Symptomatic points:* Pain increases when pressed: He Gu (LI-4), Zhong Ji (RN-3); Breast distension and pain: Gui Lai (ST-29), Tai Chong (LR-3); Severe abdominal pain: Ci Liao (BL-32); Pain is relieved when pressed: Shen Shu (BL-23), Qi Hai (RN-6).

Moxibustion Method:

- Gentle Moxa: Apply moxa to each acupoint for 6–20 minutes. Perform once daily. One treatment course consists of 5 treatments. Begin to perform moxibustion from 5 days before menstruation until menstruation occurs. Continue for 3 treatment courses. (Figure 9.2.1)

- Moxa on Ginger: Apply 5–7 moxa cones to each acupoint, using cones approximately the size of a date pit. Perform once daily. One treatment course consists of 5 treatments. (Figure 9.2.2)

- Medicinal Moxa: Take 10g of Rou Gui (Cinnamomi Cortex) and 20g each of Wu Zhu Yu (Evodiae Fructus) and Hui Xiang (Foeniculi Fructus), grind them into a powder and fry them with an appropriate amount of dry white wine. Apply the mixture to Shen Que (RN-8), and then fry again when the powder becomes cold. The temperature should be hot, but not so hot that it burns the patient's skin. Fix it in place with sticking plasters and leave for 3 days. Repeat the treatment before the following menstruation. (Figure 9.2.3)

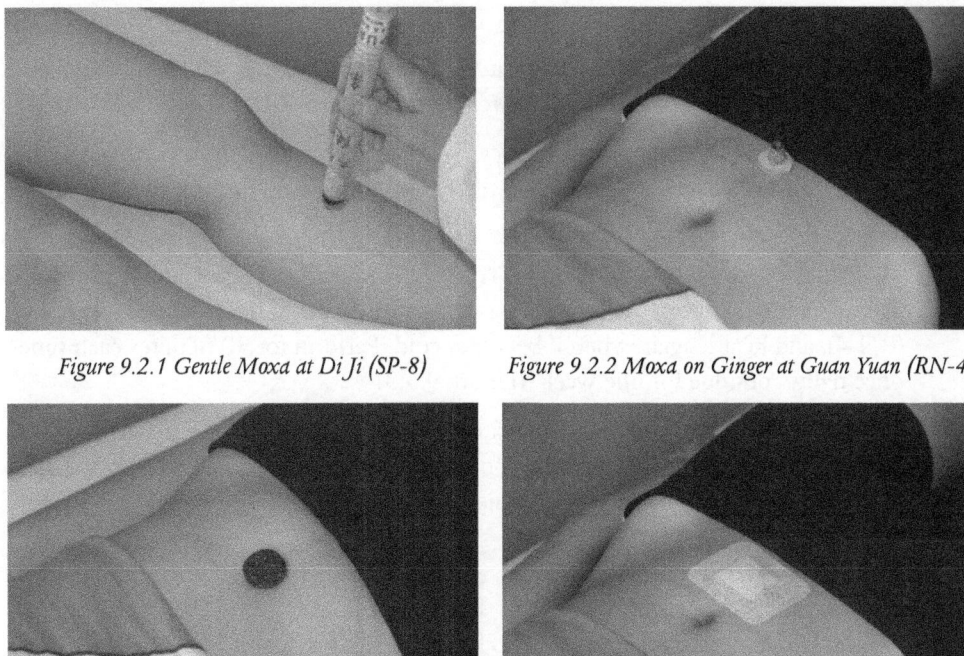

Figure 9.2.1 Gentle Moxa at Di Ji (SP-8)   *Figure 9.2.2 Moxa on Ginger at Guan Yuan (RN-4)*

Figure 9.2.3 Medicinal Moxa at Shen Que (RN-8)

3. Amenorrhoea

Amenorrhoea, also called amenia, refers to a condition in which a woman over 18 years old has not commenced menarche, or has had a stable menstrual cycle prior to menstruation ceasing for over 3 months. It usually occurs due to the following factors: insufficient constitution causing kidney qi deficiency; depletion of qi and blood due to long and serious illness; contraction of external cold or drinking cold beverages causing congealing cold in the blood; splenic transformation failure causing internal exuberant phlegm-damp; seven-affect internal damage causing inhibited qi movement. In Western medicine it is subcategorized into primary and secondary amenorrhoea.

Main Symptoms: No commencement of menarche after the age of 18, or cessation of the menstrual cycle for over 3 months, often presenting as an increase in the menstrual interval after having a stable menstrual cycle, a gradual decrease in menstrual quantity, leading to an eventual cessation.

Acupoints:

- *Primary points:* Guan Yuan (RN-4), Gui Lai (ST-29), San Yin Jiao (SP-6).

- *Symptomatic points:* Limp aching lumbar region and knees: Pi Shu (BL-20), Shen Shu (BL-23), Zu San Li (ST-36); Emotional depression and testiness: Tai Chong (LR-3), Gan Shu (BL-18), Xue Hai (SP-10), Xing Jian (LR-2).

Moxibustion Method:

- Gentle Moxa: Apply moxa to each acupoint for 6–20 minutes. Perform once daily. One treatment course consists of 10 treatments. (Figure 9.3.1)

- Moxa on Ginger: Apply 3–5 moxa cones to each acupoint, using cones approximately the size of a date pit. Perform once daily. One treatment course consists of 10 treatments. (Figure 9.3.2)

- Medicinal Moxa: Take 30g each of Yi Mu Cao (Leonuri Herba) and Yue Ji Hua (Rosae Chinensis Flos), mash into a paste then heat. Apply the paste to Guan Yuan (RN-4), and heat it again when it becomes cold. Perform for 30 minutes each time, once daily, continue for one week. (Figure 9.3.3)

- Warm Needle Moxa: Apply 1–3 moxa cones and retain the needle for 10 minutes. Perform once daily. One treatment course consists of 15 treatments, with a 2-day interval between each course of treatment. (Figure 9.3.4)

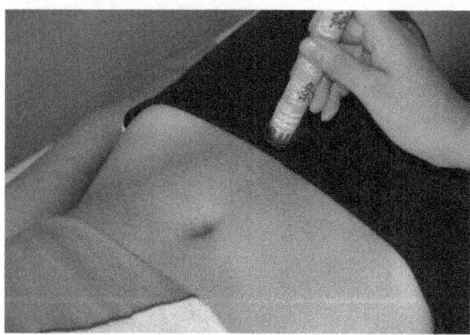

Figure 9.3.1 Gentle Moxa at Guan Yuan (RN-4)

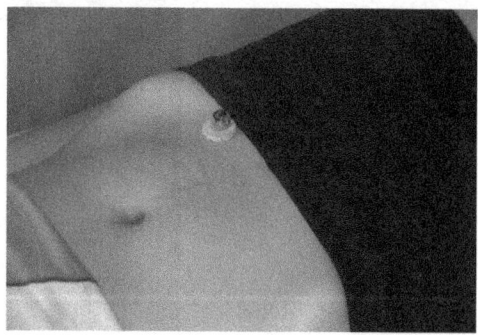

Figure 9.3.2 Moxa on Ginger at Gui Lai (ST-29)

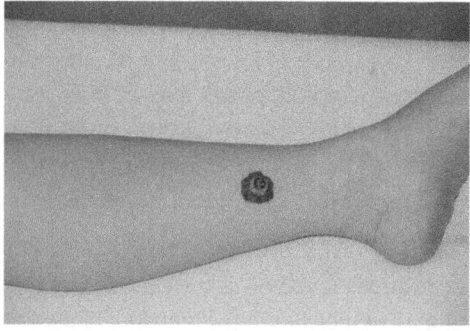

Figure 9.3.3 Medicinal Moxa at San Yin Jiao (SP-6)

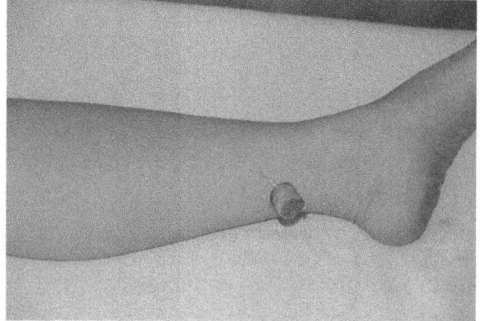

Figure 9.3.4 Warm Needle Moxa at San Yin Jiao (SP-6)

4. Flooding and Spotting

Flooding and spotting refers to non-periodic uterine bleeding; flooding refers to a fulminant downpour of blood, which comes on urgently with a large amount of haemorrhage, spotting refers to scanty dripping of blood, which comes on gradually with a small amount of haemorrhage. It is more prevalent during adolescence and menopause. It usually occurs due to the following: liver depression transforming into fire causing damage to the thoroughfare and controlling vessels; blood stasis obstruction and stagnation causing blood failing to stay in the channels; spleen qi deficiency causing a failure to control blood; kidney qi deficiency causing a failure in governing storage. The disease is mainly associated with the thoroughfare and controlling vessels, and the 3 viscera of liver, spleen and kidney. It is often seen in the case of dysfunctional uterine bleeding and secondary uterine bleeding.

Main Symptoms: Menstruation occurs beyond the normal menstrual period, which is either flooding of a large amount of haemorrhage or continual scanty dripping of red blood.

Acupoints:

- *Primary points:* Yin Bai (SP-1), Da Dun (LR-1), Guan Yuan (RN-4), San Yin Jiao (SP-6).

- *Symptomatic points:* Purple blood with clots: Xue Hai (SP-10), Tai Chong (LR-3); Fatigue and dispirited: Bai Hui (DU-20), Qi Hai (RN-6); Blood deficiency: Ge Shu (BL-17), Pi Shu (BL-20); Limp aching lumbar region and knees: Shen Shu (BL-23), Tai Xi (KI-3).

Moxibustion Method:

- Gentle Moxa: Apply moxa to each acupoint for 15–20 minutes. Perform once daily. One treatment course consists of 7 treatments. (Figure 9.4.1)

- Moxa on Ginger: Apply 7 moxa cones to each acupoint, using cones approximately the size of a date pit. Perform once every other day. One treatment course consists of 5 treatments. (Figure 9.4.2)

- Medicinal Moxa: Take equivalent amounts of Wu Zhu Yu (Evodiae Fructus) and salt, grind them into a powder and mix with an appropriate amount of yellow wine to made 3 herbal cakes the size of a coin. Apply to Shen Que (RN-8), Yin Bai (SP-1), and Pi Shu (BL-20). Apply moxa on each herbal cake, using cones approximately the size of a date pit, using 5–7 cones each time, once daily. (Figure 9.4.3)

- Pecking Sparrow Moxa: Apply moxa to each acupoint for 6–20 minutes, once daily. One treatment course consists of 7 treatments. (Figure 9.4.4)

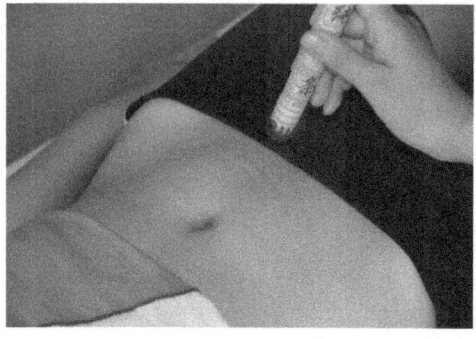
Figure 9.4.1 Gentle Moxa at Guan Yuan (RN-4)

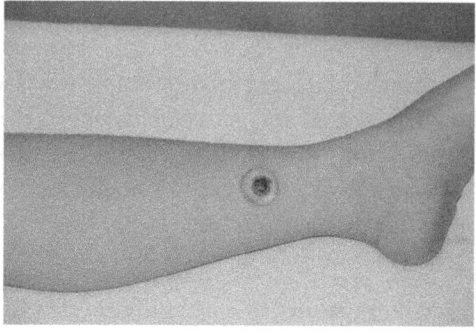
Figure 9.4.2 Moxa on Ginger at San Yin Jiao (SP-6)

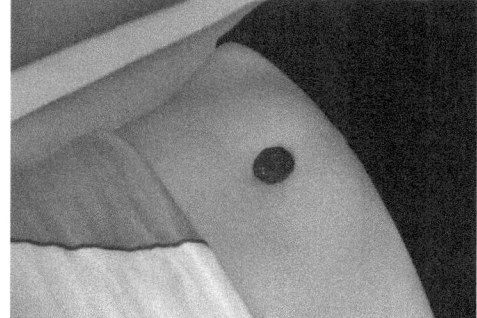
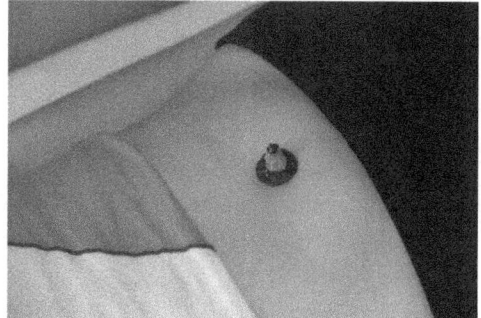

Figure 9.4.3 Medicinal Moxa at Shen Que (RN-8)

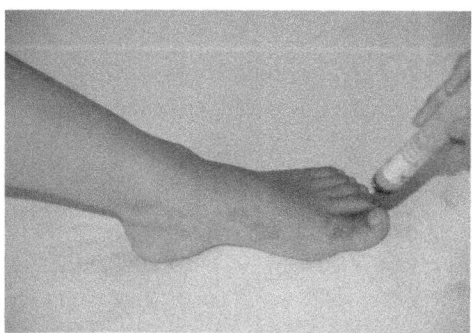
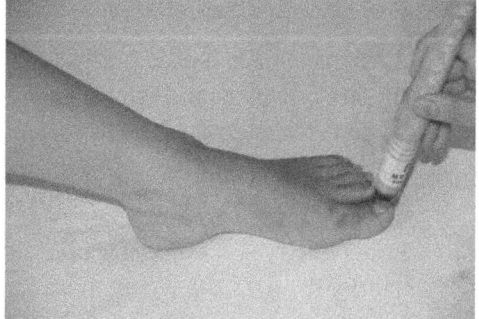

Figure 9.4.4 Pecking Sparrow Moxa at Yin Bai (SP-1)

5. Morbid Leucorrhoea

Morbid Leucorrhoea refers to a presenting symptom in which vaginal discharge increases and has an abnormal colour, quality and odour, or is accompanied by general or local symptoms. It usually occurs due to the following: contraction of external damp toxin causing damage to the thoroughfare and controlling vessels; emotional depression transforming into heat causing downpour of damp-heat; splenic damage due to food and drink or insecurity of kidney qi causing downpour of water-damp and turbid liquid. This condition is often seen in cases of vaginitis, cervicitis, pelvic inflammation and gynaecological tumour.

Main Symptoms: Sticky vaginal discharge is increased.

Acupoints:

- *Primary points:* Dai Mai (GB-26), Zhong Ji (RN-3), San Yin Jiao (SP-6), Ci Liao (BL-32).

- *Symptomatic points:* Clear thin white vaginal discharge: Pi Shu (BL-20), Ming Men (DU-4), Zu San Li (ST-36); Yellow turbid vaginal discharge: Yin Ling Quan (SP-9), Xing Jian (LR-2).

Moxibustion Method:

- Gentle Moxa: Apply moxa to each acupoint for 15–20 minutes. Perform once daily. One treatment course consists of 10 treatments. (Figure 9.5.1)

- Pecking Sparrow Moxa: Apply moxa to each acupoint for 15–20 minutes. Perform once daily. One treatment course consists of 10 treatments. (Figure 9.5.2)

- Medicinal Moxa: Take 30g each of Qian Shi (Euryales Semen) and Sang Piao Xiao (Mantidis Ootheca), add 20g of Bai Zhi (Angelicae Dahuricae Radix), grind them into a powder. Mix with vinegar to make a paste and apply an appropriate amount to the umbilical region and fix to Shen Que (RN-8) with plasters. Change the medicine once daily and continue for one week. (Figure 9.5.3)

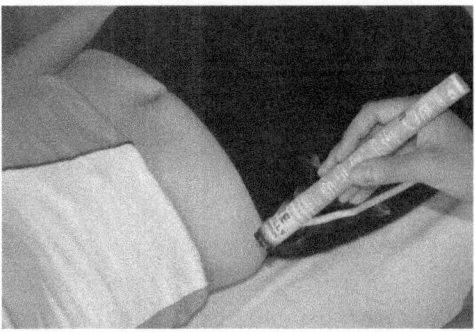

Figure 9.5.1 Gentle Moxa at Dai Mai (GB-26)

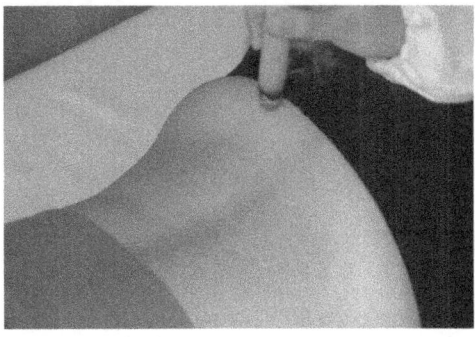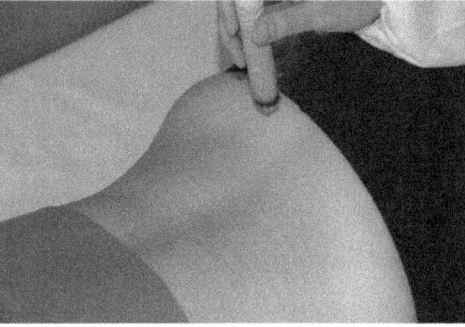

Figure 9.5.2 Pecking Sparrow Moxa at Ci Liao (BL-32)

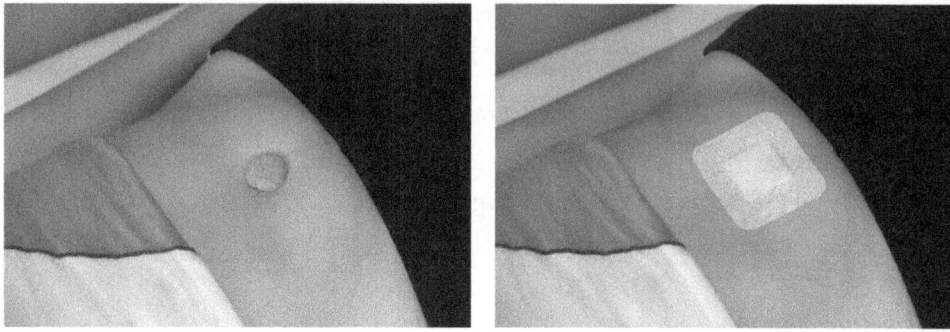

Figure 9.5.3 Medicinal Moxa at Shen Que (RN-8)

6. Infertility

Infertility, also known as childlessness, refers to the inability of a woman of child-bearing age to conceive after two or more years of normal sexual activity, assuming contraception is not used and the reproductive function of her spouse is normal; or the inability to conceive for more than two years after giving birth or having a termination when practising normal sexual activity without any contraceptive measures. The former is primary infertility, and the latter is secondary infertility. It usually occurs due to the following factors: congenital deficiency of kidney qi causing deprivation of nourishment to the uterine vessels; liver qi depression causing disharmonious flow of qi and blood; the inability to receive essences to conceive after chronic impairment of splenic movement and transformation, as well as uterine vessel obstruction. It usually occurs in cases of salpingitis, inflammation of the endometrium, cervicitis and disorders of the endocrine system.

Main Symptoms: An inability of a woman of child-bearing age to conceive after two or more years of normal sexual activity without the use of contraception, assuming the reproductive function of her spouse is normal; or the inability to conceive for more than two years after giving birth or having a termination.

Acupoints:

- *Primary points:* Guan Yuan (RN-4), Shen Shu (BL-23), Zu San Li (ST-36), San Yin Jiao (SP-6).

- *Symptomatic points:* Tending toward kidney yang deficiency: Ming Men (DU-4); Tending toward kidney yin deficiency: Tai Xi (KI-3); Liver qi depression: Gan Shu (BL-18), Tai Chong (LR-3); Spleen deficiency causing phlegm obstruction: Feng Long (ST-40), Zhong Wan (RN-12).

Moxibustion Method:

- Gentle Moxa: Apply moxa to each acupoint for 15–20 minutes. Perform once daily. One treatment course consists of 7 treatments. (Figure 9.6.1)

- Moxa on Ginger: Apply 5–7 moxa cones to each acupoint, using cones approximately the size of a date pit. Perform once every other day. One treatment course consists of 15 treatments, with a 5-day interval between 2 treatment courses. (Figure 9.6.2)

- Moxa on Fu Zi Cake: Take an appropriate amount of Fu Zi (Aconiti Radix Lateralis Praeparata), grind it into a powder and mix with yellow wine to make coin-sized herbal cakes. Apply to the primary points as well as Ming Men (DU-4) and Ci Liao (BL-32). Apply moxa on each herbal cake, using cones approximately the size of a date pit. Use 5–7 cones each time, and perform once daily. (Figure 9.6.3)

- Moxa on Salt: Fill the umbilicus with salt. Apply moxa to it, using cones approximately the size of a date pit. Use 3–5 cones each time and repeat once every other day. One treatment course consists of 10 treatments. (Figure 9.6.4)

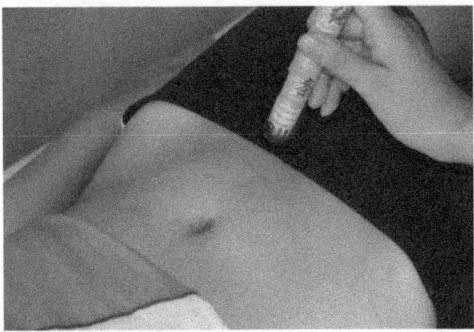

Figure 9.6.1 Gentle Moxa at Guan Yuan (RN-4)

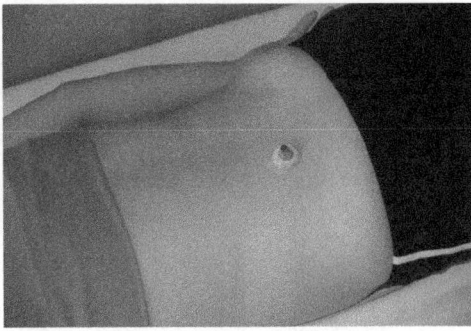

Figure 9.6.2 Moxa on Ginger at Shen Shu (BL-23)

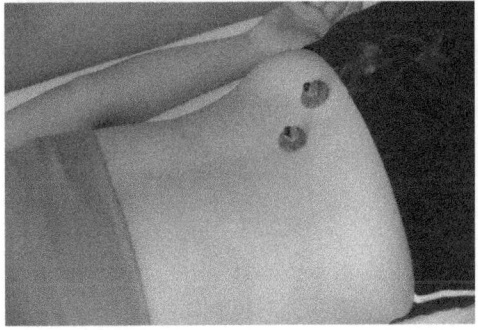

Figure 9.6.3 Moxa on Fu Zi Cake at Ming Men (DU-4) and Ci Liao (BL-32)

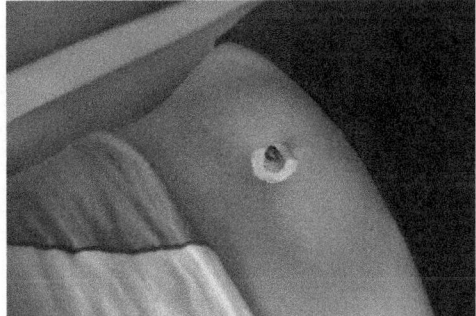

Figure 9.6.4 Moxa on Salt at Shen Que (RN-8)

7. Foetal Malposition

Malposition of the foetus refers to a state in which the foetus is either in a breech presentation, transverse presentation, occipitoposterior position or face presentation, identified in prenatal diagnosis after 30 weeks of pregnancy. The most commonly seen malposition is the breech presentation. Malposition of the foetus is usually seen in multiparas or in pregnant women with a loose abdominal wall. It occurs due to the deficiency of qi and blood failing to keep the foetus in a normal position or affect-mind ill-being causing inhibited qi movement.

Main Symptoms: The foetus is found in an abnormal position after 30 weeks of pregnancy.

Acupoints:

- *Primary point:* Zhi Yin (BL-67).

- *Symptomatic points:* Deficiency of qi and blood: Zu San Li (ST-36), Shen Shu (BL-23); Depression of qi movement: Gan Shu (BL-18), Xing Jian (LR-2).

Moxibustion Method:

- Gentle Moxa: Apply moxa to bilateral Zhi Yin (BL-67) for 15–20 minutes. Perform once daily. One treatment course consists of 10 treatments. Perform until the foetus is in a normal position. When performing moxibustion, ask the pregnant woman to lie in a supine position and loosen her waistband. (Figure 9.7.1)

- Non-scarring Moxa: Apply 3–5 moxa cones to each acupoint, using cones approximately the size of a wheat kernel. Perform once daily. One treatment course consists of 5 treatments. (Figure 9.7.2)

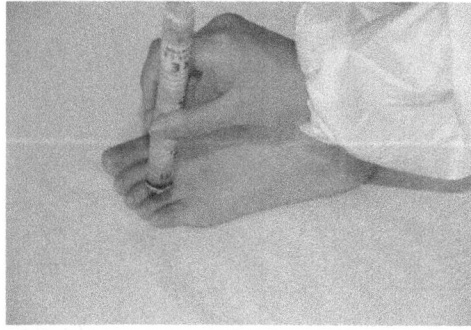
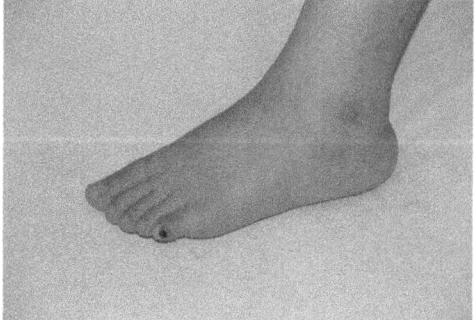

Figure 9.7.1 Gentle Moxa at Zhi Yin (BL-67)

Figure 9.7.2 Non-scarring Moxa at Zhi Yin (BL-67)

8. Protracted Labour

The process starting from the first occurrence of regular uterine contractions to complete opening of the uterine cervix is known as the first stage of labour. Protracted labour presents when this first stage of birth exceeds 24 hours. It was also known as difficult childbirth in ancient books. It usually occurs due to the following: a weak constitution and deficient right qi; premature rupture of the foetal membrane causing dried blood plasma; cold blood stagnation causing inhibited qi movement. In Western medicine it is also associated with cases of uterine inertia.

Main Symptoms: Labour has commenced and amniotic fluid has been expelled but the foetus does not achieve delivery for over 24 hours.

Acupoints:

- *Primary points:* He Gu (LI-4), San Yin Jiao (SP-6), Zhi Yin (BL-67), Jian Jing (GB-21).

- *Symptomatic points:* Deficiency of qi and blood: Zu San Li (ST-36), Qi Hai (RN-6); Qi stagnation and blood stasis: Ci Liao (BL-32), Xue Hai (SP-10).

Moxibustion Method:

- Pecking Sparrow Moxa: Apply moxa to each acupoint for 15–20 minutes. Perform continuously until the foetus is delivered. (Figure 9.8.1)

- Non-scarring Moxa: Apply moxa to Zhi Yin (BL-67), using cones approximately the size of a wheat kernel. Perform continuously until the foetus is delivered. (Figure 9.8.2)

- Warm Needle Moxa: Apply moxa to each acupoint for 15–20 minutes. Perform continuously until the foetus is delivered. The moxa cone can be changed when doing it. (Figure 9.8.3)

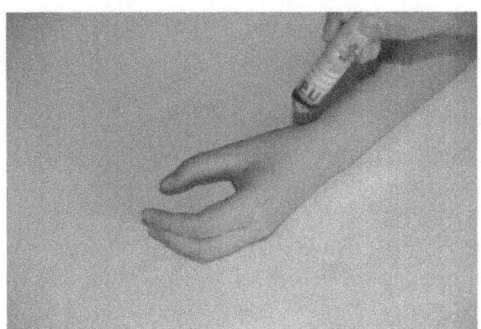 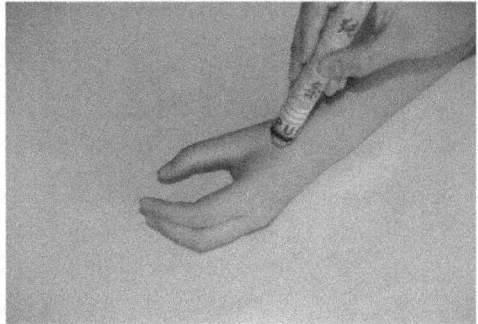

Figure 9.8.1 Pecking Sparrow Moxa at He Gu (LI-4)

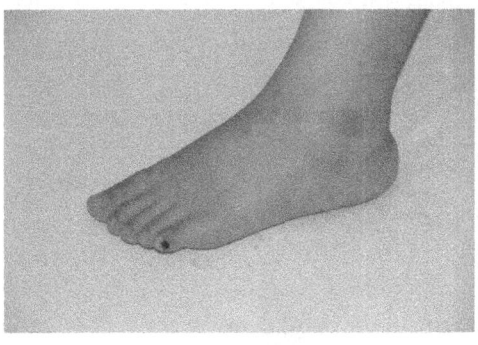 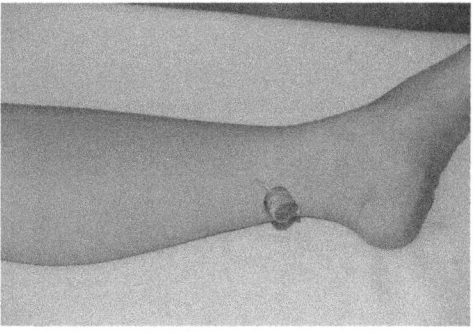

Figure 9.8.2 Non-scarring Moxa at Zhi Yin (BL-67)

Figure 9.8.3 Warm Needle Moxa at San Yin Jiao (SP-6)

9. Metroptosis

Metroptosis refers to a condition in which the uterus drops into the vagina and can protrude from the vaginal orifice, in which case the cervix becomes lower than the ischial spine. Alternatively, the vaginal wall is prolapsed and appears under examination as reddish, cockscomb-shaped or goose egg-shaped. Metroptosis usually occurs after delivery due to the following factors: a weak constitution and deficiency of middle qi; overexertion in delivery leading to collapse from qi deficiency; excessive deliveries and nursing causing damage to kidney qi. In TCM it is also known as uterine prolapse.

Main Symptoms: Uterine prolapse or protrusion from the vagina, accompanied by a sense of dropping and exacerbated by coughing, walking or fatigue.

Acupoints:

- *Primary points:* Bai Hui (DU-20), Qi Hai (RN-4), Wei Dao (GB-28), Zi Gong (EX-CA-1).

- *Symptomatic points:* Collapsing from spleen deficiency: Zu San Li (ST-36); Kidney yang deficiency: Guan Yuan (RN-4), Ming Men (DU-4); Downpour of damp-heat: Pi Shu (BL-20), Yin Ling Quan (SP-9).

Moxibustion Method:

- Gentle Moxa: Apply moxa to each acupoint for 15–20 minutes. Perform once daily. One treatment course consists of 10 treatments. (Figure 9.9.1)

- Moxa on Ginger: Apply 7 moxa cones to each acupoint, using cones approximately the size of a date pit. Perform once daily. One treatment course consists of 15 treatments, with an interval of 5 days between each treatment course. (Figure 9.9.2)

- Moxa on Salt: Fill Shen Que (RN-8) with an appropriate amount of salt. Apply moxa, using cones approximately the size of a soybean. Use 5–7 cones each time and perform once every other day. One treatment course consists of 7 treatments. (Figure 9.9.3)

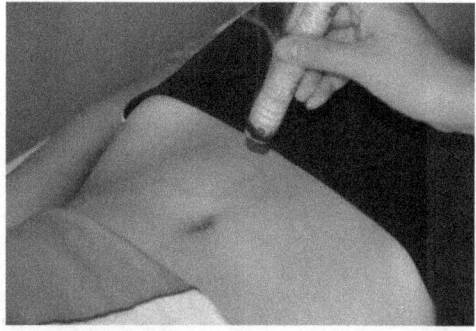

Figure 9.9.1 Gentle Moxa at Qi Hai (RN-4)

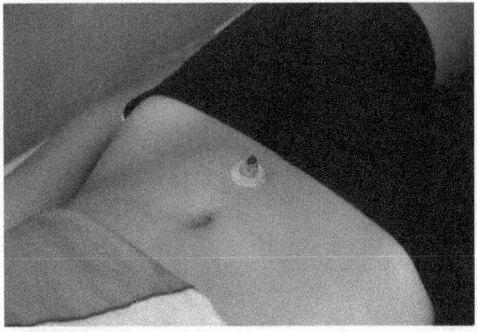

Figure 9.9.2 Moxa on Ginger at Qi Hai (RN-4)

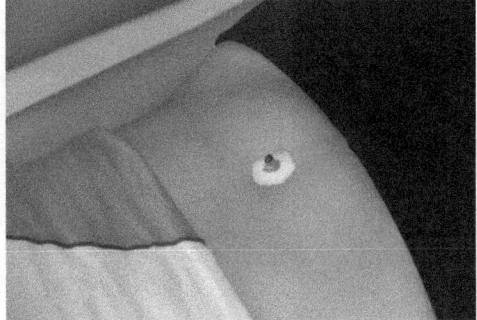

Figure 9.9.3 Moxa on Salt at Shen Que (RN-8)

10. Distending Pain in the Breasts during Menstruation

Distending pain in the breasts during menstruation refers to a syndrome that occurs before or during menstruation. It usually occurs due to the following: liver depression and qi stagnation; stomach deficiency causing phlegm stagnation; yin deficiency with effulgent fire.

Main Symptoms: Distending pain in the breasts or itching pain in the mammillae occurs before or during menstruation, in some cases the breasts are too tender to palpate. It is often accompanied by distending pain in the chest and rib cage; as well as vexation, agitation and irascibility.

Acupoints:

- *Primary points:* Dan Zhong (RN-7), Gan Shu (BL-18), Xing Jian (LR-2), Qi Hai (RN-6).

- *Symptomatic points:* Breast induration: Yang Ling Quan (GB-34); Tidal fever: Bai Lao (EX-HN-15), Gao Huang Shu (BL-43).

Moxibustion Method:

- Gentle Moxa: Apply moxa to each acupoint for 15–20 minutes. Perform once daily. One treatment course consists of 10 treatments. Cease treatment during menstruation. (Figure 9.10.1)

- Moxa on Medicinal Cake: Take equivalent amounts of Xiang Fu (Cyperi Rhizoma) and Yuan Hu (Corydalis Rhizoma), grind them into a powder for further use; take 5g of the powder and mix with tea to make a soft paste, then form into a slice 2cm in diameter. Put a slice on each acupoint, and apply 3–5 moxa cones on each slice, using cones approximately the size of a date pit. Perform once daily or every other day. One treatment course consists of 10 treatments. (Figure 9.10.2)

- Warm Needle Moxa: Apply 1–3 moxa cones to each acupoint and retain the needle for 10 minutes. Perform once daily. One treatment course consists of 10 treatments. Cease manipulation during menstruation. (Figure 9.10.3)

- Moxa on Salt: Fill Shen Que (RN-8) with an appropriate amount of salt. Apply moxa using cones approximately the size of a soybean; use 5–7 cones in total. (Figure 9.10.4)

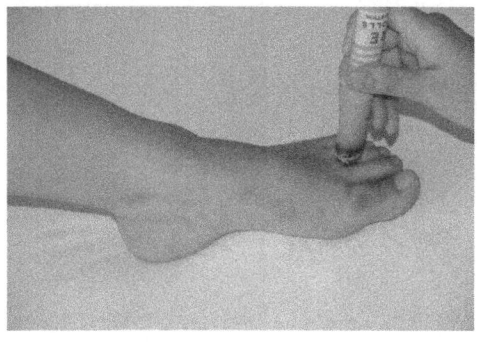

Figure 9.10.1 Gentle Moxa at Xing Jian (LR-2)

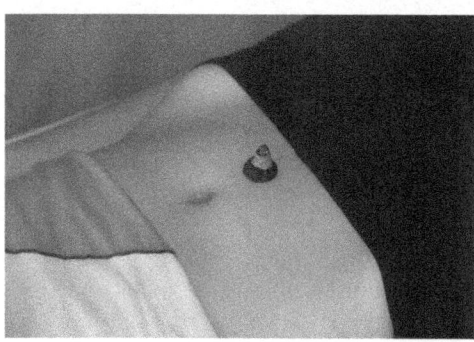

Figure 9.10.2 Moxa on Medicinal Cake at Qi Hai (RN-6)

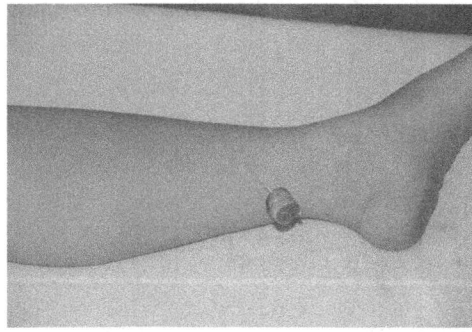

Figure 9.10.3 Warm Needle Moxa at San Yin Jiao (SP-6)

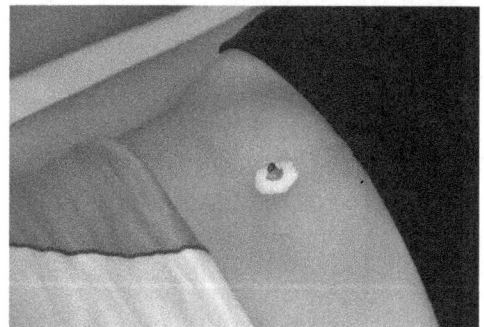

Figure 9.10.4 Moxa on Salt at Shen Que (RN-8)

11. Menopausal Syndrome

Menopausal syndrome refers to a condition in which women, aged between 45 and 55, began to terminate menstruation and suffer from a number of uncomfortable symptoms. These may occur before and after menopause and will usually last 3–5 years. In Western medicine it is called climacteric syndrome. It usually occurs due to the following: the prenatal essence will be exhausted and kidney qi decreased; deficiency of essence and blood, as well as deficiency in the thoroughfare and conception vessels; emotional depression and malnourishment of liver-wood.

Main Symptoms: Menstrual disorder; paroxysmal tidal heat and reddening of the face; vexing heat in the chest, palms and soles or dizziness and tinnitus; vexation, agitation and irascibility; insomnia and palpitations, as well as abnormal sensations in the skin.

Acupoints:

- *Primary points:* Shen Shu (BL-23), Xin Shu (BL-15), Pi Shu (BL-20), San Yin Jiao (SP-6).

- *Symptomatic points:* Vexing heat in the chest, palms and soles: Tai Xi (KI-3), Ran Gu (KI-2); Vexation, agitation and irascibility: Gan Shu (BL-18), Tai Chong (LR-3).

Moxibustion Method:

- Gentle Moxa: Apply moxa to each acupoint for 6–20 minutes. Perform once daily. One treatment course consists of 10 treatments. (Figure 9.11.1)

- Moxa on Ginger: Apply 3–5 moxa cones to each acupoint; using cones approximately the size of a date pit. Perform once every the other day. One treatment course consists of 15 treatments, conduct with a 5-day interval between 2 treatment courses. (Figure 9.11.2)

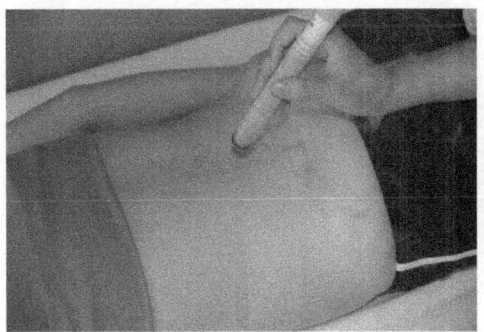
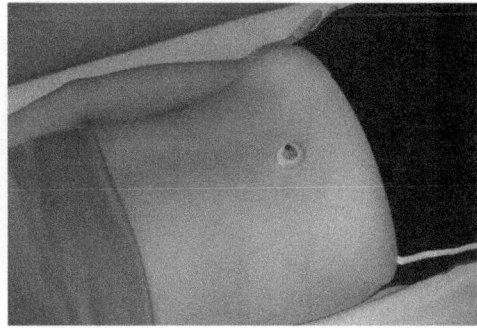

Figure 9.11.1 Gentle Moxa at Pi Shu (BL-20)   *Figure 9.11.2 Moxa on Ginger at Shen Shu (BL 23)*

12. Postpartum Hypogalactia

Postpartum hypogalactia refers to a condition in which breast milk is limited or non-existent so that it does not meet the nutritional requirements of the infant. It is usually due to the following: spleen deficiency causing insufficiency of engendering transformation; excessive bleeding leading to deficiency of the source of transformation; and affective disorders causing inhibited qi movement. It can occur not only after delivery but also during the lactation period.

Main Symptoms: Breast milk is limited or non-existent either postpartum or during the lactation period.

Acupoints:

- *Primary points:* Shao Ze (SI-1), Ru Gen (ST-18), Dan Zhong (RN-17).

- *Symptomatic points:* Deficiency of qi and blood: Zu San Li (ST-36), Pi Shu (BL 20); Liver depression and qi stagnation: Tai Chong (LR-3), Nei Guan (PC-6).

Moxibustion Method:

- Gentle Moxa: Apply moxa to each acupoint for 6–20 minutes. Perform once to twice daily. One treatment course consists of 5 treatments. (Figure 9.12.1)

- Moxa on Ginger: Apply 3–5 moxa cones to each acupoint, using cones approximately the size of a date pit. Perform once every other day. One treatment course consists of 5 treatments. (Figure 9.12.2)

- Moxa on Scallion: Take an appropriate amount of scallion whites, mash and apply to the acupoints. Apply 3–5 moxa cones to each point, using cones approximately the size of a date pit. Perform once every day. One treatment course consists of 5 treatments. (Figure 9.12.3)

- Warm Needle Moxa: Apply 3–5 moxa cones to each point. Perform once daily. One treatment course consists of 10 treatments. (Figure 9.12.4)

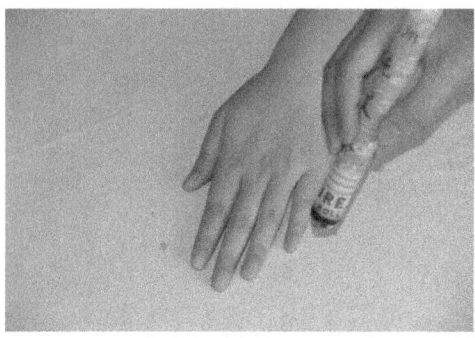

Figure 9.12.1 Gentle Moxa at Shao Ze (SI-1)

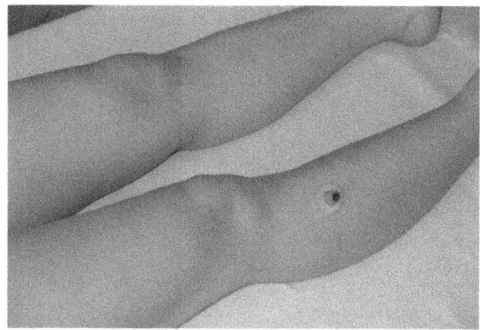

Figure 9.12.2 Moxa on Ginger at Zu San Li (ST-36)

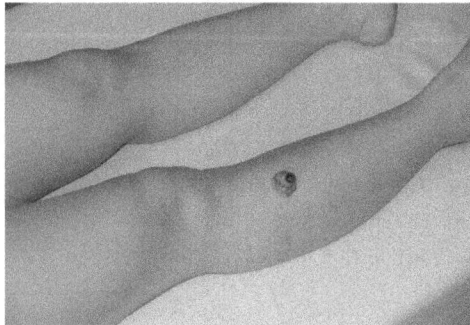

Figure 9.12.3 Moxa on Scallion at Zu San Li (ST-36)

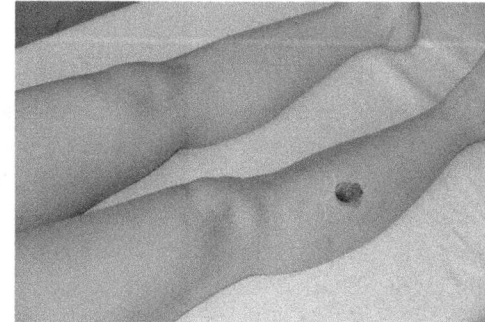

Figure 9.12.4 Warm Needle Moxa at Zu San Li (ST-36)

13. Postpartum Abdominal Pain

Postpartum abdominal pain is a normal condition in the first 3–5 days after delivery. However, it is abnormal when the pain is still severe and accompanied by increased lochia after this period. It is usually due to the following: a weak constitution causing inhibited qi and blood after delivery; contraction of cold after delivery causing congealing cold with blood stasis; liver depression and a failure to govern free-flow causing blood stasis accumulating internally.

Main Symptoms: It manifests as pain in the lower abdomen after delivery.

Acupoints:

- *Primary points:* Qi Hai (RN-6), Zu San Li (ST-36), Gui Lai (ST-29), Zhong Ji (RN-3).

- *Symptomatic points:* Dull pain in the lower abdomen: San Yin Jiao (SP-6); Stabbing pain in the lower abdomen: Xue Hai (SP-10), Di Ji (SP-8).

Moxibustion Method:

- Gentle Moxa: Apply moxa to each acupoint for 6–20 minutes. Perform once to twice daily. One treatment course consists of 5 treatments. (Figure 9.13.1)

- Moxa on Ginger: Apply 5–7 moxa cones to each acupoint, using cones approximately the size of a soybean. Perform once every other day. One treatment course consists of 5 treatments. (Figure 9.13.2)

- Warm Needle Moxa: Apply 3–5 moxa cones to each acupoint. Perform once daily. One treatment course consists of 5 treatments. (Figure 9.13.3)

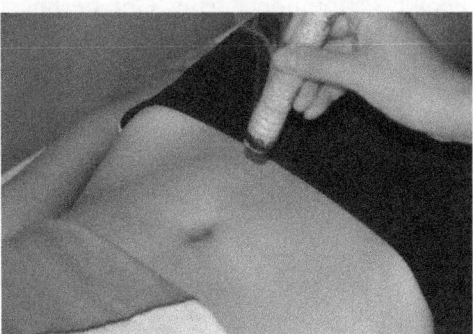

Figure 9.13.1 Gentle Moxa at Qi Hai (RN-6)

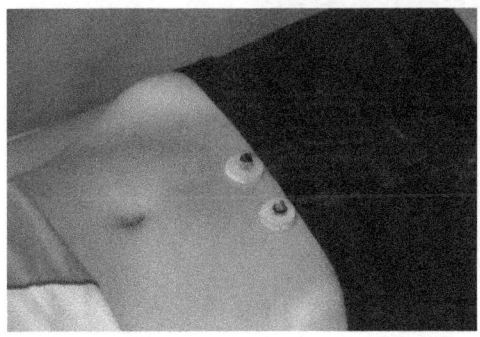
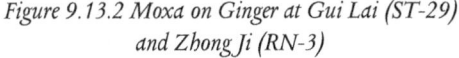
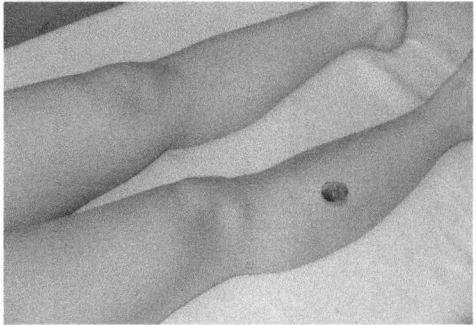

Figure 9.13.2 Moxa on Ginger at Gui Lai (ST-29) and Zhong Ji (RN-3)   *Figure 9.13.3 Warm Needle Moxa at Zu San Li (ST-36)*

14. Pruritus Vulvae

Pruritus vulvae manifests as itching of the vulva. It is a common gynaecologic disease. In Western medicine it belongs to the category of vulvitis. It usually occurs due to a downpour of damp-heat and additional contraction of wind pathogens.

Main Symptoms: Intolerable vaginal itching accompanied by a burning heat sensation or morbid leucorrhoea.

Acupoints:

- *Primary points:* Zhong Ji (RN-3), Yin Ling Quan (SP-9), Li Gou (LR-5), San Yin Jiao (SP-6).

- *Symptomatic points:* Damp-heat in the liver meridian: Qu Quan (LR-8); Genital erosion due to worm toxins: Qu Gu (RN-2), Ci Liao (BL-32); Excessive leucorrhoea: Ci Liao (BL-32).

Moxibustion Method:

- Gentle Moxa: Apply moxa to each acupoint for 15–20 minutes. Perform once to twice daily. One treatment course consists of 10 treatments. (Figure 9.14.1)

- Warm Needle Moxa: Retain the needle for 6–15 minutes after applying 1–2 moxa cones to each acupoint. Perform once daily. One treatment course consists of 10 treatments. (Figure 9.14.2)

- Moxa on Ginger: Apply 3–5 moxa cones to each acupoint, using cones approximately the size of a soybean. Perform once every other day. One treatment course consists of 15 treatments. (Figure 9.14.3)

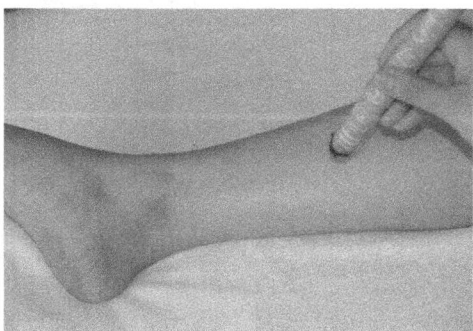

Figure 9.14.1 Gentle Moxa at Li Gou (LR-5)

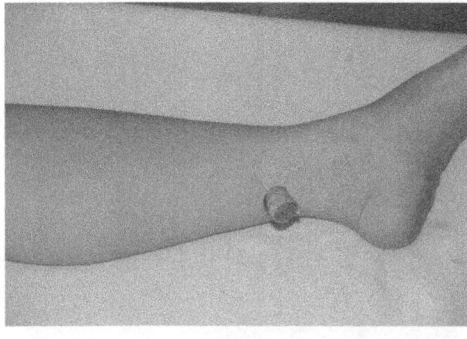

Figure 9.14.2 Warm Needle Moxa at San Yin Jiao (SP-6)

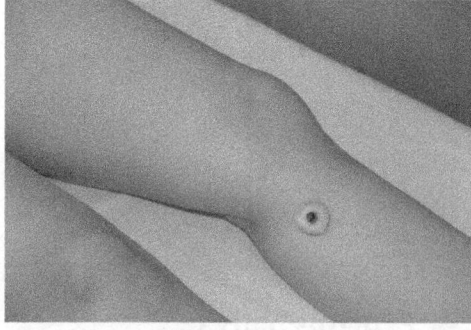

Figure 9.14.3 Moxa on Ginger at Yin Ling Quan (SP-9)

15. Leukoplakia of the Vulva

Leukoplakia of the vulva refers to white lesions on the vulva or vitiliginous vaginitis. In TCM it belongs to the category of pruritus vulvae or erosion of the vulva. It is more prevalent in middle-aged and older women. It usually occurs before or after menopause and can be due to the following: deficiency of kidney and liver causing a deprivation of nourishment to the genitals; spleen deficiency engendering damp which accumulates and transforms into heat, a downpour of damp-heat brews and steams in the vagina.

Main Symptoms: White patches or spots appear on the skin and mucosa of the vulva, the skin of the genitals becomes thin and brittle, or rough and plump. Accompanied by pruritus vulvae or even severe itching that cannot be endured, sometimes with a sensation of burning heat.

Acupoints: Ashi points, Zhong Ji (RN-3), Qu Gu (RN-2), San Yin Jiao (SP-6), Da Chang Shu (BL-25).

Moxibustion Method:

- Scarring Moxa:* Select 2 acupoints each time. Apply 5–7 moxa cones to each acupoint, using cones approximately the size of a soybean. Perform once every month. One treatment course consists of 3 treatments. (Figure 9.15.1)

- Gentle Moxa: Apply moxa to each acupoint for 10 minutes. Apply moxa to the vulva for 20–30 minutes. Perform once daily. One treatment course consists of 10 treatments.

- Moxa on Ginger: Apply 5–7 moxa cones to each acupoint, using cones approximately the size of a soybean. Perform once every other day. One treatment course consists of 10 treatments. (Figure 9.15.2)

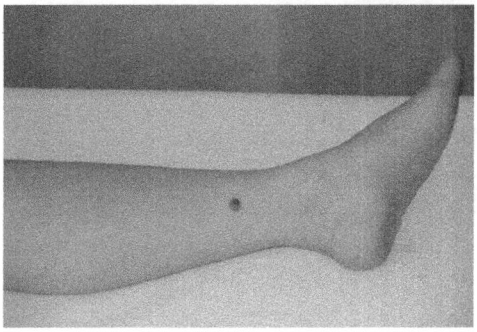
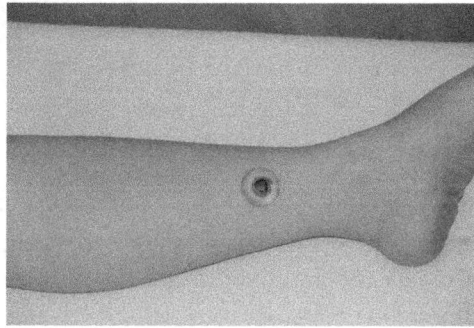

Figure 9.15.1 Scarring Moxa at San Yin Jiao (SP-6)   *Figure 9.15.2 Moxa on Ginger at San Yin Jiao (SP-6)*

CHAPTER 10

Dermatological and External Medicine Conditions

1. Herpes Zoster

Herpes zoster is a disease that manifests primarily as a sudden occurrence of a cluster of blisters distributed in a snake-like belt along one side of the body (Figure 10.1.1), accompanied by a sensation of burning and a prickling pain. In traditional Chinese medicine herpes zoster is known as twining waist dragon and girdling fire pellet, and colloquially referred to as snake pellet or spider sores. It is usually due to the following factors: excessive fire in the liver and gallbladder; internal brewing of damp-heat in the spleen channel; coagulation of the toxic heat in the skin and channels.

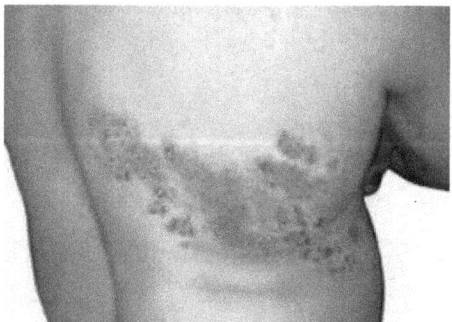

Figure 10.1.1 Herpes Zoster

Main Symptoms: Burning sensations, prickling pain and cutaneous redness occur first, succeeded by a cluster of millet-sized herpes distributed in a line along one side of the body, mainly on the waist and the hypochondrium. Painful sensations can remain after the herpes disappear.

Acupoints:

- *Primary points:* Ashi points.

- *Symptomatic points:* When the location of disease is superior to the waist: Qu Chi (LI-11), He Gu (LI-4), Wai Guan (SJ-5); When the location of disease is inferior to the waist: San Yin Jiao (SP-6), Tai Chong (LR-3), Xue Hai (SP-10).

Moxibustion Method:

- Cone Moxa: Apply a moxa cone respectively to two Ashi points; the first where the herpes first appeared, the second at the area of highest concentration. Also apply moxa to other points. After lighting the moxa, remove the unburned moxa cone once pain is felt. Use only one cone at each point, once daily. One course of treatment consists of 3 treatments. Apply moxa cone again after 5 days if the condition does not heal. (Figure 10.1.2)

- Gentle Moxa: Apply circling moxibustion until the highest temperature the patient can endure is achieved. Perform for approximately 30 minutes according to the size of the lesion area, and repeat once every day. One treatment course consists of 3 treatments. Apply moxa again after 5 days if the condition does not heal. (Figure 10.1.3)

- Juncibustion:* Take a 10–15cm long Juncus bufonius or paper string, infuse 3–4cm in ginger oil, ignite the fire and quickly touch the end to the point; after a popping sound is heard quickly remove from the point. If the sound doesn't occur, repeat. Perform once every other day. One treatment course consists of 6 treatments. (Figure 10.1.4)

- Moxa on Cotton:* Take a piece of absorbent cotton, as thin as possible, and cover the herpes with it. Ask the patient to close their eyes, ignite one end of the cotton and let it burn out. In the majority of patients their herpes will darken, lessen and disappear after only one treatment. (Figure 10.1.5)

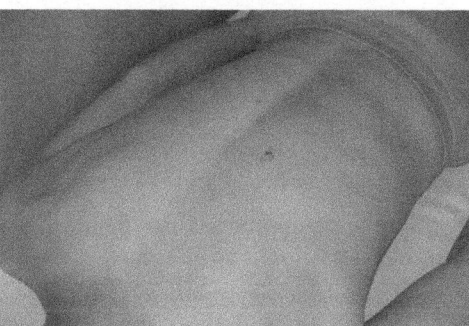

Figure 10.1.2 Cone Moxa at Ge Shu (BL-17)

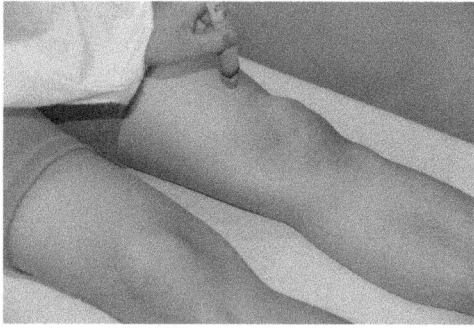

Figure 10.1.3 Gentle Moxa at Xue Hai (SP-10)

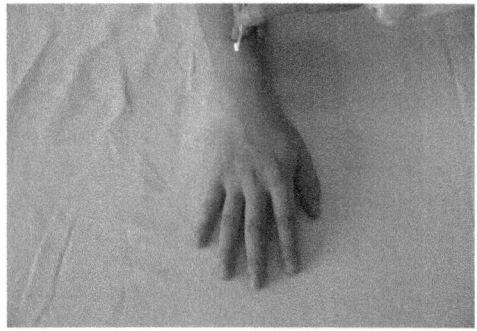
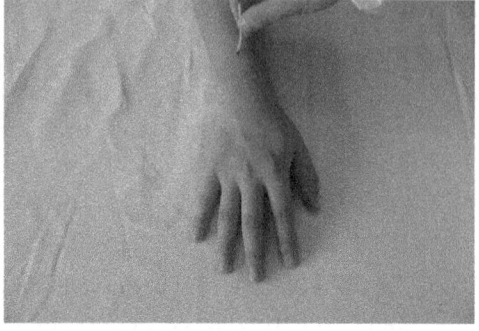

Figure 10.1.4 Juncibustion at Wai Guan (SJ-5)

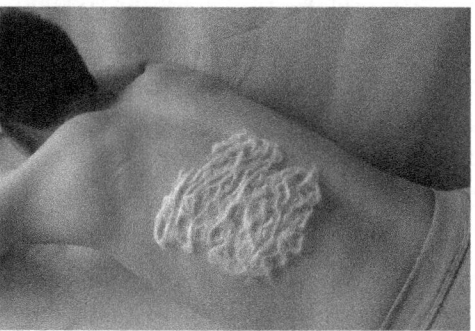

Figure 10.1.5 Moxa on Cotton

2. Eczema

Eczema is a common allergic inflammatory skin disease. It manifests as patches or a diffuse area of polymorphous rash with symmetrical distribution, severe itching and an obvious tendency to exude. It easily recurs and becomes chronic. It is usually due to the following: contraction of external damp-heat; food damageing the spleen causing spleen deficiency and a failure in transportation; constitutional damp accumulation, long-term damp depression transforming into heat, damp-heat brewing and coagulating in the skin. Chronic eczema usually develops from an uncontrolled case of acute eczema; or due to blood deficiency, strong wind and spleen dampness.

Main Symptoms: Red lumps occur over the entire body or locally on the upper and lower back, abdomen or extremities; or the skin presents with tidal redness and itching with clusters or sporadic millet-sized red papules or papular blisters; or the skin is festering with excessive exudation.

Acupoints: Pi Shu (BL-20), Yin Ling Quan (SP-9), Zu San Li (ST-36), San Yin Jiao (SP-6), Bai Chong Wo (EX-LE-3).

Moxibustion Method:

- Direct Cone Moxa: Apply 3–5 moxa cones to each acupoint, using cones approximately the size of a grain of wheat. When the patient senses burning extinguish the cone with forceps and change another point. Perform until the local skin becomes flushed but does not blister. Perform once daily. One treatment course consists of 7 treatments. (Figure 10.2.1)

- Moxa on Garlic: Cut fresh garlic, a large clove is suitable, into 0.3–0.4cm slices and puncture them. Place a slice of garlic on the point and perform moxibustion with a finger-tip-sized cone. When the patient feels a burning sensation slightly adjust the position of the garlic or remove and replace the moxa cone. Apply 7–9 cones each time, perform 1–2 times daily. One course of treatment consists of 7 treatments. (Figure 10.2.2)

- Pecking Sparrow Moxa: Apply pecking sparrow moxa to each point for 6–20 minutes, perform once daily. One treatment course consists of 7 treatments. (Figure 10.2.3)

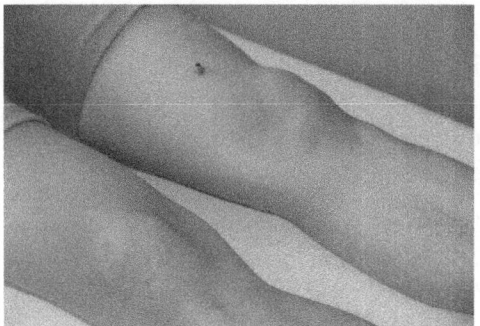

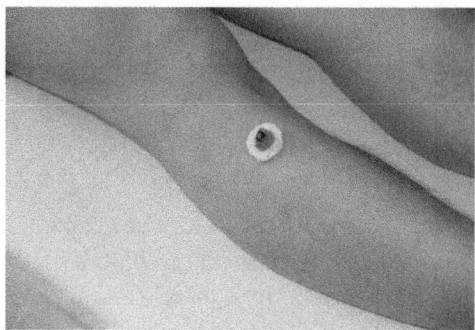

Figure 10.2.1 Direct Cone Moxa at Bai Chong Wo (EX-LE-3)

Figure 10.2.2 Moxa on Garlic at Zu San Li (ST-36)

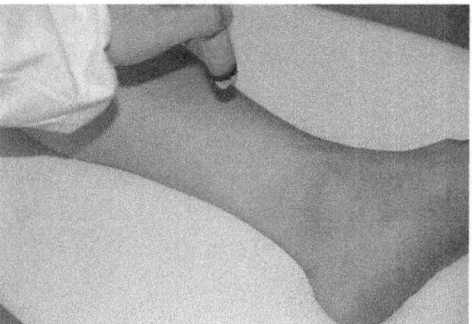

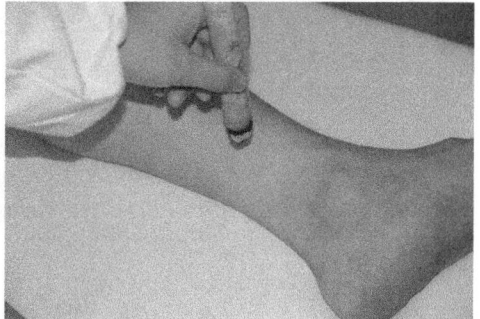

Figure 10.2.3 Pecking Sparrow Moxa at San Yin Jiao (SP-6)

3. Urticaria

Urticaria is a common disease, also known as wind wheal, nettle rash, wind knots, pomphus. The pathology can proceed in the following ways: a variety of factors causing inflammatory hyperaemia and excessive exudation of skin mucosa and vessels. This results in localized myxoedema. It itches severely and appears and disappears swiftly, and can be accompanied by fever, abdominal pain, diarrhoea and other systemic symptoms. It is classified by Western medicine into acute urticaria and chronic urticaria, and belongs to the category of hidden rash in TCM. It is usually due to the following: brewing damp-heat; a blood deficient constitution and contraction of wind-cold or damp-heat coagulating in the skin.

Main Symptoms: White or red wheals erupt on the skin, and may occur in any part of the body, disappearing from one area and rising in another, associated with severe itching. Both the appearance and disappearance of the eruptions are swift and no marks are left after wheals disappear. It may be accompanied by general symptoms such as fever, diarrhoea and abdominal pain.

Acupoints: Qu Chi (LI-11), Xue Hai (SP-10), San Yin Jiao (SP-6), Ge Shu (BL-17), Bai Chong Wo (EX-LE-3).

Moxibustion Method:

- Moxa on Ginger: Cut a piece of ginger into 0.3cm slices and puncture them several times. Place a slice of ginger on an acupoint and place a fingertip-sized moxa cone on the point. When the patient has a sensation of burning slightly adjust the position of the ginger or replace the moxa cone. Apply 3–5 cones each time, and perform 1–2 times daily. Stop when the symptoms have vanished. (Figure 10.3.1)

- Moxa on Garlic: Cut the fresh garlic, a large clove is suitable, into 0.3–0.4cm slices and puncture them several times. Place a slice of garlic on the acupoint and place a fingertip-sized moxa cone on the garlic. When the patient has a sensation of burning slightly adjust the position of the garlic or replace the moxa cone. Apply 7–9 cones each time and perform 1–2 times daily. Stop when the symptoms have vanished. (Figure 10.3.2)

- Warm Needle Moxa: Choose 1.5 *cun* (40mm) needles, and apply moxa on each point for 30 minutes. Perform once daily. One treatment course consists of 7 treatments. (Figure 10.3.3)

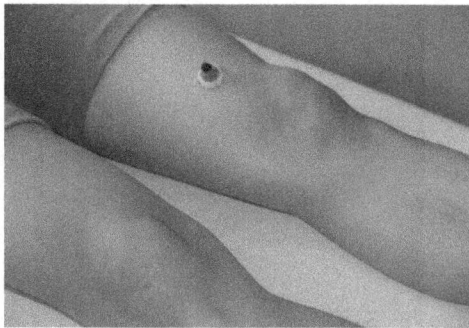

Figure 10.3.1 Moxa on Ginger at Bai Chong Wo (EX-LE-3)

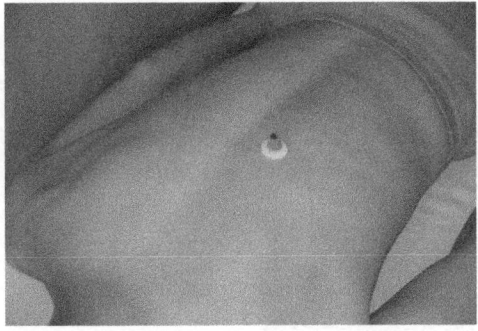

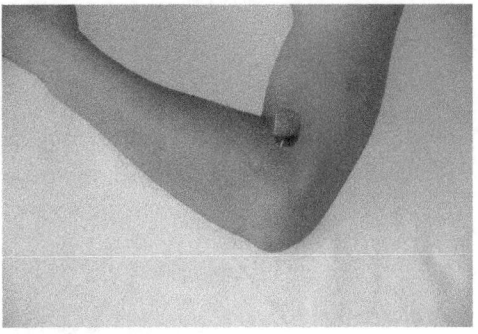

Figure 10.3.2 Moxa on Garlic at Ge Shu (BL-17)   *Figure 10.3.3 Warm Needle Moxa at Qu Chi (LI-11)*

4. Flat Wart

Flat wart is a kind of small neoplasm that grows on the surface of the skin and is often seen on the face or back of the hand in young people (Figure 10.4.1). In Western medicine, it results from a viral infection. In TCM it is also called 'flat bullseye' as it resembles a bullseye. It usually occurs due to the following: wind-heat pathogens contending and binding in the skin; liver qi depression and stagnation of qi and blood.

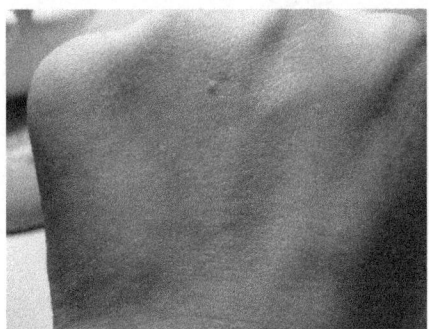

Figure 10.4.1 Flat Wart

Main Symptoms: Light brown flat papules ranging in size from a grain of rice to a soybean appear scattered in a circular, oval or polygon formation, or densely distributed in clusters just like strings of beads.

Acupoints: He Gu (LI-4), Qu Chi (LI-11), Si Bai (ST-2), San Yin Jiao (SP-6), Xue Hai (SP-10), Tai Chong (LR-3).

Moxibustion Method:

- Direct Cone Moxa: Apply 3–5 moxa cones to each acupoint, using cones approximately the size of a grain of wheat. Extinguish the cone with forceps and change to another point when the patient senses burning. Perform until the local skin becomes flushed but does not blister. Perform once daily. One course of treatment consists of 7 treatments. (Figure 10.4.2)

- Warm Needle Moxa: Choose 1.5 *cun* (40mm) needles, use reducing manipulation, and apply moxa on each point for 30 minutes. Perform once daily. One treatment course consists of 7 treatments. (Figure 10.4.3)

- Sang Zhi Moxa: Ignite the Sang Zhi (mulberry twig; Mori Ramulus) and perform moxibustion on the warts until the local skin becomes yellow or scorched. Perform once every other day. One treatment course consists of 8 treatments. (Figure 10.4.4)

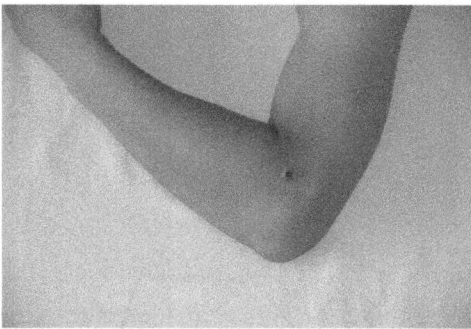

Figure 10.4.2 Direct Cone Moxa at Qu Chi (LI-11)

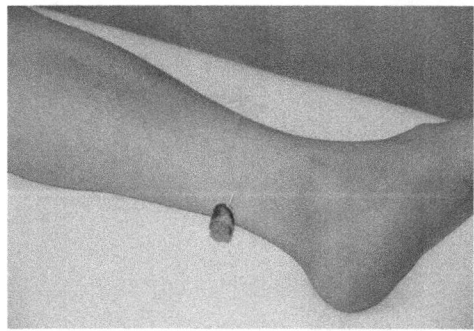
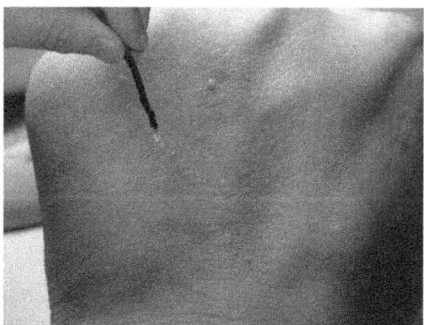

Figure 10.4.3 Warm Needle Moxa at San Yin Jiao (SP-6)   *Figure 10.4.4 Sang Zhi Moxa*

5. Neurodermitis

Neurodermitis is a common chronic skin disease manifesting as severe itching and lichenoid skin changes. It often occurs in local areas such as the neck, elbow, cubital fossa, thigh and lumbosacral area; it can also be widely distributed. It is common in young people and adults; it appears without a clear cause but is related to nervous system and mental factors. In TCM it is also called cow skin tinea, and, when it appears on the neck, neck sores. It is usually due to one of the following: wind-damp pathogens stagnating in the skin and transforming into heat; external mechanical stimulation and scratching; blood deficiency and effulgent liver fire, anxiety and upset, or deficiency of yin fluids causing deprivation of skin nourishment.

Main Symptoms: Paroxysmal severe itching and lichenoid skin.

Acupoints: Feng Chi (GB-20), Da Zhui (DU-14), Xue Hai (SP-10), Qu Chi (LI-11), Nei Guan (PC-6), Wei Zhong (BL-40), Shen Men (HT-7), Zhao Hai (KI-6), Ashi points.

Moxibustion Method:

- Gentle Moxa: Choose Ashi points and 2–3 other points, choosing different points each treatment. Ignite the moxa and hold it 3–5cm above the points. The temperature should be hot, but not so hot that it burns the patient's skin. Apply moxa to every point for 5–7 minutes until the local skin becomes flushed. Perform once daily. One treatment course consists of 10 treatments. (Figure 10.5.1)

- Cone Moxa: Apply moxa cone on Ashi points, using wheat kernel-sized moxa cones. The distance between the points should be 1.5cm. Spread some oil on the points before moxibustion to fix the cone; after the cone burns out sweep away the moxa ash, clean the skin with saline solution, and cover with a dressing. One can press and extinguish the fire with a tongue depressor and pat the skin to relieve pain before the cone burns out. Apply only 1 cone each time, 2 times a week, and change the points to apply moxa until the skin becomes normal. If blisters occur, puncture, drain and apply gentian violet; if there is pus, spread anti-inflammatory ointment; no scar will remain. (Figure 10.5.2)

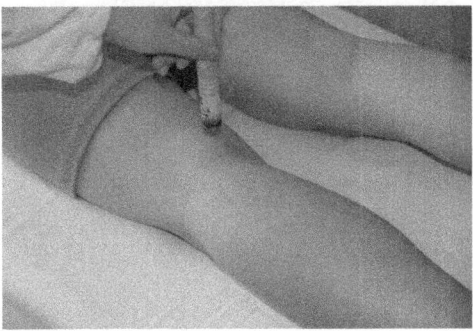

Figure 10.5.1 Gentle Moxa at Wei Zhong (BL-40)

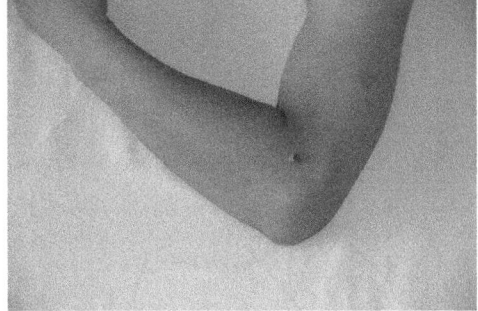

Figure 10.5.2 Cone Moxa at Qu Chi (LI-11)

6. Common Wart

Common warts, also called rigid warts, are a kind of papilliform neoplasm that occurs on the surface of the skin. It is more prevalent in children and young people and usually occurs on areas such as the fingers, dorsum of the hand, as well as the head and face. It is caused by the papilloma virus, infection through others or autoinoculation. The latent period is from several months to 1 year. In TCM common wart is also called 'wart-eye' and 'thousand day sore', and the popular name for it is 'upright flesh'. It can occur due to one of the following: contraction of external wind pathogens and toxic heat; internal liver fire flaming upwards; effulgent liver fire and blood dryness; stagnation of qi and blood.

Main Symptoms: Keratotic papula the size of rice grains occur, gradually enlarge, and are flesh coloured or greyish-brown.

Acupoints: Ashi point, Tai Chong (LR-3), He Gu (LI-4), Zhong Zhu (SJ-3), Qu Chi (LI-11), Feng Chi (GB-20), Xing Jian (LR-2), Jia Xi (GB-43).

Moxibustion Method:

- Gentle Moxa: Choose 2–3 points and alternate with each treatment. Ignite the moxa and hold it 3–5cm over the point. The temperature should be hot, but not so hot that it burns the patient's skin. Apply moxa to every point for 5–7 minutes until the local skin reddens. Perform once daily. One course of treatment consists of 10 treatments. (Figure 10.6.1)

- Cone Moxa: Choose 2–3 points and alternate with each treatment. First apply moxa directly on the warts, using moxa cones the size of a grain of wheat; sweep away the moxa ash, clean the skin with saline solution and cover with a dressing after the cone has burnt out. Apply only 1 cone each time, and alternate points until the skin becomes normal. (Figure 10.6.2)

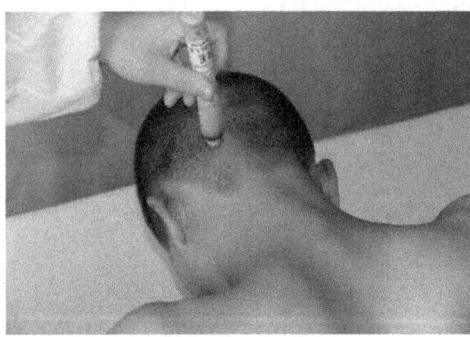
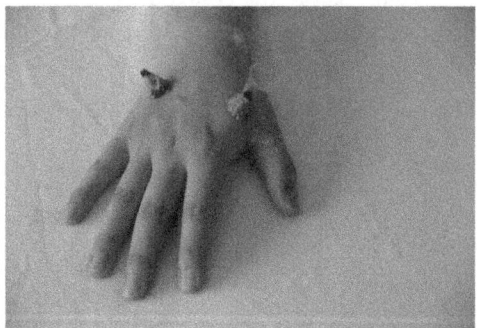

Figure 10.6.1 Gentle Moxa at Feng Chi (GB-20)

Figure 10.6.2 Cone Moxa at He Gu (LI-4) and Zhong Zhu (SJ-3)

7. Leukoderma

Leukoderma is an acquired disease involving regional skin pigment loss. It is considered to have a complex pathogenesis in TCM: contraction of external wind pathogens, traumatic injury, moodiness, blood collapse and loss of essence leading to qi and blood disharmony or qi stagnation and blood stasis so that the blood cannot nourish the skin.

Main Symptoms: Regional skin pigment loss of different sizes with clear margins, no sensations of burning or itching after exposure to the sun, the hair in the lesion can also become white.

Acupoints: Ashi points, Feng Chi (GB-20), Xue Hai (SP-10), San Yin Jiao (SP-6), Guan Yuan (RN-4).

Moxibustion Method:

- Medicinal Moxa: Disinfect with alcohol, apply a thin layer of Jin Huang Ointment, and then perform moxa stick circling moxibustion for 30 minutes. If the leukoderma is widely spread, one area can be treated each time. Clean the affected area after moxibustion. Perform once daily. One treatment course consists of 12 treatments. (Figure 10.7.1)

- Gentle Moxa: Apply moxa stick circling moxibustion to a temperature that the patient can comfortably endure. Perform for 30 minutes each time until the skin becomes dark red, and repeat 1–2 times daily. One course of treatment lasts for 4 weeks. (Figure 10.7.2)

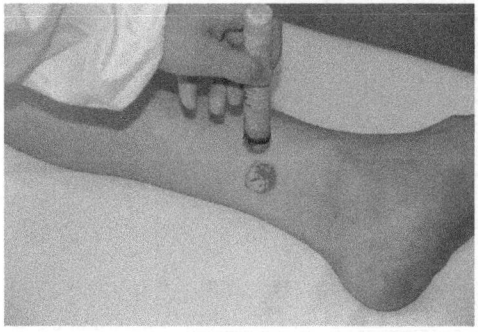
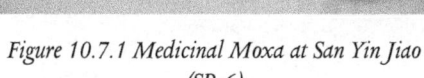
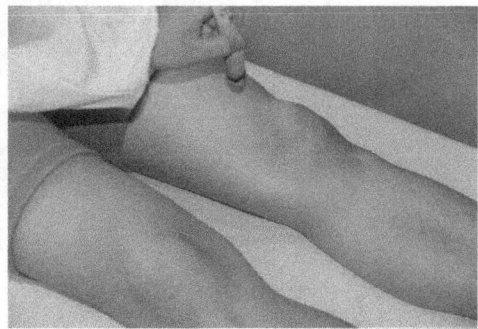

Figure 10.7.1 Medicinal Moxa at San Yin Jiao (SP-6)

Figure 10.7.2 Gentle Moxa at Xue Hai (SP-10)

8. Chloasma

Chloasma, also commonly known as liver spots, is a disease involving abnormal pigment metabolism. It tends to occur on the face and is more prevalent in young women and children, especially in pregnant women (cyasma). It is usually due to one of the following: external pathogens and toxins stagnating in the skin causing blockage of the channels; unclean food causing internal worm accumulation, worm toxins and stagnation of qi in the skin.

Main Symptoms: Yellow brown spots of different sizes, shapes and depth of colour, usually symmetrical, without accompanying symptoms.

Acupoints: Si Bai (ST-2), Ying Xiang (LI-20), Gan Shu (BL-18), Pi Shu (BL-20), Shen Shu (BL-23), Qi Hai (RN-6), Zu San Li (ST-36), San Yin Jiao (SP6), Tai Xi (KI-3), brown spot areas.

Moxibustion Method:

- Direct Cone Moxa: Apply moxa cones on the brown spot, using cones approximately the size of a grain of wheat. When the patient feels burning extinguish the cone with forceps and change to another point. Continue until the local skin becomes flushed but does not blister. Use 3–5 cones each time and repeat once daily. One treatment course consists of 7 treatments. (Figure 10.8.1)

- Pecking Sparrow Moxa: Choose 2–3 points; apply moxa on each point for 6–20 minutes. Perform once daily. One treatment course consists of 7 treatments. (Figure 10.8.2)

- Warm Needle Moxa: Using 1.5 *cun* (40mm) needles and reducing manipulation, apply moxa on each point for 30 minutes. Perform once daily. One treatment course consists of 7 treatments. (Figure 10.8.3)

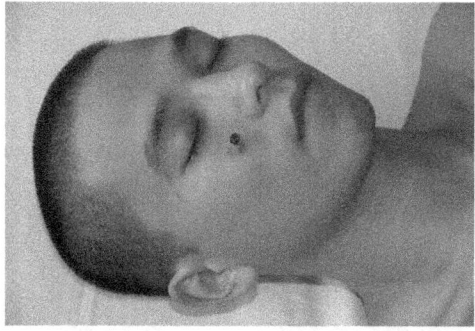

Figure 10.8.1 Direct Cone Moxa at Si Bai (ST-2)

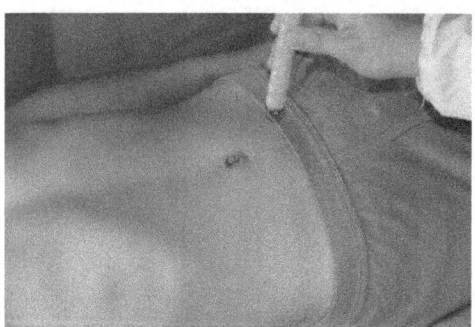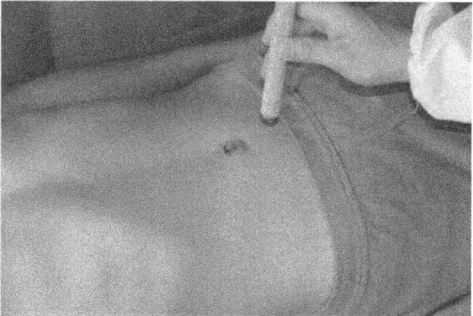

Figure 10.8.2 Pecking Sparrow Moxa at Qi Hai (RN-6)

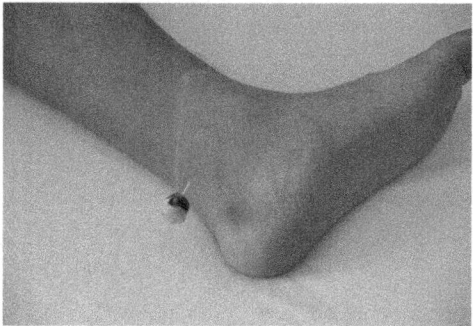

Figure 10.8.3 Warm Needle Moxa at Tai Xi (KI-3)

9. Psoriasis

Psoriasis is a common agnogenic erythroderma desquamativum without infectivity (Figure 10.9.1). It can occur in men and women, children and the old, but is more prevalent in young men. It usually occurs and becomes severe in winter, and is relieved or naturally recovers in summer. If the course of disease is protracted it will have an inconspicuous seasonal nature. Psoriasis is also commonly called cow skin tinea, white crust, or coin wind in TCM. It usually occurs due to the following: at first external pathogenic wind, cold, heat and damp accumulate and are retained in the skin and block the channels, and in the long term causes blood deficiency and wind dryness. The skin is deprived of nourishment, and therefore becomes rough and desquamative.

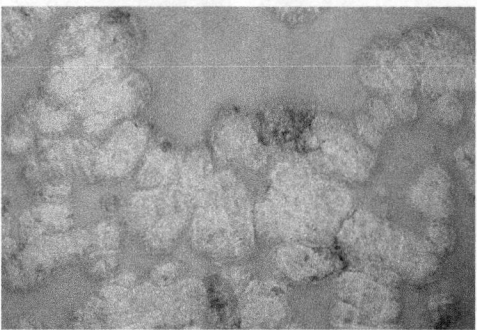

Figure 10.9.1 Psoriasis

Main Symptoms: Reddish infiltrating spot skin lesions the size of or larger than a coin covered with silver scales and with clear margins. If the scales are removed the skin presents with a stearic shine; if more flesh is removed cribriform bleeding will occur. It occurs repeatedly all over the body, especially on the extensor aspect of the extremities.

Acupoints: Ashi points, Qu Chi (LI-11), Xue Hai (SP-10), Feng Chi (GB-20), Shen Shu (BL-23), San Yin Jiao (SP-6).

Moxibustion Method:

- Gentle Moxa: Choose 2–3 points, ignite the moxa and hold it 3–5cm over the point. The temperature should be hot, but not so hot that it burns the patient's skin. Apply at every point for 5–7 minutes until the local skin becomes flushed. Perform once daily. One treatment course consists of 7 treatments, with a 3-day rest between courses. (Figure 10.9.2)

- Burning Cotton Therapy:* Perform cutaneous needling at Ashi points with moderate stimulation until there is a little bleeding; then spread a little absorbent cotton and flatten it on the lesioned skin; ignite the cotton and quickly let it burn out then extinguish it, change the cotton and repeat the manipulation 3–4 times until the skin becomes flushed. Perform once every 3–4 days. One course of treatment consists of 5 treatments. (Figure 10.9.3)

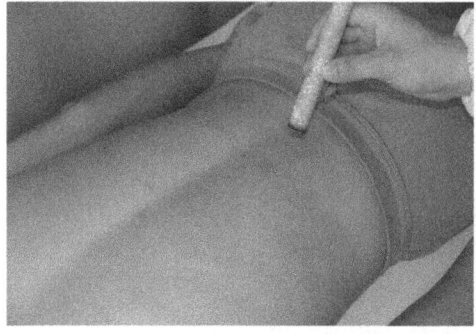

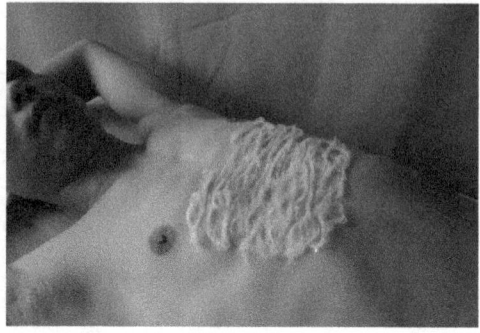

Figure 10.9.2 Gentle Moxa   *Figure 10.9.3 Burning Cotton Therapy*

10. Trichomadesis

Trichomadesis refers to the phenomenon of hair loss. Normal hair loss occurs at the catagen or telogen phase. As hair in the catagen and anagen phases is in constant dynamic balance, hair can maintain normal quantity. That is called physiological trichomadesis. Pathologic trichomadesis refers to abnormal or excessive hair loss. In traditional Chinese medicine, this condition is related to dual deficiency of qi and blood, insufficiency of the liver and kidney and blood stasis in the hair orifice. Hair is indicative of blood condition; if qi vacuity is unable to engender blood, hair roots are deprived of nourishment, which leads to a loss of hair; liver stores blood and kidney stores essence, insufficiency of essence and blood deprive hair of the source of growth; blockage of blood pathways impedes the nourishment of hair, causing hair loss.

Main Symptoms: The onset is sudden with patches of hair loss or complete hair loss, even including the eyebrow, beard and underarm hair.

Acupoints: Bai Hui (DU-20), Tou Wei (ST-8), Ashi points, Sheng Fa (in the centre of a line between Feng Shi and Feng Fu), Fang Lao (1 *cun* behind Bai Hui), Jian Nao (0.5 *cun* beneath Feng Chi).

Moxibustion Method:

- Gentle Pole Moxa: Apply moxa to 2–3 points in turn, 5–7 minutes per point or until reddening occurs, once per day. Seven treatments comprise one course of treatment, with a 3-day interval between each course. (Figure 10.10.1)

- Moxa on Ginger: Apply moxa to 2–3 points in turn, 3–5 cones per acupoint, once or twice per day. Seven treatments comprise one course of treatment, with a 3-day interval between each course. (Figure 10.10.2)

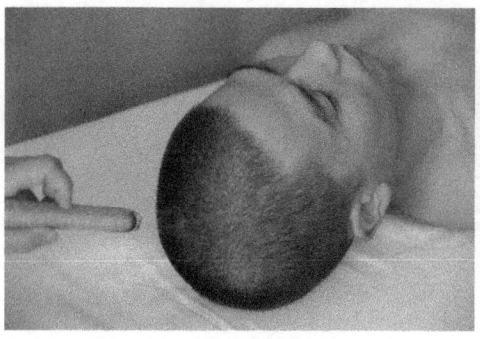

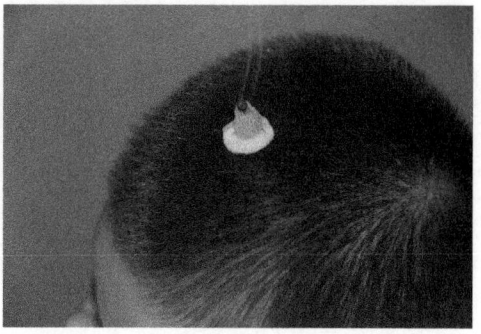

Figure 10.10.1 Gentle Pole Moxa at Bai Hui (DU-20)

Figure 10.10.2 Moxa on Ginger at Bai Hui (DU-20)

11. Acne

Acne usually occurs during puberty, and presents especially on the facial area. It also occurs on the superior part of the chest, back and scapular region. Acne is usually caused by one of the following: lung heat or blood heat accumulating in the muscle and skin; surfeit of fat, rich food causing retention of heat in the spleen and stomach, brewing the skin; insecurity of the interstices and cosmetic irritation; or adherence of oil to the skin.

Main Symptoms: In the early stage small pimples shaped like millet or blackhead pimples are dispersed primarily along follicular orifices. The surrounding skin is red, swollen and painful, and a grainy liquid can be squeezed out using the fingers. Some appear with a pustule at the top, and some can form adipoma or furuncle. The course of disease is lingering, and can disappear and reappear sporadically.

Acupoints: Qu Chi (LI-11), He Gu (LI-4), Xue Hai (SP-10), Zu San Li (ST-36), San Yin Jiao (SP-6).

Moxibustion Method:

- Pecking Sparrow Moxa: Apply moxa to 2–3 points, 10–20 minutes per point, once per day. Seven treatments comprise one course of treatment. (Figure 10.11.1)

- Non-scarring Moxa: Use moxa cones the size of a wheat-grain. Apply moxa to 2–3 points, 3–5 cones per point, once per day. Seven treatments comprise one course of treatment. (Figure 10.11.2)

- Moxa on Ginger: Apply moxa to 2–3 points in turn, 3–5 cones per acupoint, once or twice per day. Seven treatments comprise one course of treatment. (Figure 10.11.3)

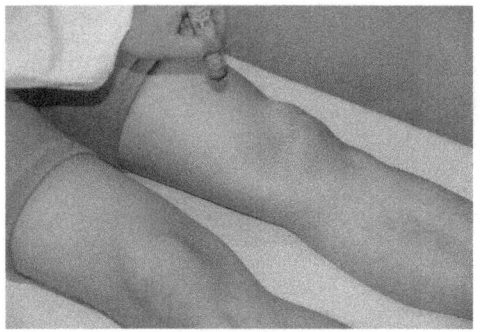
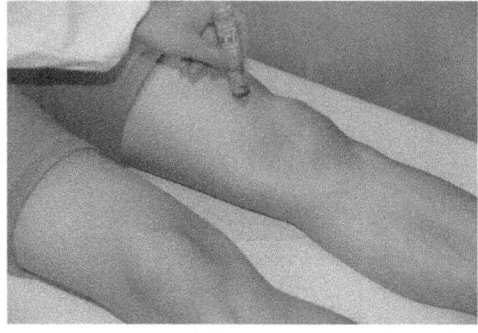

Figure 10.11.1 Pecking Sparrow Moxa at Xue Hai (SP-10)

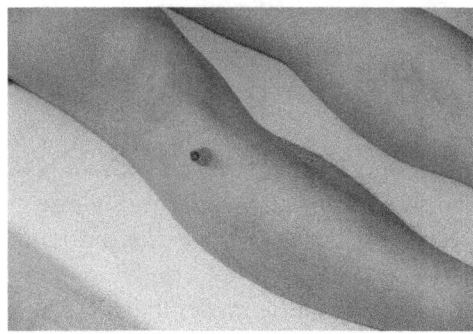
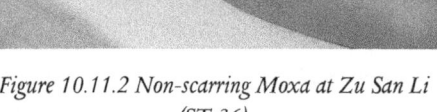
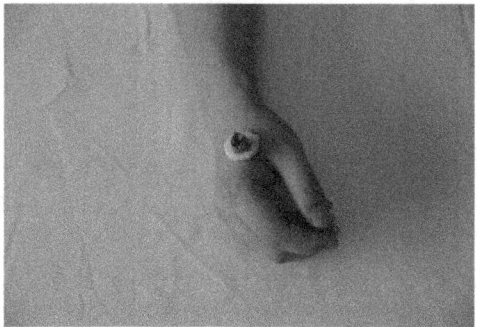

Figure 10.11.2 Non-scarring Moxa at Zu San Li (ST-36)

Figure 10.11.3 Moxa on Ginger at He Gu (LI-4)

12. Osmidrosis

Osmidrosis is also known as hircismus or bromhidrosis. This disease is often seen under the arm and most often occurs in young people, especially in females. It is usually caused by damp-heat depressed internally or due to heredity factors.

Main Symptoms: Sweat is especially odorous. In mild cases there is no odour when not sweating; in severe cases even the areola mammae, belly button, inguinal region and pudenda is odorous.

Acupoints: Axilla (black point), Ji Quan (HT-1).

Moxibustion Method:

- Non-scarring Moxa: First shave the armpit, and then mix starch into a paste with an appropriate amount of water, applying it to the underarm. A needle-like black point will appear on the surface of starch paste; this is the area of a large sweat gland. Put a small moxa cone on the black point and perform direct moxa, 3–5 cones each time, 2 or 3 times per week.

- Pole Medicinal Moxa: Use 12g of Mi Tuo Seng (Lithargyrum) powder and an appropriate amount of flour and water to mix into a paste, put the paste on Ji Quan (HT-1), light the moxa stick and perform suspended moxa for 5–10 minutes. Perform treatment 3 times per day. Seven treatments comprise one course of treatment.

13. Eczema of the Scrotum

Eczema of the scrotum is the most common type of eczema. It is localized to the skin of the scrotum, sometimes spreads to the area around the anus, and can also spread to the penis. This patient experiences severe pruritus. The papules are pantomorphic and liable to recur. It has the following causes: long-term sitting in a humid environment and being invaded by damp, which becomes depressed and transforms to heat; or in the case of damp-heat in the lower burner, pathogenic wind attacks externally, causing wind, damp and heat pathogens to settle in the scrotum.

Main Symptoms: Pruritus scroti, flowing yellow exudate and scabs after scratching; then the skin thickens and tuberculum occurs, or even becomes infected and suppurates.

Acupoints: Xue Hai (SP-10), Zu San Li (ST-36), Shen Shu (BL-23), Yong Quan (KI-1), Tai Xi (KI-3).

Moxibustion Method:

- Pecking Sparrow Moxa: Apply moxa to 2–3 points, 6–20 minutes per point, once per day. Seven treatments comprise one course of treatment. (Figure 10.13.1)

- Gentle Pole Moxa: Apply moxa to 2–3 points in turn, 5–7 minutes per point, once per day. Seven treatments comprise one course of treatment, with a 3-day interval between the courses. (Figure 10.13.2)

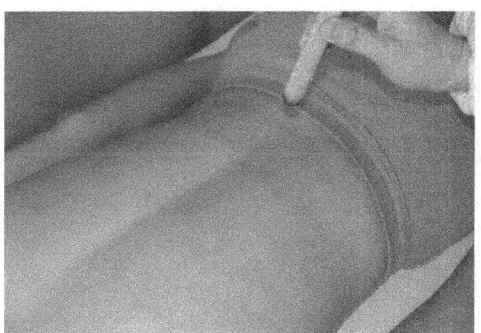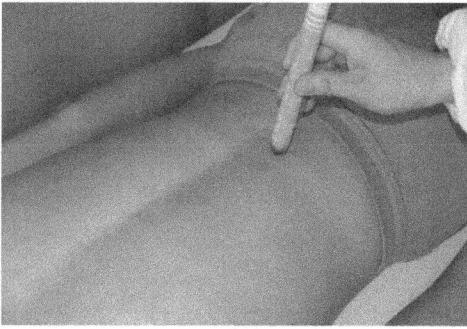

Figure 10.13.1 Pecking Sparrow Moxa at Shen Shu (BL-23)

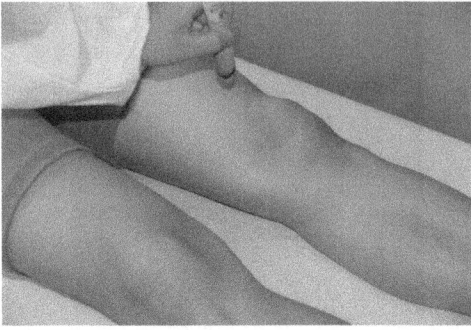

Figure 10.13.2 Gentle Pole Moxa at Xue Hai (SP-10)

14. Frostbite

Frostbite is a common disease in winter. Patients usually have a constitutional tendency toward frostbite and it recurs in the same location every winter. In Chinese medicine, frostbite is usually caused by one of the following: an inability of yang qi to defend the fleshy exterior, with additional invasion of cold pathogens causing an inhibited flow of qi and blood, and obstructed meridians and vessels. This brings about congealing and stagnation of the qi and blood of the skin.

Main Symptoms: Oedematous erythema appears on the affected region, as well as water blisters and even ulcers; accompanied by itching and pain that becomes aggravated by heat.

Acupoints: Ashi points.

Moxibustion Method:

- Pecking Sparrow Moxa: Light the moxa stick and use the pecking sparrow moxa technique to quickly tap the glowing tip of the stick on Ashi points, 2 or 3 times per second. The affected part feels a mild burning pain or burning sensation but will not scar. Perform treatment for 5–10 minutes, once per day or every other day. Seven treatments comprise one course of treatment.

- Moxa on Ginger: Apply 3–5 cones on each part, once per day. Five treatments comprise one course of treatment.

15. Appendicitis

In Chinese medicine, appendicitis falls within the definition of an intestinal welling abscess, which is one of the most common acute abdominal diseases seen in clinical practice. Appendicitis is caused by appendix obstruction and secondary infection, and an important physical sign is tenderness in the right lower abdominal quadrant. Appendicitis is usually caused by one of the following factors: eating and drinking without temperance, excessive cold or warmth, or urgent running causing qi stagnation and blood stasis, meridian vessel obstruction and binding depression of damp-heat.

Main Symptoms: The first symptom is paroxysmal pain in the mid-upper abdomen or around the umbilicus. After several hours, the pain radiates to the right lower quadrant. Lasting dull pain or paroxysmal colic accompanies mild chills and fever, nausea and vomiting.

Acupoints: Lan Wei Xue (EX-LE 7), Ashi points, right Tian Shu (ST-25), Guan Yuan (RN-4), Zhong Wan (RN-12), Qi Hai (RN-6), Ge Shu (BL-17), Xue Hai (SP-10), Da Chang Shu (BL-25).

Moxibustion Method:

- Non-scarring Moxa: Use moxa cones the size of a wheat-grain on 2–3 points in turn. Apply 3–5 cones per point, once per day. Seven treatments comprise one course of treatment. (Figure 10.15.1)

- Pecking Sparrow Moxa: Apply moxa to 2–3 points in turn. Light the moxa stick, use pecking sparrow moxa and quickly tap the glowing tip of the stick on Ashi points, 2 or 3 times per second. The affected part feels a mild burning pain or a burning sensation but does not scar. Perform treatment for 5–10 minutes, once per day or every other day. Seven treatments comprise one course of treatment. (Figure 10.15.2)

- Gentle Pole Moxa: Apply moxa to 2–3 points in turn, 5–7 minutes per point, once per day. Seven treatments comprise one course of treatment, with a 3-day interval between the courses. (Figure 10.15.3)

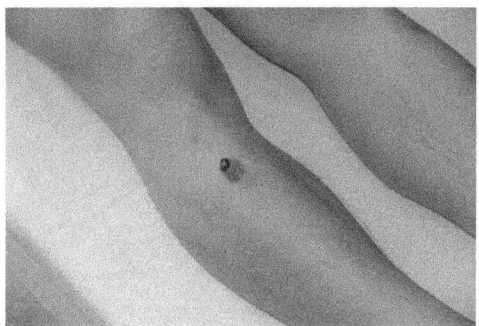

Figure 10.15.1 Non-scarring Moxa at Lan Wei Xue (EX-LE-7)

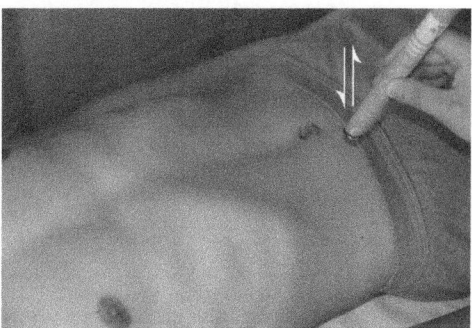

Figure 10.15.2 Pecking Sparrow Moxa at Right Tian Shu (ST-25)

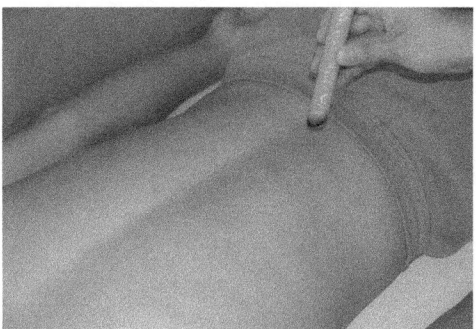

Figure 10.15.3 Gentle Pole Moxa at Da Chang Shu (BL-25)

16. Multiple Furuncles

Multiple furuncles are an acute purulent disease occurring on the superficial skin. There are several different types: a furuncle with a 'head' is called a folliculus pili furuncle while a headless furuncle is called a sweat gland furuncle, and summer suppurative boils occur between summer and autumn. Multiple furuncles attack recurrently and stay unresolved for a long time or if they are not treated properly will result in perforated folliculitis. This disease is often seen on the head, face and nape. It can occur in any individual but is most common in children.

Main Symptoms: Several furuncles appear that are red, swollen, hot and painful, protruding and with swollen potential; they may be accompanied by exterior syndrome or systemic symptoms; the course of disease is lingering and attacks recurrently.

Acupoints: Ling Tai (DU-10), Shen Zhu (DU-12), He Gu (LI-4), Wei Zhong (BL-40), Wai Guan (SJ-5), Ashi points.

Moxibustion Method:

- Moxa on Garlic: Apply moxa to 2–3 points in turn. Slice fresh large garlic cloves into pieces approximately 0.3–0.4cm and puncture the middle of each slice with a pin. Apply 7–9 cones every time, once or twice per day. (Figure 10.16.1)

- Gentle Pole Moxa: Apply moxa to 2–3 points in turn, for 5–7 minutes per point, once per day. Seven treatments comprise one course of treatment, with a 3-day interval between each course. It is applicable at the early stages of the disease. (Figure 10.16.2)

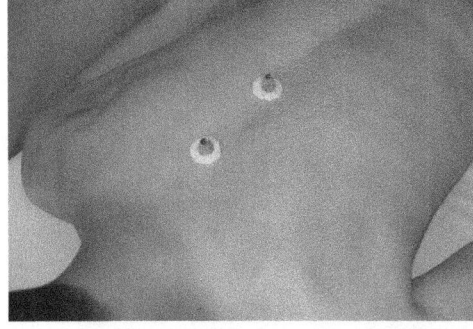 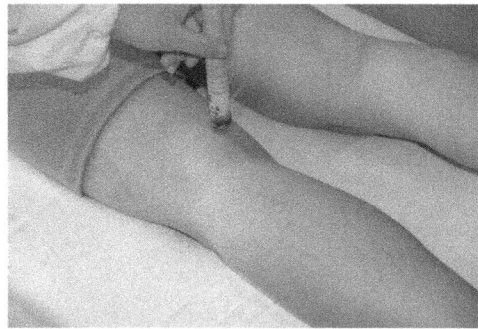

Figure 10.16.1 Moxa on Garlic at Ling Tai (DU-10) and Shen Zhu (DU-12)   *Figure 10.16.2 Gentle Pole Moxa at Wei Zhong (BL-40)*

- Juncibustion:* 2–3 Ashi points, once per day, repeated every other day. (Figure 10.16.3)

- Non-scarring Moxa: Apply moxa cones the size of a wheat-grain to 2–3 points in turn. Apply 3–5 cones per point, once per day. Three treatments comprise one course of treatment. (Figure 10.16.4)

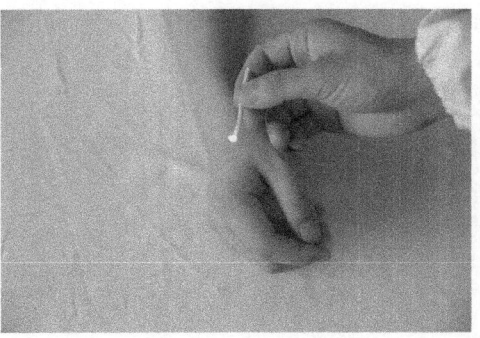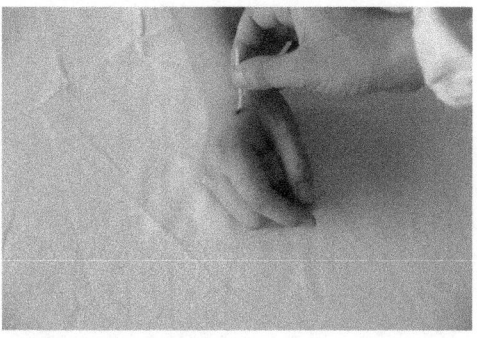

Figure 10.16.3 Juncibustion at He Gu (LI-4)

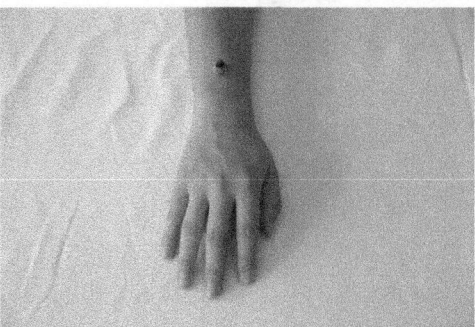

Figure 10.16.4 Non-scarring Moxa at Wai Guan (SJ-5)

17. Furunculosis

Furunculosis is a common emergency condition seen in the surgical department. It is small and has a deep, nail-like hard root. Furunculosis is usually caused by external contraction of wind pathogens and toxic fire, or traumato-infection. This disease is often seen on the face, limbs and torso.

Main Symptoms: In the early stages it appears as a millet-sized boil of a pustular shape and of various colours (yellow, white, purple or yellow-white). The root is hard, swollen, itchy and painful; it is usually accompanied by alternating cold and heat patterns, and maybe resulting from septicemic furunculosis, following ulceration and suppuration.

Acupoints: Shen Zhu (DU-12), Ling Tai (DU-10), He Gu (LI-4), Wei Zhong (BL-40), Ashi points.

Moxibustion Method:

- Moxa on Garlic: Apply moxa to 2–3 points in turn. Slice fresh garlic (large cloves) into pieces approximately 0.3–0.4cm and puncture the middle of each slice with a pin. Apply 7–9 cones every time, once or twice per day. Seven treatments comprise one course of treatment. (Figure 10.17.1)

- Gentle Pole Moxa: Apply moxa to 2–3 points in turn, for 5–7 minutes per point, once per day. Seven treatments comprise one course of treatment, with a 3-day interval between courses. (Figure 10.17.2)

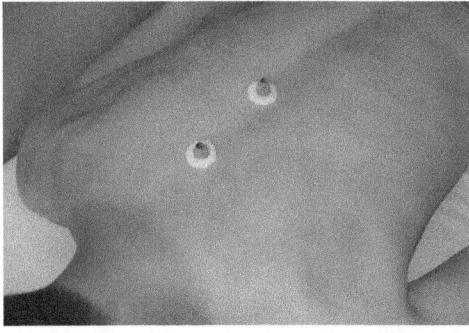

Figure 10.17.1 Moxa on Garlic at Shen Zhu (DU-12) and Ling Tai (DU-10)

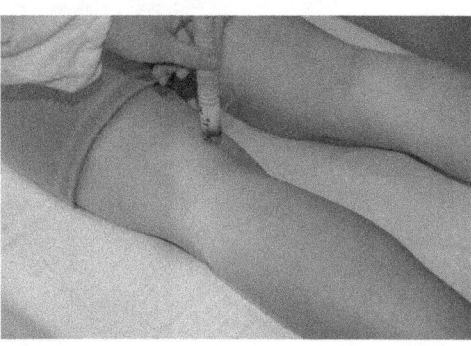

Figure 10.17.2 Gentle Pole Moxa at Wei Zhong (BL-40)

18. Angileucitis

Angileucitis refers to inflammation of absorbent vessels and the surrounding tissue (Figure 10.18.1), which is caused by pathogenic bacteria spread into adjacent absorbent vessels via damaged skin or the focus of infection. It is often seen on the limbs. Superficial layer angileucitis appears as one or more red lines at the proximum of the wound, which are stiff and tender. This is accompanied by heat effusion, a fear of cold and general weakness.

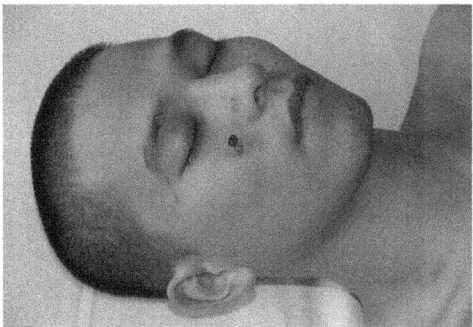

Figure 10.18.1 Angileucitis

Main Symptoms: Red ecphyma in the shape of lines appears on local skin. They effuse heat, and are tough and tender when palpated, so are also commonly known as red-thread clove sores.

Acupoints: Ashi points (at the head and root of red lines), acupoints which are adjacent or on both sides of red lines (3–5 points).

Moxibustion Method:

- Gentle Pole Moxa: Apply moxa slowly along red lines from the head to the root for 5–10 minutes, then 10–20 minutes per point, once per day. Three treatments comprise one course of treatment.

- Juncibustion:* Apply moxa on Ashi points, once per day, repeated every other day.

19. Mastitis

Acute mastitis is a kind of acute breast inflammation caused by bacterial infection. It often occurs in lactating women from 2 to 6 weeks post partum. The key symptoms are as follows: pain, swelling and distension of the affected mammary glands; regional stiffening, red skin with tenderness; enlargement of lymph nodes in the affected axillary region. The affected mammary glands often suppurate a few days after onset. This can be accompanied by a high fever, shivering, fatigue and a poor appetite. Mastitis falls within the scope of breast abscesses in TCM, which is an acute purulent disease.

Main Symptoms: Swelling and pain in the breast with or without a regional mass, white or red skin; scorching redness, swelling and pain followed by putridity, ulceration and suppuration in severe cases.

Acupoints: Jian Jing (GB-21), Ru Gen (ST-18), Qu Chi (LI-11), Zu San Li (ST-36), Ashi points.

Moxibustion Method:

- Gentle Moxa: Choose 2–3 acupoints in turn each time, moxa for 5–7 minutes per acupoint until local skin turns rosy, once daily, and 7 days for a course of treatment. (Figure 10.19.1)

- Pu Gong Ying Application: Mash an appropriate amount of Pu Gong Ying (Taraxaci Herba) into a paste. Apply the paste on acupoints or the affected areas and fix with gauze, once or twice a day. (Figure 10.19.2)

- Pole Moxa on Garlic Paste: In the initial stage of the disease, mash garlic into a paste and apply it to the acupoints. Apply hanging moxa for 6–20 minutes, once or twice a day. (Figure 10.19.3)

- Moxa on Fu Zi Cake: Apply the Fu Zi (Aconiti Radix Lateralis Praeparata) medicinal cake to Ashi points and then put moxa cones on the cake. Apply 3–5 cones per acupoint, once daily. (Figure 10.19.4)

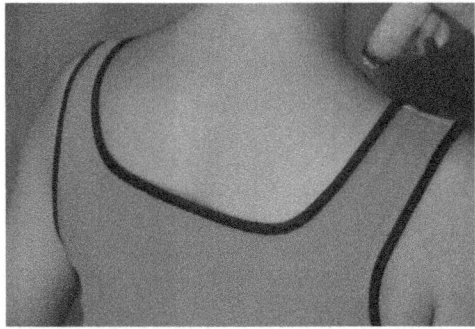

Figure 10.19.1 Gentle Moxa at Jian Jing (GB-21)

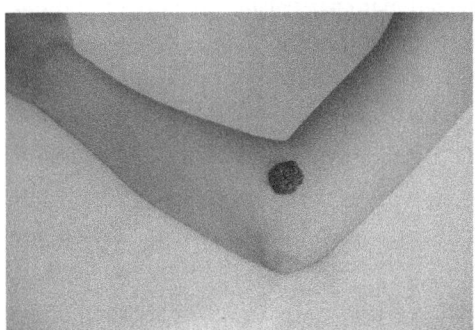
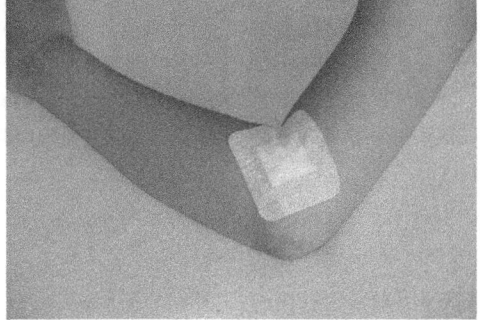

Figure 10.19.2 Pu Gong Ying Application at Qu Chi (LI-11)

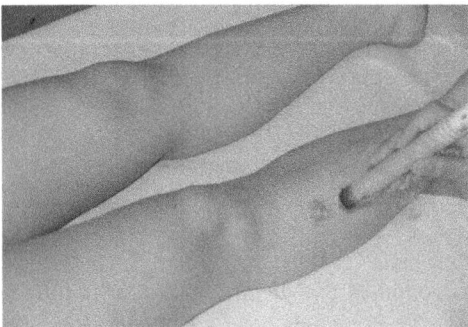
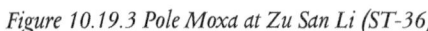
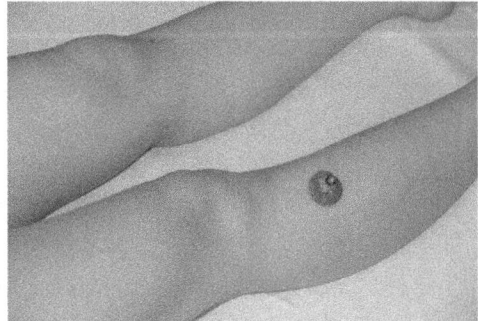

Figure 10.19.3 Pole Moxa at Zu San Li (ST-36)   *Figure 10.19.4 Moxa on Fu Zi Cake at Zu San Li (ST-36)*

20. Hyperplasia of the Mammary Gland

Hyperplasia of the mammary gland, also called cystic hyperplasia of the breast, is a breast stroma benign hypertrophic disease. The key symptoms are periodic aggravated distending pain in the breast and multiple breast lumps. The disease occurs or is aggravated during the premenstrual period. It often occurs in women between the ages of 25–40. This disease usually has the following causes: affect-mind internal damage causing liver depression, congealing phlegm gathering in the breast and the network vessels of the stomach; excessive thought damageing the spleen and depressed anger damageing the liver resulting in disharmony of the thoroughfare and controlling vessels, qi stagnating and congealing phlegm.

Main Symptoms: Breast lumps that are hard and like an egg in shape, periodic distending pain that is aggravated during the premenstrual period and is relieved or disappears at the postmenstrual stage; many soft or tough nodes of various sizes with clear margin and no adhesion. The nodes are mobile, and round or oval in shape without tenderness. No diabrosis and nipple retraction occurs. During pregnancy the lumps will grow rapidly, and some of them may turn malignant.

Acupoints: Ru Zhong (ST-17) (affected side), Zu San Li (ST-36), Tai Chong (LR-3), Qi Hai (RN-6), Tai Xi (KI-3).

Moxibustion Method:

- Pole Moxa: Apply stick moxa for 20–40 minutes each time, once daily, 10 times for a course of treatment. Repeat after 3 days. (Figure 10.20.1)

- Warm Needle Moxa: Choose the needles as long as 40mm (1.5 *cun*). Perform acupuncture using the draining method, manipulate the needles every 5 minutes and retain the needles with moxa cones for 30 minutes, once daily, 7 times for a course of treatment. (Figure 10.20.2)

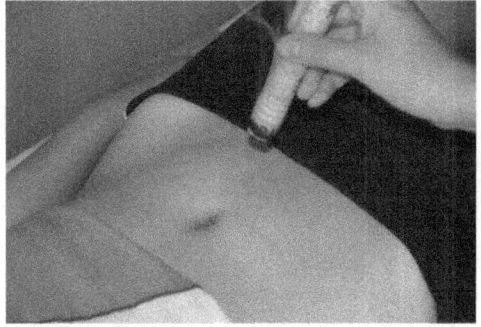
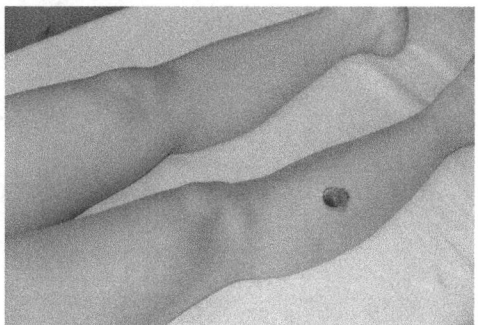

Figure 10.20.1 Pole Moxa at Qi Hai (RN-6)

Figure 10.20.2 Warm Needle Moxa at Zu San Li (ST-36)

21. Prostatitis

Prostatitis is an acute or chronic disease that is often seen in adult males. Chronic prostatitis is more common and marked by frequent and difficult urination, dribbling after voiding; or white urine, sagging distension in the perineum; or seminal emissions, premature ejaculation, impotence, accompanied by some constitutional symptoms such as dizziness and a lack of strength. The causes can be reduced to two key patterns: deficiency and excess. Deficiency refers to kidney qi and kidney essence depletion caused by insufficiency of congenital constitution or excessive damage to the acquired constitution; while excess refers to damp-heat in the lower energizer. Prostatitis falls within the category of seminal emissions, strangury patterns and dribbling urinary block in TCM.

Main Symptoms: Frequent and difficult urination, dribbling after voiding; white urine and sagging distension in the perineum; seminal emissions, premature ejaculation and impotence, accompanied by some constitutional symptoms such as dizziness and a lack of strength.

Acupoints: Guan Yuan (RN-4), Qi Hai (RN-6), Shen Shu (BL-23), San Yin Jiao (SP-6), Zhong Ji (RN-6).

Moxibustion Method:

- Gentle Moxa: Choose 2–3 acupoints in turn each time; apply moxa to each acupoint for 5–7 minutes until local skin turns rosy. Perform once daily, 7 days for a course of treatment. (Figure 10.21.1)

- Moxa on Ginger: Apply 3–5 cones per acupoint, once or twice a day, 7 days for a course of treatment. (Figure 10.21.2)

- Moxa on Garlic: Apply 7–9 cones per acupoint, once or twice a day, 7 days for a course of treatment. (Figure 10.21.3)

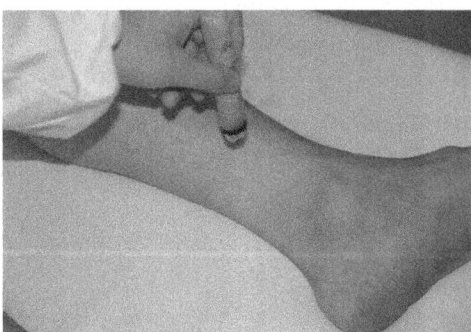

Figure 10.21.1 Gentle Moxa at San Yin Jiao (SP-6)

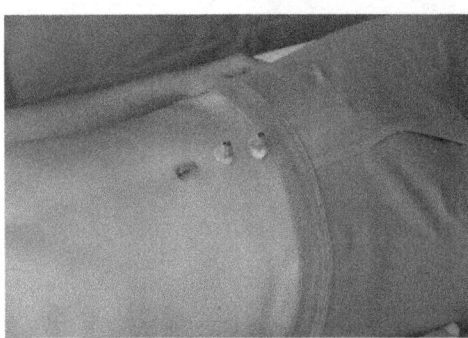

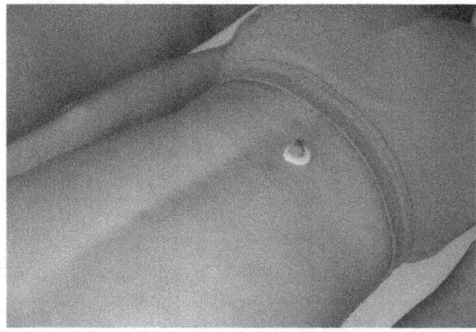

Figure 10.21.2 Moxa on Ginger at Guan Yuan (RN-4) and Qi Hai (RN-6)

Figure 10.21.3 Moxa on Garlic at Shen Shu (BL-23)

22. Haemorrhoids

Haemorrhoids are soft haemangioma consisting of dilated and varicose veins of the distal rectal submucosa and peripheral anal subcutis. According to the location, haemorrhoids are classified into three types: the internal, external and mixed haemorrhoids. When haemorrhoid pain attacks, the key symptoms are bloody stools, pain, prolapse of the rectum and sagging distension. The disease is also called haemorrhoids in TCM. The pathogenic basis of haemorrhoids is considered to be root vacuity of the viscera and bowels, depletion of qi and blood. This disease usually has the following causes: disharmony of yin-yang, inhibited movement of qi and blood, obstruction of meridian and collateral, dry heat arising internally, blood and heat contending with each other, obstruction of the meridians and collaterals, which are induced by affect-mind internal damage, excessive taxation, perennial constipation, dietary irregularities and pregnancy.

Main Symptoms: Sarcoid protuberance in the anorectal area with pain, swelling and distension; sometimes bloody stools. Internal haemorrhoids are located inside the anus (above the dentate line); external haemorrhoids are located outside the anus (below the dentate line); mixed haemorrhoids are found inside and outside the anus. Anaemia caused by perennial bloody stools can result with some new symptoms such as dizziness, blurred vision and a lack of strength.

Acupoints: Ba Liao (BL-31~34), Shen Que (RN-8).

Moxibustion Method:

- Pole Moxa: Apply circling moxa for 10 minutes, then apply pecking sparrow moxa for 3–5 minutes until the patient feels scorching heat. Perform once every other day, 10 times for a course of treatment. (Figure 10.22.1)

- Moxa on Ginger: Apply 3–5 cones per acupoint, once or twice a day, until the symptoms disappear. (Figure 10.22.2)

- Moxa on Salt: Apply 7–10 cones per acupoint, once daily, 3 days for a course of treatment. (Figure 10.22.3)

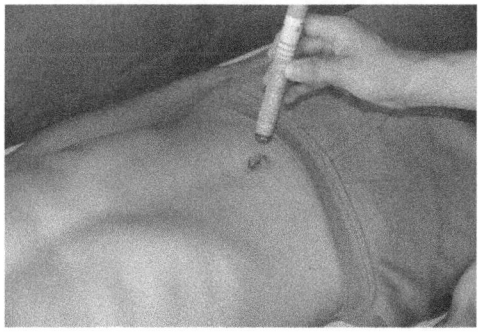

Figure 10.22.1 Pole Moxa at Shen Que (RN-8)

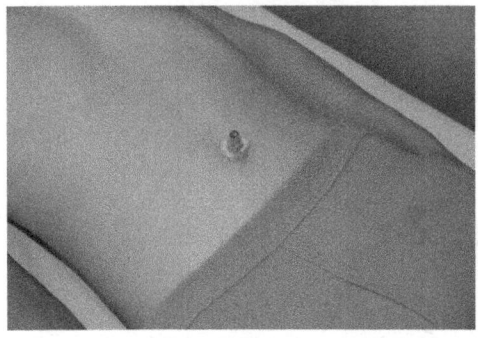

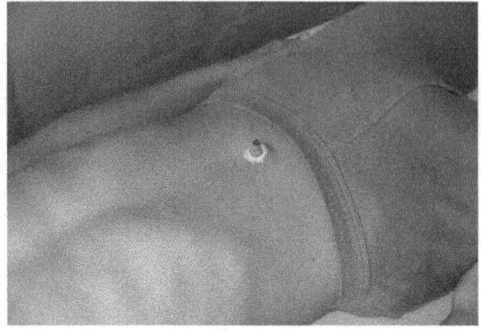

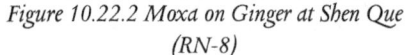

Figure 10.22.2 Moxa on Ginger at Shen Que (RN-8)

Figure 10.22.3 Moxa on Salt at Shen Que (RN-8)

23. Thecal Cyst

Thecal cysts are a manifestation caused by degenerated connective tissue around a joint capsule (Figure 10.23.1). It is characterized by soft, removable and dome-like cysts under the skin, which are often found in the centre of the wrist. The cyst under the skin is plump with fluctuation, accompanied by weakness of the wrist with discomfort, pain or dysfunction. The disease is known as a sinew tumour in TCM. This condition usually has the following causes: taxation detriment or injury causing qi stagnation and blood stasis, blood failing to nourish the sinews and gathering phlegm-stasis.

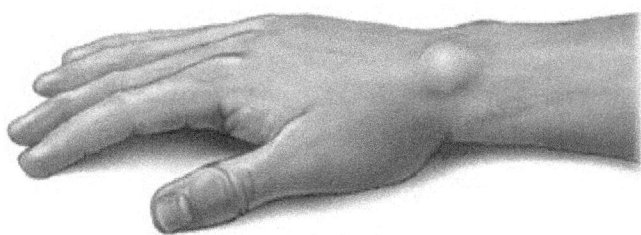

Figure 10.23.1 Thecal Cyst

Main Symptoms: Small lumps that are round or oval in shape, and soft with slight fluctuation at first; then the lumps will become smaller and harder after fibrosis. The patient will feel an aching pain or weakness when the lumps are pressed.

Acupoints: Ashi points (at the cyst).

Moxibustion Method:

- Moxa on Ginger: Apply 3–5 cones per acupoint, once or twice a day, until the symptoms disappear.

- Gentle Moxa: Choose 2–3 acupoints in turn each time; apply moxa to each acupoint for 5–7 minutes until the local skin turns rosy. Perform once daily, 7 days for a course of treatment.

24. Proctoptosis

Proctoptosis is a chronic condition characterized by the downward displacement of the rectal mucosa, anal tube, rectum and some parts of the sigmoid colon, with external prolapse of the anus. The key symptoms are rectal mucosal prolapse and painful sagging of the lower abdomen when performing bowel movements. Symptoms also include congestion of the rectal mucosa, oedema, ulcers and bleeding in severe cases. The disease is known as prolapse of the rectum in TCM. This condition usually has the following causes: insufficiency of qi and blood, downward movement due to qi deficiency and damp-heat descending into the large intestine.

Main Symptoms: Rectal mucosal prolapse, painful sagging of the lower abdomen, incomplete bowel movements; congestion of rectal mucosa, oedema, ulcers and bleeding in severe cases.

Acupoints: Bai Hui (DU-20), Chang Qiang (DU-1), Da Chang Shu (BL-25), Shang Ju Xu (ST-37), Pi Shu (BL-20), Shen Shu (BL-23), Qi Hai (RN-6), Guan Yuan (RN-4).

Moxibustion Method:

- Pole Moxa: Apply moxa to each acupoint for 5–7 minutes until local skin turns rosy. Once daily, 7 days for a course of treatment. Repeat after 3 days. (Figure 10.24.1)

- Moxa on Ginger: Mainly used in infantile proctoptosis and on Bai Hui (DU-20) only. Ask the parents to encourage the child to sit up. Rub the acupoint until it feels hot and apply moxa on ginger. The ginger slice should be approximately 2.5cm thick, and the cones should be as small as a mung bean. Apply 2–4 cones, once daily, repeat for 3 days. (Figure 10.24.2)

- Moxa on Bi Ma Ren Cake: Put a Bi Ma Ren (Ricini Semen) cake on the acupoint, then apply 3–5 cones as large as wheat kernels, once every other day, 8 days for a course of treatment. (Figure 10.24.3)

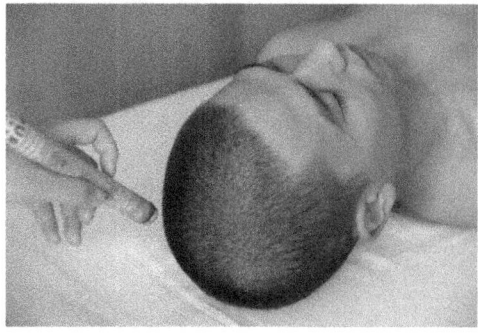

Figure 10.24.1 Pole Moxa at Bai Hui (DU-20)

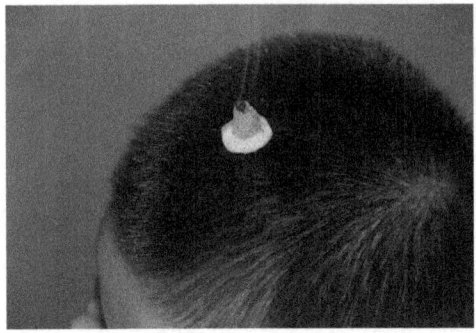

*Figure 10.24.2 Moxa on Ginger at Bai Hui
(DU-20)*

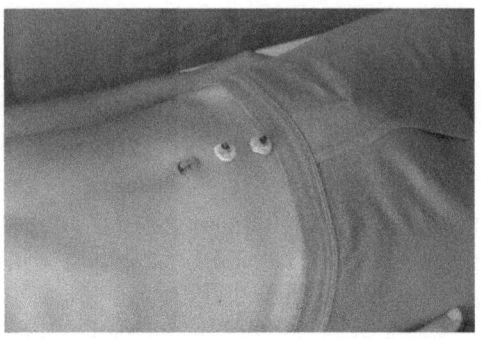

*Figure 10.24.3 Moxa on Bi Ma Ren Cake at Qi Hai
(RN-6) and Guan Yuan (RN-4)*

25. Cholelithiasis

Cholelithiasis is a disease caused by stones in the biliary duct and gall bladder. The key symptoms are severe abdominal pain, jaundice and fever. It is the most common disease of the biliary tract, and falls within the scope of gallbladder distension, lateral rib pain and jaundice. This disease usually has the following causes: spleen-stomach vacuity resulting in damp-phlegm obstruction of qi movement; internal collection of stasis which transforms into heat to decoct bile; coagulation of phlegm and static blood to form stones.

Main Symptoms: Severe gripping pain in the gall bladder area, nausea and vomiting accompanied by various degrees of jaundice and high fever.

Acupoints: Dan Shu (BL-19), Gan Shu (BL-18), Ri Yue (GB-24), Qi Men (LR-14), Yang Ling Quan (GB-34), Dan Nang Xue (EX-LE-6), Tai Chong (LR-3).

Moxibustion Method:

- Pole Moxa: Choose 2–3 acupoints in turn for each treatment. Apply moxa to each acupoint for 5–7 minutes until the local skin turns rosy. Perform once daily, 7 days for a course of treatment. Repeat after 3 days. (Figure 10.25.1)

- Non-scarring Moxa: Choose 2–3 acupoints in turn for each treatment. Apply 3–5 cones to each acupoint, once daily, 3 days constitutes a course of treatment. (Figure 10.25.2)

- Juncibustion:* Choose 1–2 acupoints in turn for each treatment. Apply juncibustion once daily or every other day, 3 times for a course of treatment. (Figure 10.25.3)

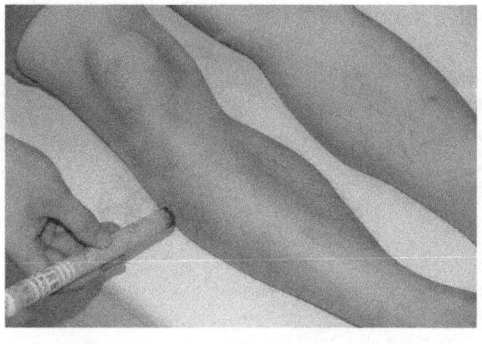

Figure 10.25.1 Pole Moxa at Dan Nang Xue (EX-LE-6)

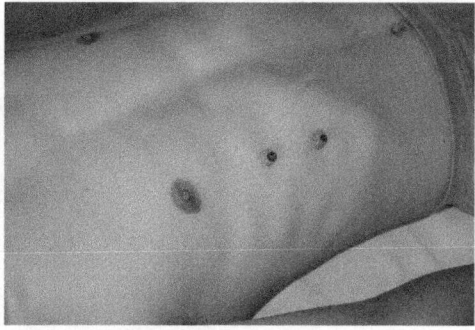

Figure 10.25.2 Non-scarring Moxa at Ri Yue (GB-24) and Qi Men (LR-14)

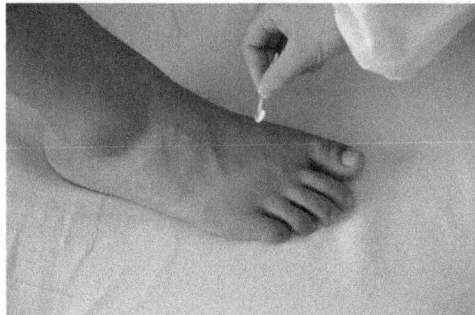

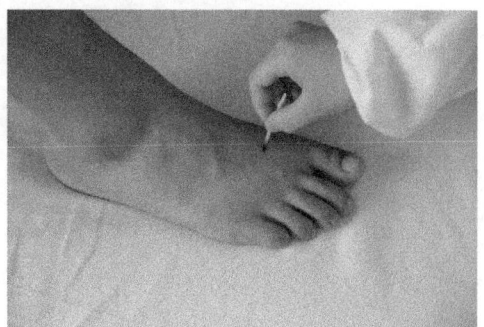

Figure 10.25.3 Juncibustion at Tai Chong (LR-3)

26. Urinary Calculus

Urinary calculus is a common condition of the urinary system. It can occur in any part of the urinary system, but usually originates in the kidney. The onset is sudden with severe lumbar pain that is continuous or intermittent, radiating to the iliac fossa, perineum and scrotum along the ureter. Other symptoms include bloody urine, pyuria, dysuria or urinary stoppage. Urinary calculus is known as stone strangury in TCM. This disease usually has the following causes: damp-heat brewing and binding in the lower burner, long-term storage of urine causing impurities in the urine to coagulate to form stones.

Main Symptoms: Sudden onset with severe lumbar pain which is either continuous or intermittent, radiating to the iliac fossa, perineum and scrotum along the ureter; bloody urine, pyuria, dysuria or urinary stoppage.

Acupoints: Shen Shu (BL-23), Guan Yuan (RN-4), Yin Ling Quan (SP-9).

Moxibustion Method:

- Gentle Pole Moxa: Choose 2–3 acupoints in turn for each treatment, then apply moxa for 5–7 minutes per acupoint until local skin turns rosy, once daily; 7 days comprise a course of treatment. (Figure 10.26.1)

- Moxa on Ginger: Apply 3–5 cones per acupoint, once or twice a day; 7 days comprise a course of treatment. (Figure 10.26.2)

- Moxa on Garlic: Apply 7–9 cones per acupoint, once or twice a day; 7 days comprise a course of treatment. (Figure 10.26.3)

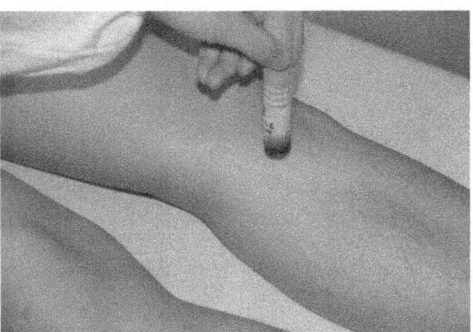

Figure 10.26.1 Gentle Pole Moxa at Yin Ling Quan (SP-9)

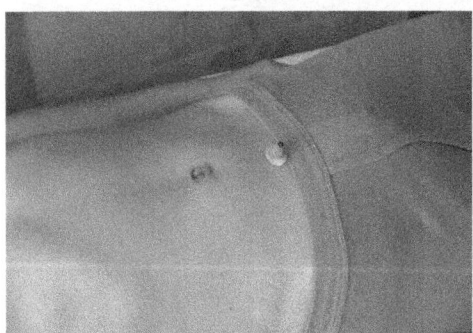

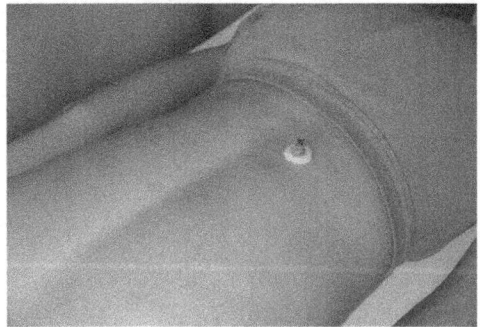

Figure 10.26.2 Moxa on Ginger at Guan Yuan (RN-4)

Figure 10.26.3 Moxa on Garlic at Shen Shu (BL-23)

CHAPTER 11

Ear, Nose and Throat Diseases

1. Conjunctivitis

Conjunctivitis refers to all kinds of inflammatory reactions of the conjunctiva caused by pathogenic factors from either the environment or the body itself. The manifestations are as follows: conjunctival hyperaemia induced by infection, allergy or trauma; effusion, papillary hypertrophy or follicles. The main cause of the disease is inflammation induced by exposure of the conjunctiva to various microbes, dust particles, physical and chemical toxicants. It is called 'heaven-current red eye' in TCM, and also commonly known as 'pinkeye'.

Main Symptoms: Sudden conjunctival congestion, burning and itching, with excessive secretions and no effect on vision. On examination, other symptoms include red and swollen eyelids, conjunctival congestion, hyperplasia of the follicular papilla, peripheral congestion of bulbar conjunctiva and sometimes subconjunctival haemorrhage and secretions in the conjunctival sac.

Acupoints: He Gu (LI-4), Feng Chi (GB-20), Tai Yang (EX-HN-5), Shao Shang (LU-11).

Moxibustion Method:

- Hanging Moxa: Apply moxa for 5–15 minutes per acupoint, once daily. Three days comprise a course of treatment. (Figure 11.1.1)

- Gentle Moxa: Apply moxa for 5–15 minutes per acupoint, once daily. Three days comprise a course of treatment. (Figure 11.1.2)

- Pecking Sparrow Moxa: Apply moxa for 5–15 minutes per acupoint, once daily. Three days comprise a course of treatment. (Figure 11.1.3)

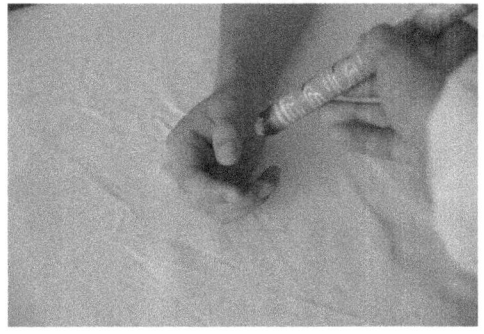

Figure 11.1.1 Hanging Moxa at Shao Shang (LU-11)

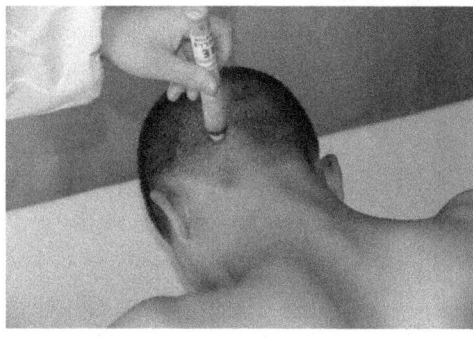

Figure 11.1.2 Gentle Moxa at Feng Chi (GB-20)

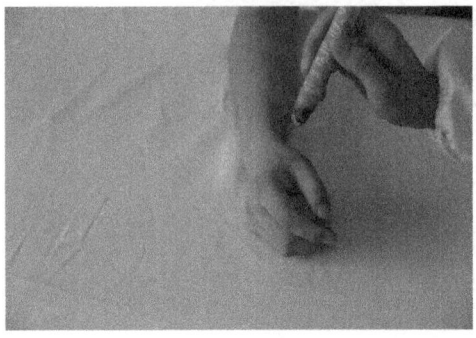 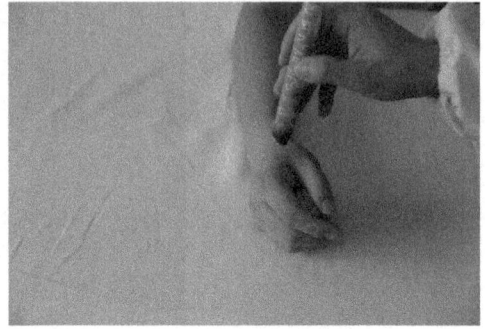

Figure 11.1.3 Pecking Sparrow Moxa at He Gu (LI-4)

- Moxa on Garlic: Apply 5–10 cones, the size of a jujube pit, per acupoint, 3 times constitutes a course of treatment. (Figure 11.1.4)

- Moxa on Mao Gen: Apply Mao Gen (Ranunculi Japonici) to the normal eye. If both eyes are infected, apply medication to both. Retain the herb for 5–15 minutes per acupoint, and perform once daily. Three days comprise a course of treatment. (Figure 11.1.5)

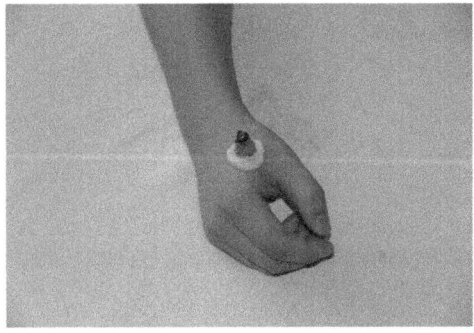 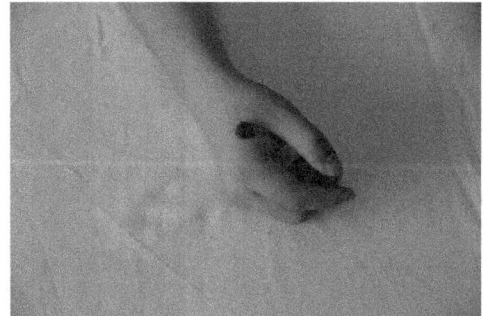

Figure 11.1.4 Moxa on Garlic at He Gu (LI-4)   *Figure 11.1.5 Moxa on Mao Gen at He Gu (LI-4)*

2. Keratitis

There are two types of keratitis; ulcerative keratitis (keratohelcosis) and non-ulcerative keratitis (deep keratitis). External injury causing trauma to the cornea and allowing bacteria and virus to invade the corneal epithelium is the most common causative factor for this condition.

Main Symptoms: Subjective sensation of a foreign object in the eye, a stabbing pain and burning; mixed congestion on the surface of bulbar conjunctiva, with photophobia, lacrimation, visual defects and increased secretion.

Acupoints: Cuan Zhu (BL-2), Si Zhu Kong (SJ-23), Tai Yang (EX-HN-5), Tong Zi Liao (GB-1), He Gu (LI-4), Zu San Li (ST-36).

Moxibustion Method:

- Warm Needle Moxa: Apply 3–5 cones (or for 15–20 minutes) per acupoint, once daily, 7 days constitute a course of treatment. (Figure 11.2.1)

- Moxa on Garlic: Choose 1–2 acupoints each time; apply 3–5 cones on the acupoints of the healthy side. If both eyes are infected, apply moxa cones to both sides. Once daily, 7 days constitute a course of treatment. (Figure 11.2.2)

- Pecking Sparrow Moxa: Apply moxa 6–15 minutes per acupoint, once or twice a day, 7 times for a course of treatment. (Figure 11.2.3)

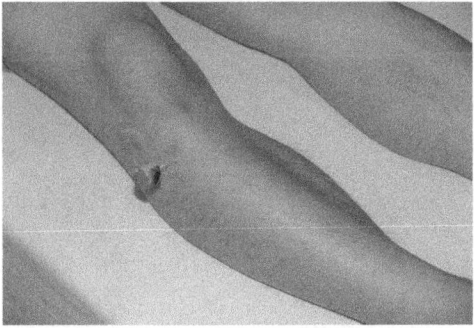 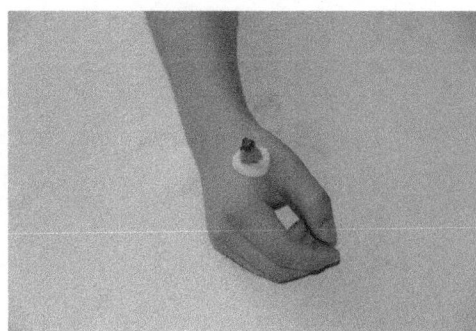

Figure 11.2.1 Warm Needle Moxa at Zu San Li (ST-36)   *Figure 11.2.2 Moxa on Garlic at He Gu (LI-4)*

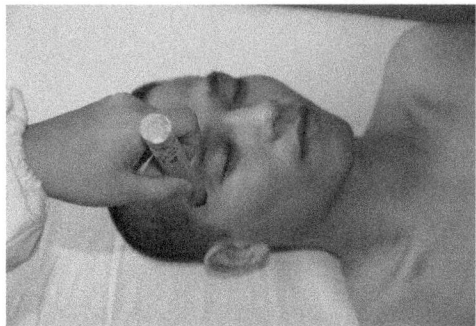 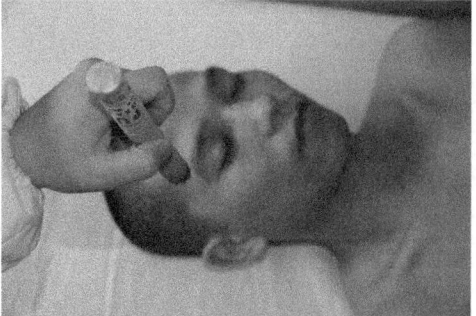

Figure 11.2.3 Pecking Sparrow Moxa at Tai Yang (EX-HN-5)

3. Myopia

Myopia is a condition characterized by impaired long-distance vision with unimpaired vision at close range. The main causes of the disease are as follows: excessive reading, writing or working for long periods in poor lighting or with incorrect posture. TCM asserts that the liver stores blood and opens into the eyes; the eyes require sufficient blood to function properly. Persistent or excessive use of the eyes or a lack of the nourishment of blood can cause myopia.

Main Symptoms: Impaired long-distance vision with unimpaired vision at close range. The diminution of vision and myopic degree are out of proportion. Additional symptoms may include exotropia or asthenopia. Pathological myopia may be associated with retinopathy.

Acupoints: Tai Yang (EX-HN-5), Yang Bai (GB-14), Zu San Li (ST-36), Guang Ming (GB-37).

Moxibustion Method:

- Gentle Moxa: Apply moxa for 5–15 minutes per acupoint, once every other day, 10 times constitute a course of treatment. (Figure 11.3.1)

- Moxa on He Tao Pi (Juglandis Semen): Apply 3–9 cones to the eye area, once every other day, 10 times constitute a course of treatment. (Figure 11.3.2)

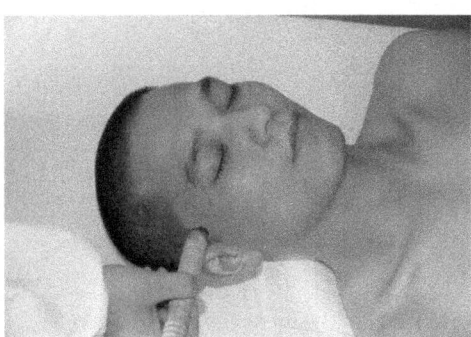

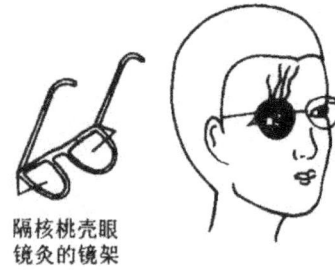

隔核桃壳眼
镜灸的镜架

Figure 11.3.1 Gentle Moxa at Tai Yang (EX-HN-5)   *Figure 11.3.2 Moxa on He Tao Pi on the Eye Area*

4. Hyperopia (Farsightedness)

Hyperopia is an ametropic ocular condition that often occurs in youngsters and children. This condition usually has the following causes: blastocolysis caused by inherent and external environmental factors, an abnormal length of the axis oculi, or a low degree of surface curvature of any of the refractive bodies that are necessary for ocular refraction.

Main Symptoms: In severe cases, the patient cannot see any peripheral objects, so the visual symptoms are obvious. Whereas mild cases present with refractive defects that can be overcome by regulation, there may be no visual symptoms. Teenagers have strong abilities to self-regulate and may present with no visual symptoms even in moderate cases.

Acupoints:

- *Primary points:* Jing Ming (BL-1), Yu Yao (EX-HN-4), Tai Yang (EX-HN-5).

- *Symptomatic points:* Blurred vision: Gan Shu (BL-18); limp aching lumbar region and knees: Shen Shu (BL-23).

Moxibustion Method:

- Gentle Moxa: Apply moxa for 5–15 minutes per acupoint, once every other day, 10 times constitute a course of treatment. (Figure 11.4.1)

- Medicinal Moxa: Grind 20g of Jue Ming Zi (Cassiae Semen) and 10g of Zhen Zhu Fen (Margarita Pulverata) into a fine powder, and then mix well with an appropriate amount of vinegar. Apply the paste to Gan Shu (BL-18) and Shen Shu (BL-23) and fix with gauze, once every other day. (Figure 11.4.2)

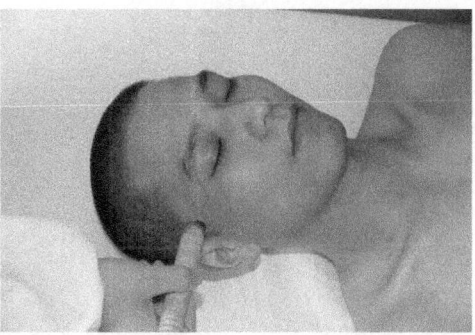

Figure 11.4.1 Gentle Moxa at Tai Yang (EX-HN-5)

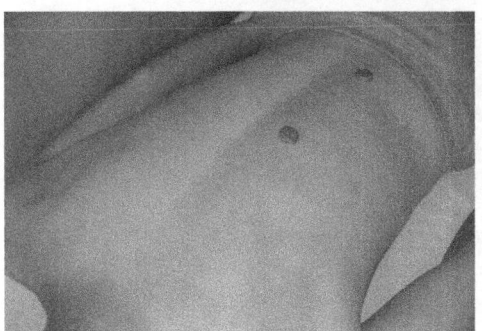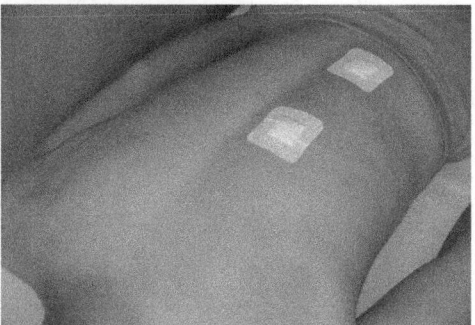

Figure 11.4.2 Medicinal Moxa at Gan Shu (BL-18) and Shen Shu (BL-23)

5. Wind Induced Tearing

Wind induced tearing manifests as an increased number of tears when exposed to cold wind. This condition usually has the following causes: liver-kidney yin deficiency, failure of the kidney to receive qi and external stimulation of cold wind. Tears are one of the five humours of the human body. Excessive tearing can cause blurred vision and severe loss of vision.

Main Symptoms: In some cases, there are no abnormal phenomena, red eyes, swelling or itching. However, when exposed to wind, the patient experiences an involuntary production of excessive tears, resulting in blurred vision.

Acupoints: Gan Shu (BL-18), Shen Shu (BL-23), Gao Huang Shu (BL-43), Zhong Ji (RN-3), Zu San Li (ST-36).

Moxibustion Method:

- Pecking Sparrow Moxa: Apply moxa for 5–10 minutes per acupoint, once daily, 10 treatments constitute a course of treatment. (Figure 11.5.1)

- Moxa on Ginger: Apply 5–10 cones the size of a jujube pit per acupoint, once daily, 10 treatments constitute a course of treatment. (Figure 11.5.2)

- Warm Needle Moxa: Apply 3–5 cones (or 15–20 minutes) per acupoint, once every other day, 7 times for a course of treatment. (Figure 11.5.3)

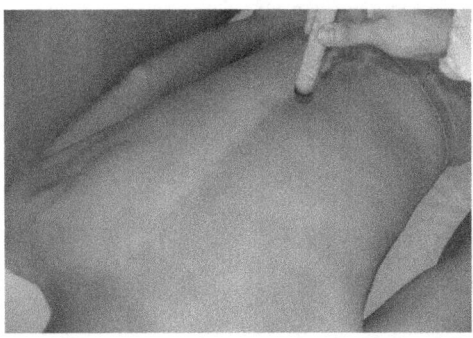
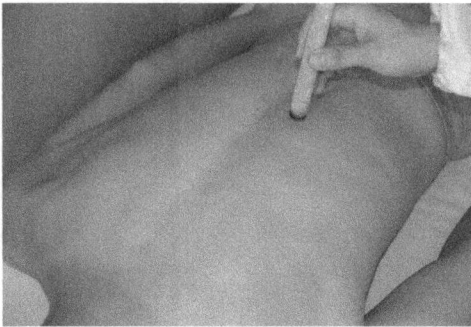

Figure 11.5.1 Pecking Sparrow Moxa at Gan Shu (BL-18)

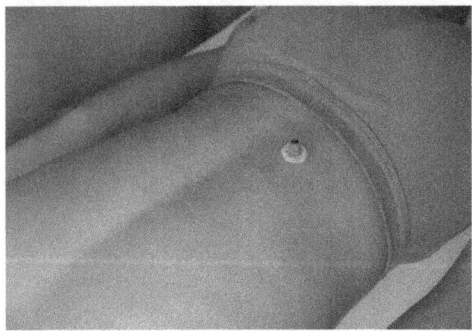
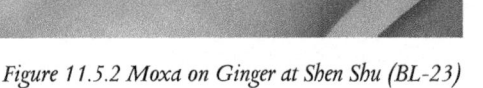
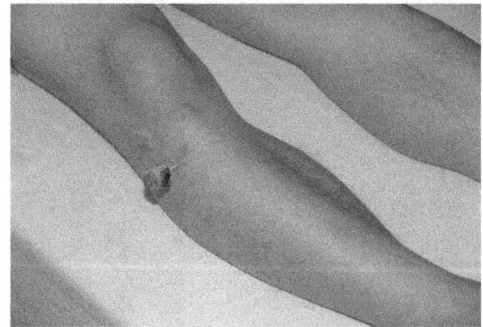

Figure 11.5.2 Moxa on Ginger at Shen Shu (BL-23)   *Figure 11.5.3 Warm Needle Moxa at Zu San Li (ST-36)*

6. Ptosis

Ptosis refers to a drooping of the eyelid due to palpabralis dysfunction or other reasons. The condition can be divided into congenital or acquired ptosis. The congenital form is mainly caused by dysplasia of the oculomotor nucleus or palpabralis, which is an autosomal dominant condition. The acquired type is induced by oculomotor nerve palsy, palpabralis injury, sympathetic nerve disease, myasthenia gravis or mechanical open eyelid movement disorders.

Main Symptoms: Partial or complete ptosis resulting in impaired vision. In congenital cases amblyopia can occur. Where the ptosis occurs in one eye, the patient will often frown in order to see clearly resulting in an increase in contralateral fissurae palpebrae. When ptosis occurs bilaterally the patient has to raise their head to see.

Acupoints: Bai Hui (DU-20), Yong Quan (KI-1), Yang Bai (GB-14), Zu San Li (ST-36), San Yin Jiao (SP-6).

Moxibustion Method:

- Moxa on Ginger: Apply moxa for 6–20 minutes per acupoint, twice a day, 10 treatments constitute a course of treatment. (Figure 11.6.1)

- Non-scarring Moxa: Apply 5 cones the size of a soybean per acupoint, once daily, 10 treatments constitute a course of treatment. Repeat after one week. (Figure 11.6.2)

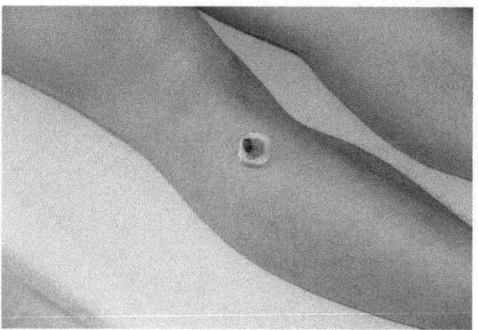
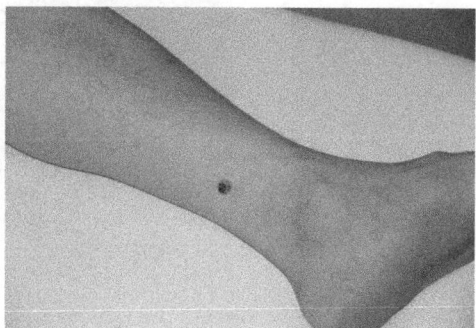

Figure 11.6.1 Moxa on Ginger at Zu San Li (ST-36)

Figure 11.6.2 Non-scarring Moxa at San Yin Jiao (SP-6)

7. Tinnitus and Deafness

Tinnitus is characterized by a ringing sound in the ears resembling the chirp of a cicada or the ocean tide. Deafness refers to either complete hearing loss or various degrees of hearing loss. Tinnitus can accompany deafness and deafness can originate from tinnitus. The conditions usually have the following causes: sudden violent anger, fright or fear, liver-gallbladder wind-fire surging upward resulting in obstruction of meridian qi; externally contracted wind-cold causing congestion in the clear orifices; or kidney qi deficiency leading to a failure of essential qi to reach the ears.

Main Symptoms: Deafness manifested as hearing difficulties in public areas. Tinnitus can be accompanied by deafness and dizziness that can spontaneously disappear or continue for months, years or even a lifetime.

Acupoints: Yi Feng (SJ-17), Tai Xi (KI-3), Yang Ling Quan (GB-34), Ting Gong (SI-19), Da Zhui (DU-14), Zhong Zhu (SJ-3).

Moxibustion Method:

- Non-suppurative Moxa: Apply 1–3 cones on Yi Feng (SJ-17), Ting Gong (SI-19), Da Zhui (DU-14) and Zhong Zhu (SJ-3), and 3–7 cones on Yang Ling Quan (GB-34) and Tai Xi (KI-3). Execute once daily; 10 treatments constitute a course of treatment. Repeat the treatment course after 5–7 days. (Figure 11.7.1)

- Gentle Moxa: Apply moxa for 5–10 minutes per acupoint, once daily, 10 times for a course of treatment. Repeat the treatment course after 5–7 days. (Figure 11.7.2)

- Moxa on Ginger: Apply 5–7 cones per acupoint, once daily or every other day, 10 treatments constitute a course of treatment. Repeat after 3–5 days. (Figure 11.7.3)

- Moxa on Cang Zhu (Rhizoma Atractylodis): Apply 5–7 cones per acupoint, once daily or every other day, 10 times for a course of treatment. Repeat after 3–5 days. (Figure 11.7.4)

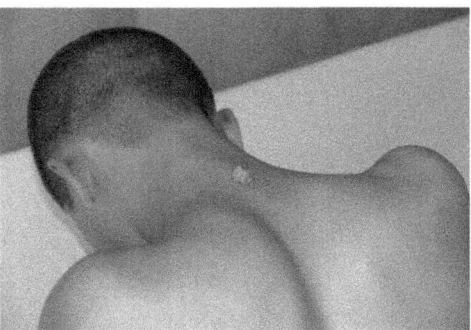

Figure 11.7.1 Non-suppurative Moxa at Da Zhui (DU-14)

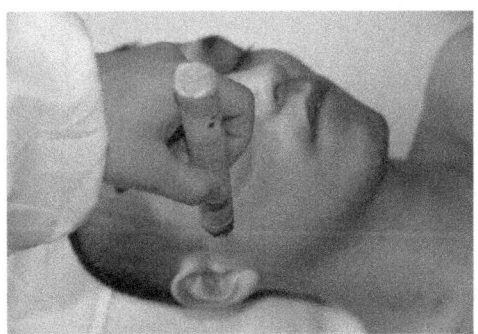

Figure 11.7.2 Gentle Moxa at Ting Gong (SI-19)

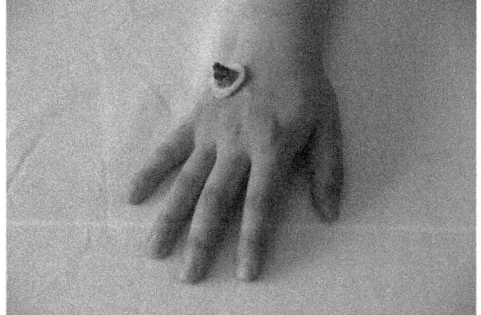

Figure 11.7.3 Moxa on Ginger at Zhong Zhu (SJ-3)

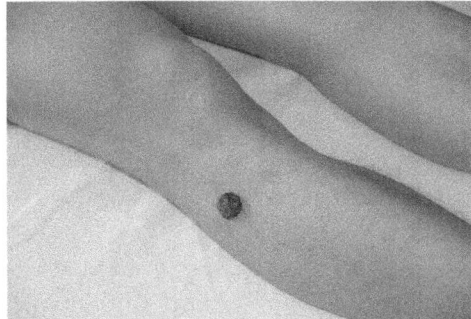

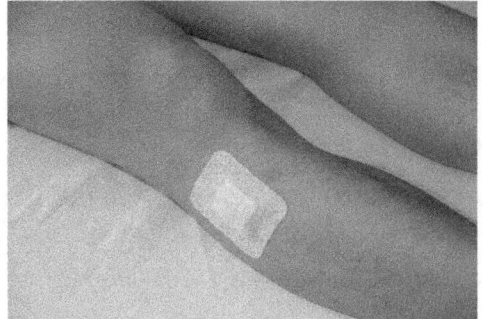

Figure 11.7.4 Moxa on Cang Zhu at Yang Ling Quan (GB-34)

8. Aural Vertigo

Aural vertigo, also known as Meniere's disease refers to vertigo caused by dysfunction of the vestibular labyrinth. The condition usually has the following causes: kidney qi deficiency causing a disturbance of qi transformation and a flooding upwards of water-dampness to the clear orifices; insufficiency of kidney yin resulting in a failure of water to moisten wood and vacuous yang harassing the upper body; affect-mind ill-being causing binding depression of liver qi, liver wind-fire harassing the clear orifices.

Main Symptoms: Paroxysmal vertigo, dysacusis, tinnitus, nausea, vomiting, a sombre white facial complexion and sweating. In severe cases nystagmus may occur. When it occurs, the surroundings seem to spin and the patient may have difficulty walking steadily while maintaining consciousness.

Acupoints: Bai Hui (DU-20), Nei Guan (PC-6), Xing Jian (LR-2), Tai Xi (KI-3), Zu San Li (ST-36), San Yin Jiao (SP-6).

Moxibustion Method:

- Direct Moxa: Apply moxa cones the size of a soybean, mung bean or kernel for 5–10 minutes per acupoint, once every other day, 3 treatments constitute a course of treatment. (Figure 11.8.1)

- Moxa on Ginger: Apply 5–20 cones the size of a jujube pit or soybean per acupoint, once daily or every other day, 3 treatments constitute a course of treatment. (Figure 11.8.2)

- Warm Needle Moxa: Apply moxa for 6–20 minutes per acupoint, once daily, 5 days constitute a course of treatment. (Figure 11.8.3)

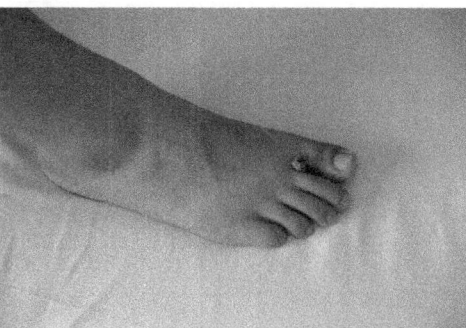

Figure 11.8.1 Direct Moxa at Xing Jian (LR-2)

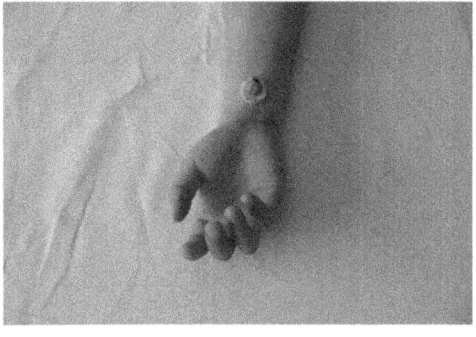

Figure 11.8.2 Moxa on Ginger at Nei Guan (PC-6)

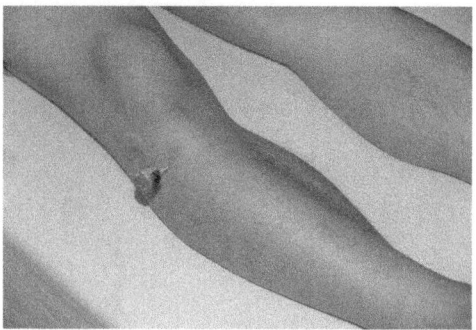

Figure 11.8.3 Warm Needle Moxa at Zu San Li (ST-36)

9. Toothache

Toothache is a common symptom in oral diseases. Toothache occurs in various diseases, such as dental caries, acute and chronic pulpitis, acute apical periodontitis, acute and chronic periodontitis, wisdom tooth pericoronitis, acute and chronic gingivitis, dentin hypersensitivity and dental trauma. It falls within the scope of gum atrophy, maxillary osteomyelitis, bleeding gums or ulcerative gingivitis in TCM. TCM asserts that the kidney governs the bones and teeth are the surplus of the bones, therefore, toothache is significantly related to kidney deficiency. The stomach meridian travels through the gums, so toothache can be caused by excessive gastrointestinal heat or retained heat in the liver meridian.

Main Symptoms: Toothache can be induced or aggravated by a variety of stimuli such as cold, heat, acidic or sweet foods, and may be relieved after the stimulation is removed. Signs and symptoms can include a continuous toothache radiating to the ear and temporal region that is aggravated by contact with the teeth or chewing, crackles in the teeth, accompanied by red and swollen gums or loose teeth.

Acupoints: He Gu (LI-4), Nei Ting (ST-44), Tai Xi (KI-3), Zhao Hai (KI-6), San Yin Jiao (SP-6), Jia Che (ST-6), Xia Guan (ST-7).

Moxibustion Method:

- Non-suppurative Moxa: Apply 3–9 cones per acupoint, once daily or every other day, 3 treatments constitute a course of treatment. (Figure 11.9.1)

- Moxa on Fu Zi (Aconiti Radix Lateralis Praeparata): Apply 7–9 cones per acupoint, once daily or every other day, 3 treatments constitute a course of treatment. (Figure 11.9.2)

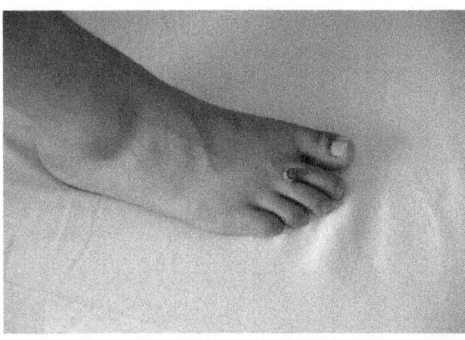
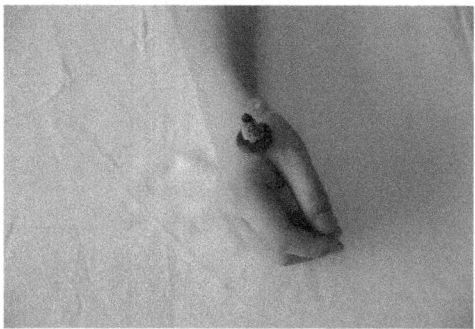

Figure 11.9.1 Non-suppurative Moxa at Nei Ting (ST-44)

Figure 11.9.2 Moxa on Fu Zi at He Gu (LI-4)

- Juncibustion:* Apply moxa once per acupoint when toothache occurs. (Figure 11.9.3)

- Moxa on Garlic: When toothache occurs, apply 5–7 cones the size of a jujube pit or soybean per acupoint, once daily or every other day. (Figure 11.9.4)

- Moxa on Ginger: When toothache occurs, apply 5–7 cones the size of a jujube pit or soybean per acupoint, once daily or every other day. (Figure 11.9.5)

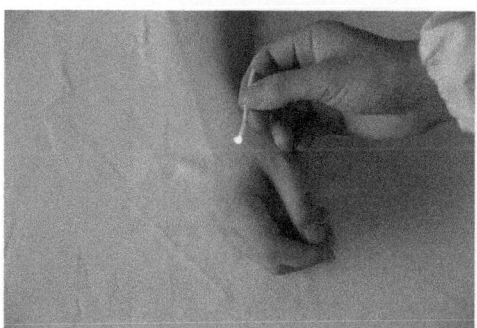
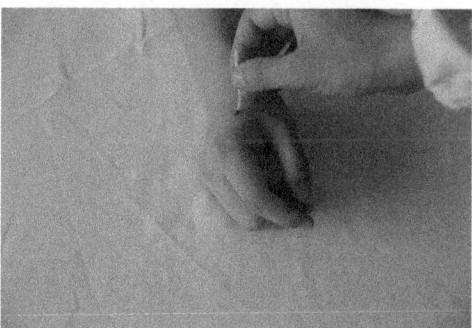

Figure 11.9.3 Juncibustion at He Gu (LI-4)

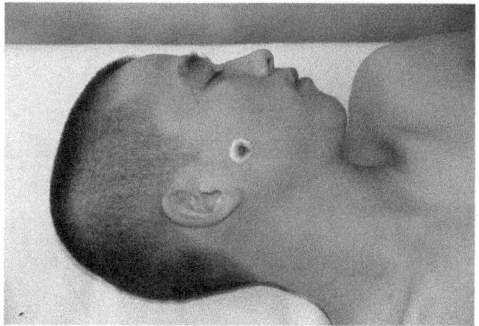
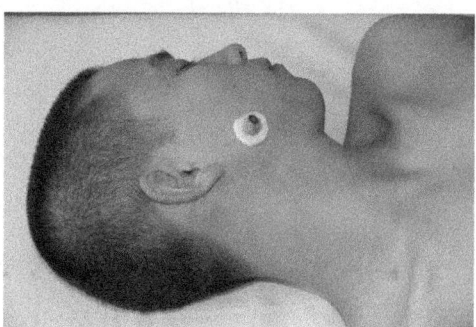

Figure 11.9.4 Moxa on Garlic at Xia Guan (ST-7)   *Figure 11.9.5 Moxa on Ginger at Jia Che (ST-6)*

10. Allergic Rhinitis

Allergic rhinitis is caused by increased sensitivity of the body to certain allergens. It manifests as oedematous nasal mucosa, proliferated muciparous glands and infiltration with eosinophilia. The disease is often induced by lung qi deficiency, insecurity of exterior qi or externally contracted wind-cold.

Main Symptoms: Paroxysmal intranasal itching, spastic sneezing, nasal congestion, excessive nasal discharge and olfaction disorders, which often occurs when the patient wakes in the morning.

Acupoints: Fei Shu (BL-13), Jing Ming (BL-1), Ying Xiang (LI-20), Yin Tang (EX-HN-3), He Gu (LI-4).

Moxibustion Method:

- Gentle Moxa: Apply moxa for 15–30 minutes per acupoint, once or twice a day, 7–10 treatments constitute a course of treatment. Repeat after 3–5 days. (Figure 11.10.1)

- Moxa on Ginger: Apply 3–7 cones the size of a jujube pit or soybean per acupoint, once daily, 7–10 treatments constitute a course of treatment. (Figure 11.10.2)

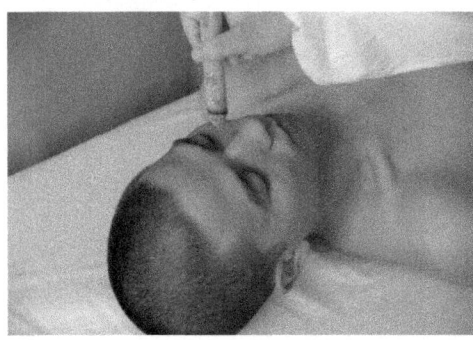
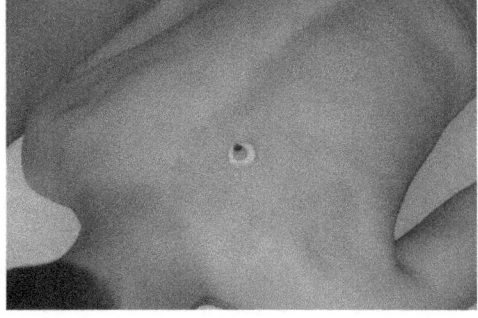

Figure 11.10.1 Gentle Moxa at Yin Tang (EX-HN-3)

Figure 11.10.2 Moxa on Ginger at Fei Shu (BL-13)

- Thunder-Fire Hanging Moxa: Apply moxa 60 times travelling from Shang Xing (DU-23) to Su Liao (DU-25), and from Yin Tang (EX-HN-3) to Ying Xiang (LI-20), taking approximately 1 second to complete each circuit. Then apply pecking sparrow moxa on Yin Tang (EX-HN-3), Jing Ming (BL-1), Ying Xiang (LI-20), Shang Xing (DU-23), bilateral He Gu (LI-4) and the nostrils 30 times, 7 days constitutes a course of treatment. (Figure 11.10.3)

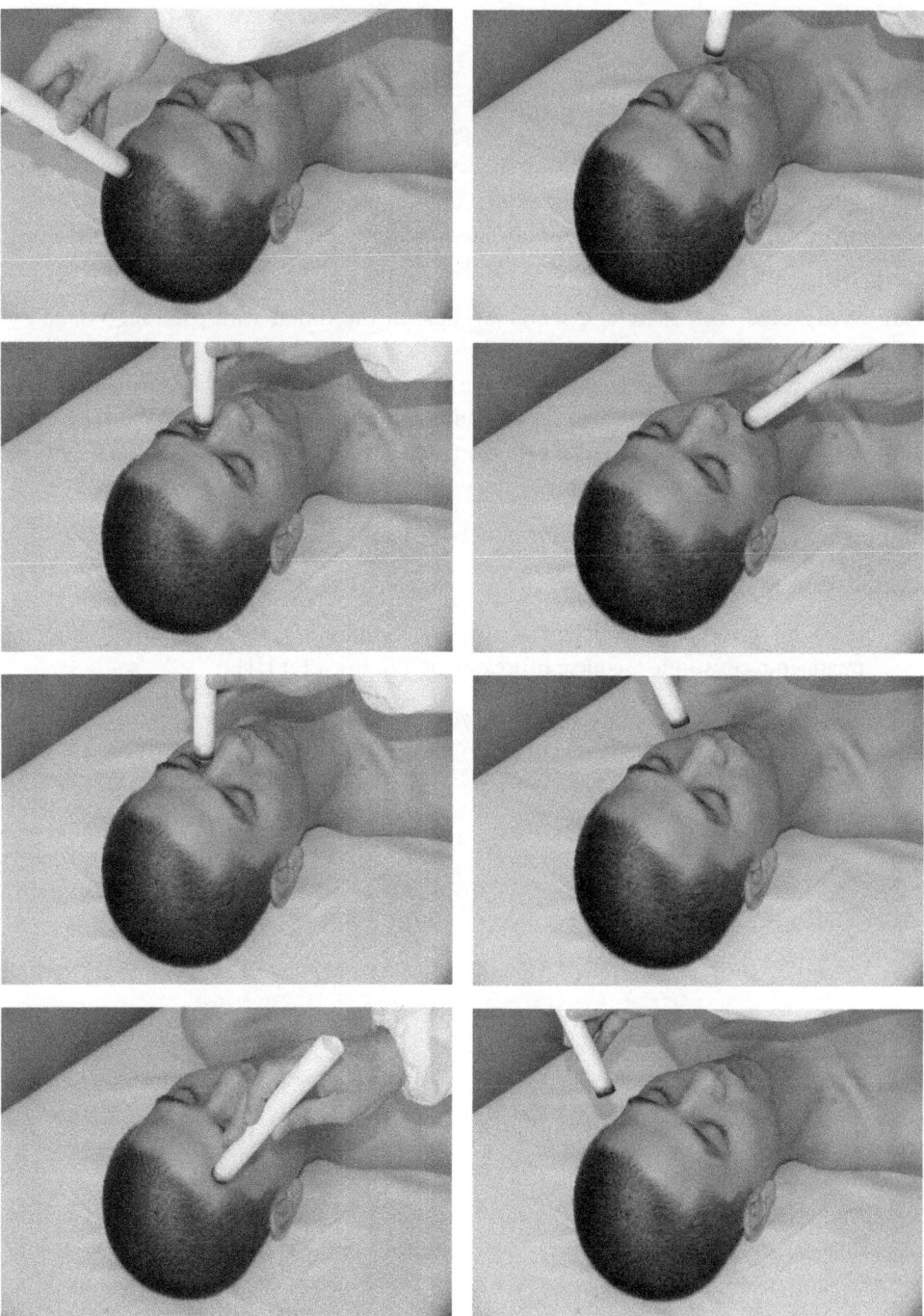

Figure 11.10.3 Thunder-Fire Hanging Moxa

11. Pharyngolaryngitis

Pharyngolaryngitis is a condition induced by bacteria. It is divided into acute and chronic pharyngolaryngitis. Acute pharyngolaryngitis is mainly caused by viruses, and secondly by bacteria. It can be induced by cold, fatigue, long-term stimulation by chemical gas or dust, or excessive smoking. Chronic pharyngolaryngitis often originates from acute pharyngolaryngitis, which attacks repeatedly and has not been treated appropriately. The following causes can also induce chronic pharyngolaryngitis: various rhinopathies causing obstruction of the nasal orifices, physical and chemical factors, and neck radiotherapy.

Main Symptoms: Dry itchy and scorching heat in the throat with pain aggravated by swallowing, increased secretion of saliva, obvious earache when the lateral pharyngeal band is involved. Discomfort in the throat with dryness, itching, swelling, scorching pain and increased secretions may also occur. Other symptoms include nausea, a sensation of a foreign body that is not easily expectorated or swallowed. The symptoms may be aggravated by excessive consumption of spicy food, fatigue or weather variations.

Acupoints: Tian Tu (RN-22), Lian Quan (RN-23), Fu Tu (LI-18), He Gu (LI-4).

Moxibustion Method:

- Hanging Moxa: Apply moxa for 15–20 minutes per acupoint, once daily, 10 treatments constitute a course of treatment. (Figure 11.11.1)

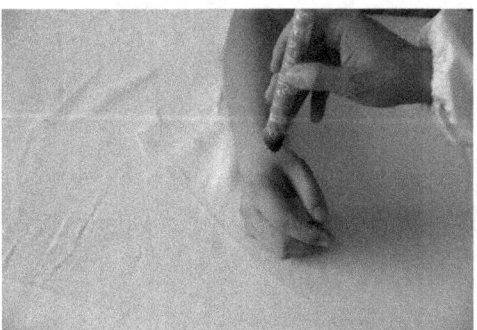

Figure 11.11.1 Hanging Moxa at He Gu (LI-4)

12. Oral Ulcer

Oral ulcer, also known as aphtha, is a kind of superficial ulcer on the oral mucosa. The ulcers may vary in size from that of a rice grain to as large as a soybean, and are round or ovoid. Ingestion of spicy foods can cause pain. The ulcers can recover spontaneously in one to two weeks. The specific cause is still unknown, but possible causative factors may include immune abnormalities, digestive diseases, endocrine changes, psychic factors, inherent causes or infective agents.

Main Symptoms: Pitting ulcers of a regular shape, round or ovoid; clear boundary between ulcers and normal mucosa.

Acupoints: Shen Que (RN-8), Da Zhu (BL-11).

Moxibustion Method:

- Gentle Moxa: Apply moxa for 15–20 minutes per acupoint, once daily, 5 treatments constitute a course of treatment. (Figure 11.12.1)

- Moxa on Salt: Place some Da Qing Yan (Halitum) on the umbilicus, and apply moxa using a moxa box until the patient feels heat in approximately 30 minutes. Perform once daily, 5 days constitute a course of treatment. (Figure 11.12.2)

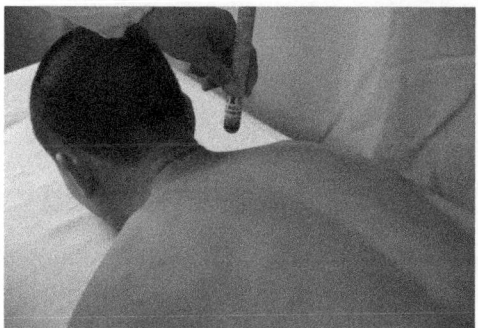
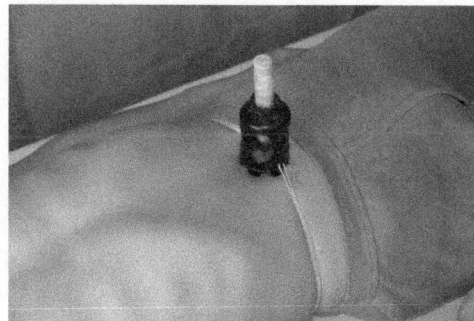

Figure 11.12.1 Gentle Moxa at Da Zhu (BL-11)   *Figure 11.12.2 Moxa on Salt at Shen Que (RN-8)*

CHAPTER 12

Acute Diseases

1. Syncope (Fainting)

Syncope is a common clinical condition that can be caused by numerous different diseases. The key symptoms are sudden and temporary loss of consciousness, accompanied by a loss of ability to stand. Its characteristics are sudden dizziness, a lack of strength, a sudden loss of consciousness, falling, and recovery several seconds or minutes later. Syncope falls within the scope of reversal pattern and qi desertion pattern in TCM. This condition usually has the following causes: original qi vacuity resulting in an inability of qi and blood to rise and fill the brain; abnormal emotions and a chaotic menstrual cycle causing a disturbance to the clear orifices. This pattern is often seen in transient ischemic attack, postural hypotension, hypoglycemia, cerebral vasospasm and hysterical coma.

Main Symptoms: Subjective dizziness and weakness, transient loss of vision, nausea, followed by sudden fainting and loss of consciousness.

Acupoints:

- *Primary points:* Shui Gou (DU-26), Zhong Chong (PC-9), Bai Hui (DU-20), Nei Guan (PC-6).

- *Symptomatic points:* Vacuity pattern: Qi Hai (RN-6), Guan Yuan (BL-26); Repletion Pattern: He Gu (LI-4), Tai Chong (LR-3).

Moxibustion Method:

- Pecking Sparrow Moxa: Apply moxa to each point for 3–5 minutes. Continue until the patient revives. (Figure 12.1.1)

- Direct Moxa: Use moxa cones the size of a soybean. Apply 3–5 cones per acupoint or for 6–15 minutes. Continue until the patient revives. (Figure 12.1.2)

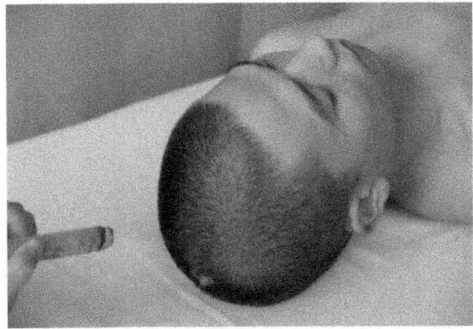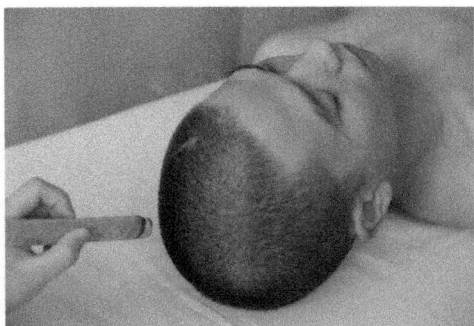

Figure 12.1.1 Pecking Sparrow Moxa at Bai Hui (DU-20)

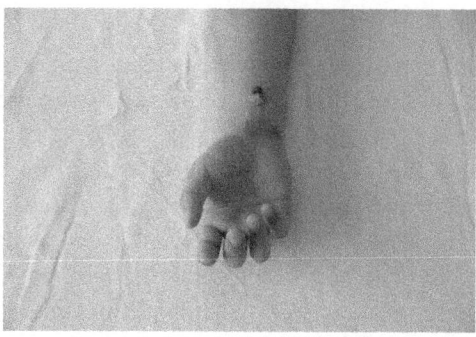

Figure 12.1.2 Direct Moxa at Nei Guan (PC-6)

2. Vacuity Qi Desertion

Vacuity qi desertion is a critical pattern. The key symptoms are a pale complexion, apathetic expression or stupor, sweating, cold extremities and a drop in blood pressure. This condition usually has the following causes: major blood loss; severe vomiting, diarrhoea and sweating; external contraction of the six excesses or internal damage by the seven affects; drug allergy or poisoning; debilitation caused by chronic illness resulting in an inability of qi and blood to support the whole body. This disease includes shock caused by various factors in modern medicine.

Main Symptoms: A sombre white or blue facial complexion, reversal cold of the limbs, profuse perspiration, haziness of the spirit, torpor or stupor; or irritability and restlessness, a fall of blood pressure; fine and weak pulse.

Acupoints: Guan Yuan (RN-4), Shen Que (RN-8).

Moxibustion Method:

- Cone Moxa: Apply large moxa cones on Guan Yuan (RN-4). Continue until the limbs become warm. (Figure 12.2.1)

- Moxa on Salt: Large moxa cones on salt are used on Guan Yuan (RN-4) and Shen Que (RN-8). Continue until the patient revives. (Figure 12.2.2)

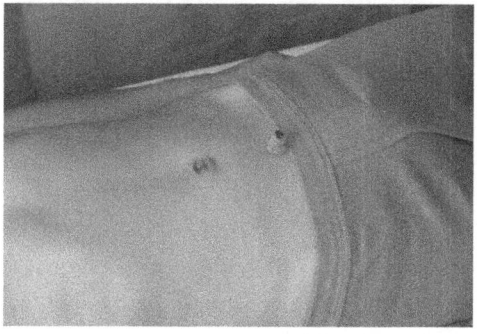

Figure 12.2.1 Cone Moxa at Guan Yuan (RN-4)

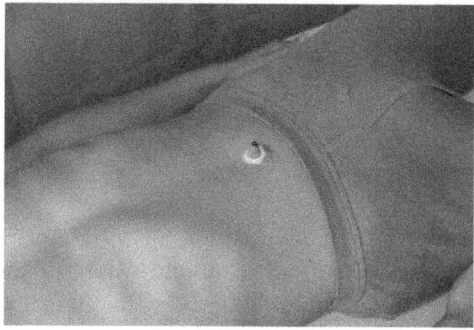

Figure 12.2.2 Moxa on Salt at Shen Que (RN-8)

3. Muscle Spasm

Muscle spasm is a common critical acute condition manifesting as rigidity of the neck and back, convulsions of the limbs, opisthotonus and clenched jaw caused by sinew dystrophy. It falls within the scope of convulsion pattern in TCM. This condition usually has the following causes: invasion of an external pathogen leading fire heat to transform into wind; wind-yang and phlegm turbidity obstructing the vessels; kidney yin deficiency causing sinew dystrophy; toxic wind invading the vessels after trauma. This disease includes muscle spasm caused by infantile convulsions, tetanus, seizures, hysteria, craniocerebral trauma, cerebral tumour and various types of meningitis in modern medicine.

Main Symptoms: Convulsions of the limbs, rigidity of the neck and nape, opisthotonus and clenched jaw, and, in severe cases, accompanied by coma.

Acupoints: Shui Gou (DU-26), Bai Hui (DU-20), Dai Zhui (DU-14), Guan Yuan (RN-4), He Gu (LI-4), Zu San Li (ST-36).

Moxibustion Method:

- Non-scarring Moxa: Prick blood at Shi Xuan (EX-UE 11) with a fine needle first, then apply 3–5 cones at Shui Gou (DU-26) and Bai Hui (DU-20). If the symptoms persist, perform moxa at Da Zhui (DU-14), Guan Yuan (RN-4), He Gu (LI-4) and Zu San Li (ST-36) until the local area turns warm and red, and the convulsions cease. (Figure 12.3.1)

- Warm Needle Moxa: Used during remission: moxa 2–3 acupoints, 3–5 cones of moxa per acupoint (or for 6–15 minutes), once a day, 5 treatments constitute a course of treatment. (Figure 12.3.2)

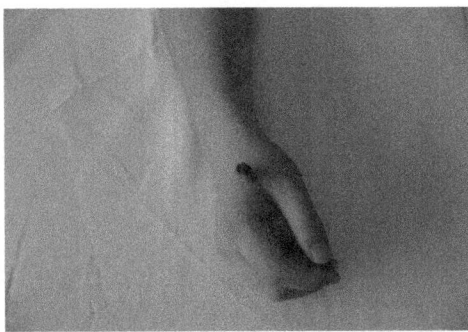
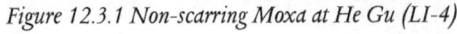
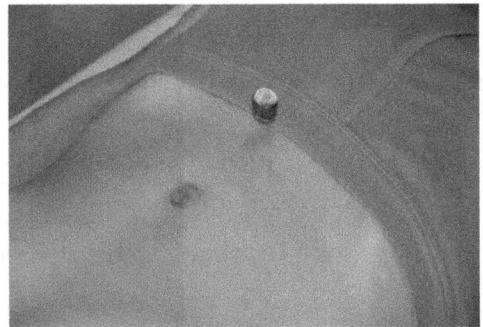

Figure 12.3.1 Non-scarring Moxa at He Gu (LI-4)   *Figure 12.3.2 Warm Needle Moxa at Guan Yuan (RN-4)*

4. Angina Pectoris

Angina pectoris is a syndrome manifesting as paroxysmal chest pain induced by coronary artery insufficiency, abrupt and short-term ischemia and myocardial hypoxia. This condition usually has the following causes: vacuity of normal qi and obstructed chest yang; emotional depression causing qi stagnation and blood stasis; dietary irregularities resulting in phlegm clouding the pericardium; deficiency of nutrients and blood causing heart vessel dystrophy. It falls within the scope of chest pain, heart pain, reversal heart pain, and true heart pain in TCM.

Main Symptoms: Sudden oppression in the chest, left thoracic precordium pain, palpitations, shortness of breath, heart pain radiating to the back and hasty panting with an inability to lie down.

Acupoints:

- *Primary points:* Nei Guan (PC-6), Yin Xi (HT-6), Dan Zhong (RN-I7), Xin Shu (BL-15), Jue Yin Shu (BL-14).

- *Symptomatic points:* Congealing Cold in Heart Vessels: Shen Que (RN-8); Qi Stagnation and Blood Stasis: Xue Hai (SP-10), Ge Shu (BL-17), Tai Chong (LR-3); Internal Damp-Phlegm Obstruction: Zhong Wan (RN-12), Feng Long (ST-40); Heart Yin Vacuity: Shen Men (HT-7), Tai Xi (KI-3); Heart Yang Vacuity: Qi Hai (RN-6), Guan Yuan (RN-4).

Moxibustion Method:

- Gentle Moxa: Moxa for 6–20 minutes per acupoint until the local skin turns rosy, once daily; 5 treatments constitute a course of treatment. (Figure 12.4.1)

- Warm Needle Moxa: Choose 4–5 acupoints each treatment; apply 5 cones per acupoint (for 20 to 30 minutes), once daily or every two days; 7–10 treatments constitute a course of treatment. Repeat after 3 days. (Figure 12.4.2)

- Moxa on Fu Zi Cake: Grind an appropriate amount of Fu Zi (Aconiti Radix Lateralis Praeparata) into a fine powder, mix well with rice wine, and make into a drug cake as large as a coin. Patch the drug cake on primary points as well as Nei Guan (PC-6) and Dan Zhong (RN-I7), and then put a jujube pit-sized moxa cone on the cake. Apply 5–7 cones per acupoint, once daily; 10 treatments constitute a course of treatment. (Figure 12.4.3)

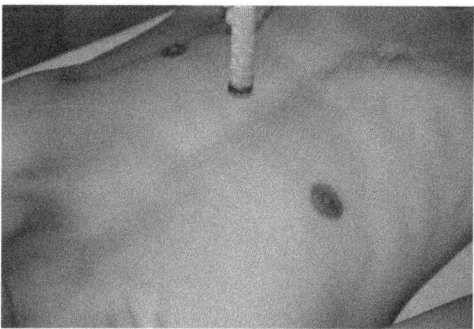

Figure 12.4.1 Gentle Moxa at Dan Zhong (RN-17)

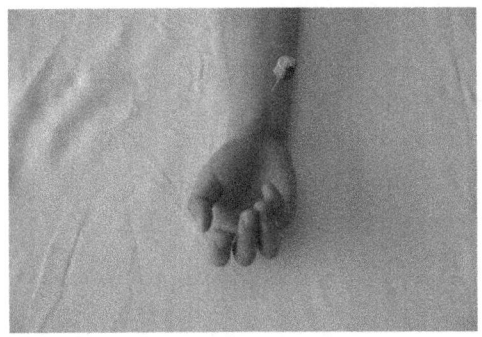

Figure 12.4.2 Warm Needle Moxa at Nei Guan (PC-6)

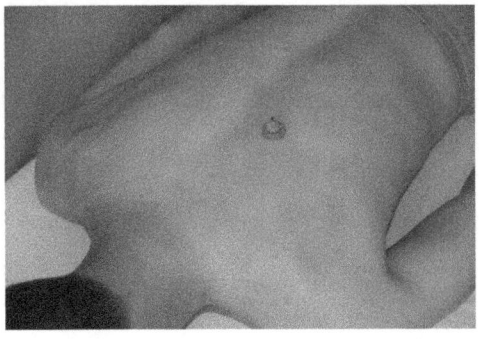

Figure 12.4.3 Moxa on Fu Zi Cake at Xin Shu (BL-15)

5. Cholecystalgia

Cholecystalgia is a common acute abdominal condition manifesting as paroxysmal aggravated or continual gripping pain in the right upper quadrant of the gallbladder area. This disease usually has the following causes: frustration causing hepatobiliary qi stagnation; dietary irregularities harming the spleen and stomach; damp-phlegm congestion transforming into heat and calculi. It falls within the scope of hypochondriac pain in TCM. This disease is often seen in cholecystitis, angiocholitis, cholelithiasis and biliary ascariasis.

Main Symptoms: Sudden severe pain in the right upper quadrant of the abdomen, continual gripping pain that is paroxysmaly aggravated.

Acupoints:

- *Primary points:* Dan Nang Xue (EX-LE 6), Yang Ling Quan (GB-34), Dan Shu (BL-19), Ri Yue (GB-24), Qi Men (LR-14).

- *Symptomatic points:* Vomiting: Nei Guan (PC-6), Gong Sun (SP-4); Icterus: Zhi Yang (DU-9), Yin Ling Quan (SP-9); Binding of phlegm-heat: Feng Long (ST-40); Biliary Ascariasis: Ying Xiang (LI-20), Si Bai (ST-2).

Moxibustion Method:

- Non-scarring Moxa: Choose 3–5 acupoints and apply 3–5 cones per point until the pain is relieved. Repeat once daily, and 5–10 times for a course of treatment. (Figure 12.5.1)

- Gentle Moxa: Apply 3–5 cones per acupoint or for 15–20 minutes until the pain is relieved. Repeat once daily or every other day, and perform 5–10 times for a course of treatment. (Figure 12.5.2)

- Juncibustion:* Perform once per acupoint, once daily or every other day, until the pain is relieved. (Figure 12.5.3)

- Moxa on Garlic: Apply 3–5 cones at Gan Shu (BL-18) or at painful points, once daily, 10 treatments constitute a course of treatment. (Figure 12.5.4)

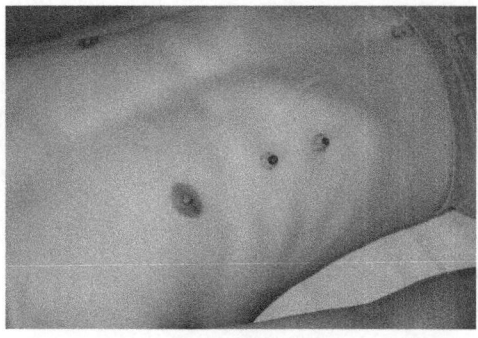

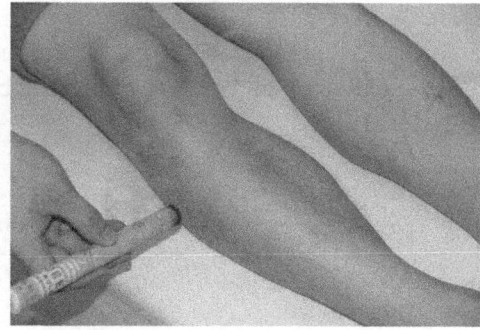

Figure 12.5.1 Non-scarring Moxa at Ri Yue (GB-24) and Qi Men (LR-14)

Figure 12.5.2 Gentle Moxa at Dan Nang Xue (EX-LE-6)

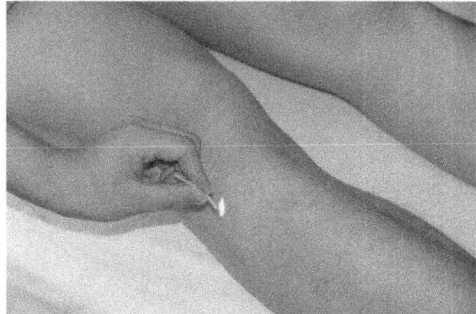

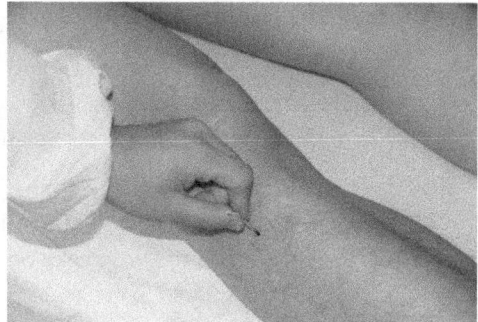

Figure 12.5.3 Juncibustion at Yang Ling Quan (GB-34)

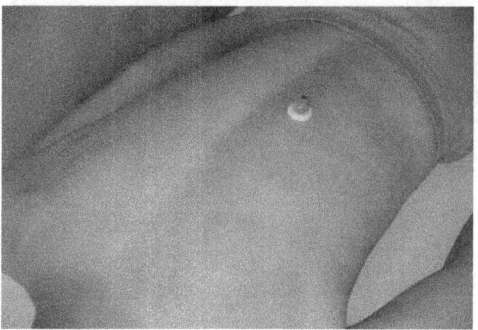

Figure 12.5.4 Moxa on Garlic at Dan Shu (BL-19)

6. Renal Colic

Renal colic is a pain syndrome induced by calculi in the urinary system. Its characteristics are paroxysmal severe gripping pain in the lumbar region or side of the abdomen radiating upward or downward along the ureter, accompanied by painful urination and bloody urine. This disease usually has the following causes: excessive consumption of hot-spicy acrid foods causing brewing and binding of damp-heat; frustration inhibiting bladder qi transformation; kidney qi vacuity inducing a lack of warmth in the bladder. It falls within the scope of lumbago, stone strangury, sand strangury and blood strangury in TCM.

Main Symptoms: Continuous or intermittent acute swelling stabbing pain in the lower abdomen and core, or stabbing pain in the lumbar region radiating to the bladder, external genitals and inner thighs, accompanied by bloody urine, dysuria and percussion pain in the renal region.

Acupoints:

- *Primary points:* Xia Wan (RN-10), Guan Yuan (RN-4), Zhong Ji (RN-3).

- *Symptomatic points:* Bloody urine: Xue Hai (SP-10), Ge Shu (BL-17); Damp-heat predominating: Yin Ling Quan (SP-9); Kidney Qi Vacuity: Yao Yang Guan (DU-3).

Moxibustion Method:

- Direct Moxa: Apply 3–5 moxa cones the size of a kernel of wheat per acupoint (or for 6–15 minutes), once daily. Repeat 10 treatments for a course of treatment. (Figure 12.6.1)

- Warm Needle Moxa: Apply 3–5 moxa cones per acupoint (or 15–20 minutes), once daily, 7 times for a course of treatment. (Figure 12.6.2)

- Moxa on Fu Zi Cake: Grind an appropriate amount of Fu Zi (Aconiti Radix Lateralis Praeparata) into a fine powder, then lightly stir-fry, and make into a drug cake the size of a coin. Patch the drug cake on Yao Yang Guan (DU-3) and Ming Men (DU-4), and then put a moxa cone as large as a jujube pit on the cake. Apply 5–7 cones per acupoint and perform the treatment once daily. (Figure 12.6.3)

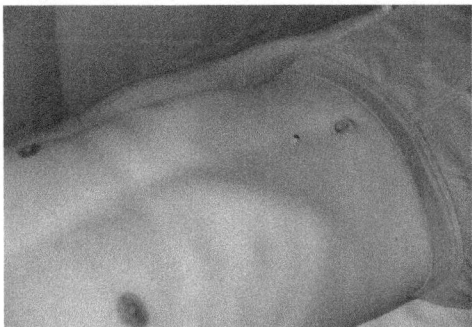

Figure 12.6.1 Direct Moxa at Xia Wan (RN-10)

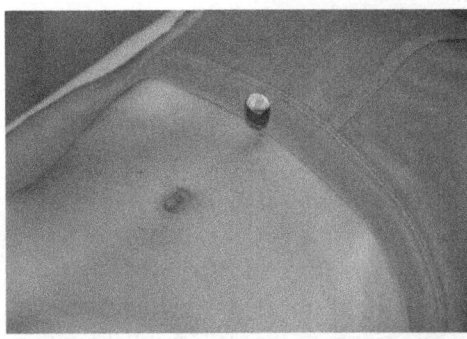

Figure 12.6.2 Warm Needle Moxa at Guan Yuan (RN-4)

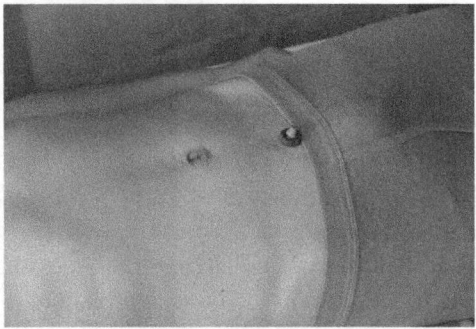

Figure 12.6.3 Moxa on Fu Zi Cake at Guan Yuan (RN-4)

7. Epistaxis (Spontaneous External Bleeding)

Epistaxis is a bleeding condition manifesting as spontaneous bleeding from the nose, gingiva, ears, tongue and skin without trauma. A common acute syndrome is rhinorrhagia. Rhinorrhagia is a nosebleed that, in mild cases, manifests as minor bleeding that ceases spontaneously. However, in severe cases the bleeding is copious and does not cease. This condition usually has the following causes: nasal vessels damaged by lung heat, stomach fire and liver fire resulting in frenetic movement of the blood; deficient qi failing to control the blood and yin deficiency with effulgent fire damageing nasal vessels.

Main Symptoms: Minor bleeding: blood in the sputum. Excessive bleeding: blood flowing from bilateral nostrils.

Acupoints: Shao Shang (LU-11), He Gu (LI-4).

Moxibustion Method:

- Juncibustion:* Choose bilateral Shao Shang (LU-11) and He Gu (LI-4), and use 'bao' juncibustion once. (Figure 12.7.1)

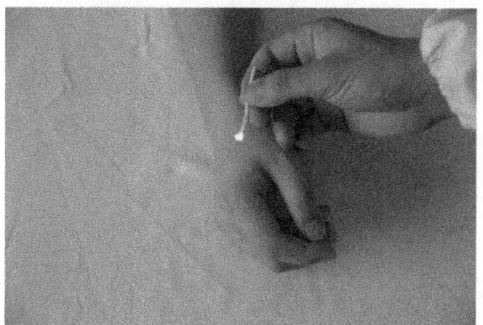 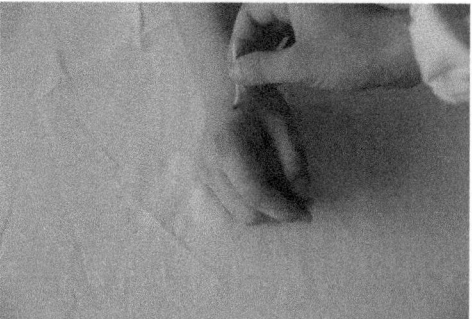

Figure 12.7.1 Juncibustion at He Gu (LI-4)

8. Hematochezia (Bloody Stool)

Hematochezia manifests as excretion of blood with the stool; it may be excreted before bowel movements, mixed with stool or independently of bowel movements. This condition usually has the following causes: external contraction of the six excesses, internal damage by the seven affects, dietary irregularities, or excessive taxation resulting in disharmony of qi and blood, disturbance to organ function, vessel damage, a failure of blood to stay in the channels and haemorrhage.

Main Symptoms: Fresh red, dull-red, dark purple or even black stools; increased stool frequency.

Acupoints:

- *Primary points:* Chang Qiang (DU-1), Cheng Shan (BL-57), Shang Ju Xu (ST-37), Ci Liao (BL-32).

- *Symptomatic points:* Internal damage by taxation fatigue: Bai Hui (DU-20), Guan Yuan (BL-26), Ming Men (DU-4); Damp-heat pouring downward: Tai Bai (SP-3), Yin Ling Quan (SP-9).

Moxibustion Method:

- Gentle Moxa: Apply moxa for 15–20 minutes per acupoint, once daily, each course of treatment consists of 7 treatments. (Figure 12.8.1)

- Moxa on Ginger: Apply 5–10 cones the size of a jujube pit per acupoint, once daily, each course of treatment consists 7 treatments. (Figure 12.8.2)

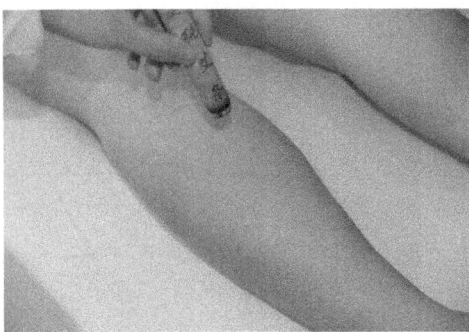

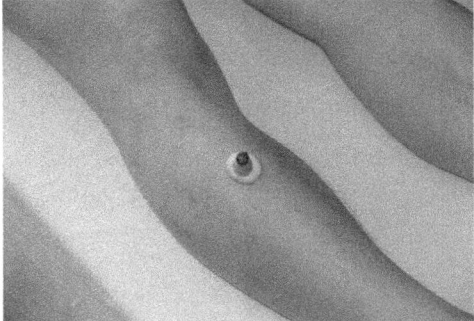

Figure 12.8.1 Gentle Moxa at Cheng Shan (BL-57)

Figure 12.8.2 Moxa on Ginger at Shang Ju Xu (ST-37)

9. Haematuria (Bloody Urine)

Haematuria manifests as blood in the urine without significant pain; it is also commonly known as bloody urine. In mild cases, the blood can only be identified by microscopic examination; in severe cases, urine mixed with blood or even complete haematuria can be observed with the naked eye. The disease is often caused by external contraction or internal damage resulting in accumulation of heat in the kidney and bladder damageing vessels.

Main Symptoms: Light red, bright red or dark brown urine mixed with blood or blood clots.

Acupoints:

- *Primary points:* Shen Shu (BL-23), Pang Guang Shu (BL-28), Xue Hai (SP-10), Yin Ling Quan (SP-3), San Yin Jiao (SP-6).

- *Symptomatic points:* Spleen-stomach vacuity: Guan Yuan (BL-26), Zu San Li (ST-36); Descending damp-heat: Zhong Ji (RN-3), Xing Jian (LR-2); Hyperactive heart fire: Da Lin (PC-7), Shen Men (HT-7).

Moxibustion Method:

- Gentle Moxa: Choose 3–5 acupoints and apply moxa for 15–20 minutes per acupoint, once daily or every other day; 7 treatments constitute a course of treatment. (Figure 12.9.1)

- Non-scarring Moxa: Choose 3–5 acupoints and apply 3–5 moxa cones per acupoint, once daily; 7 treatments constitute a course of treatment. (Figure 12.9.2)

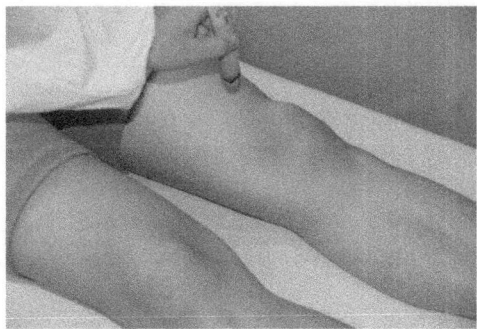
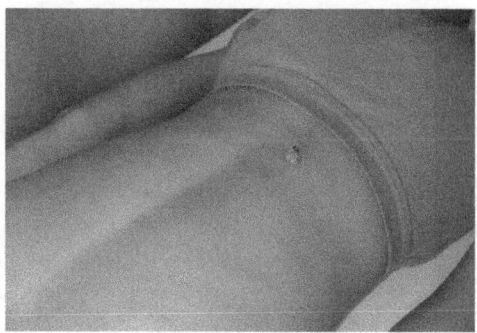

Figure 12.9.1 Gentle Moxa at Xue Hai (SP-10)   *Figure 12.9.2 Non-scarring Moxa at Shen Shu (BL-23)*

CHAPTER 13

Other Diseases

1. Chronic Fatigue Syndrome

Chronic fatigue syndrome refers to a group of clinical symptoms that mainly involve chronic fatigue lasting for or recurrently attacking for more than 6 months, sometimes accompanied by non-specific symptoms including a low-grade fever, headache, sore throat, myosalgia and psychiatric symptoms. It is usually caused by one of the following: overwork, excessive mental activity, an unbalanced lifestyle and mental stimulation.

Main Symptoms: Poor sleep quality, due, for example to insomnia or excessive dreaming, memory loss, alopecia and leukotrichia, a decline in cognitive functions and some somatic symptoms such as lumbago and general back pain, dizziness and headache, tinnitus, chest distress, palpitations and a decline in sexual function.

Acupoints:

- *Primary points:* Guan Yuan (RN-4), Zu San Li (ST-36), Shen Que (RN-8).

- *Supporting points:* Qi Hai (RN-6), San Yin Jiao (SP-6).

Moxibustion Method:

- Gentle Pole Moxa: Apply moxa to each point for 6–20 minutes. Perform treatment once per day; 15 treatments comprise one course of treatment. Three courses may be required to see an effect and consolidation therapy should be applied for a period of time after fatigue is eliminated. (Figure 13.1.1)

- Non-scarring Moxa: Using moxa cones the size of a grain of wheat, apply 4–5 cones to each acupoint. Perform once every other day. Ten treatments comprise one course of treatment. (Figure 13.1.2)

- Moxa on Medicinal Cake: Mix Ba Zhen Wan (Eight-Gem Pill) into a paste with water and shape into a cake the diameter of 2cm and thickness of 0.8cm. Cut a 1.5cm moxa pole and put it on the medicinal cake. Perform treatment 3 times per week; 10 treatments comprise one course of treatment, 3 courses are required in total. (Figure 13.1.3)

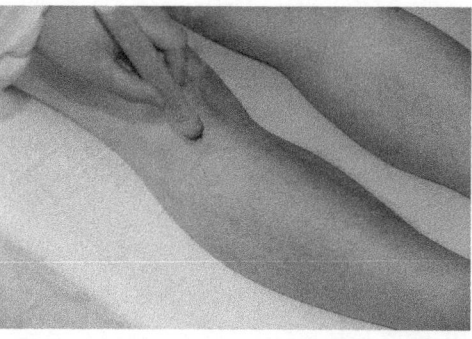

Figure 13.1.1 Gentle Pole Moxa at Zu San Li (ST-36)

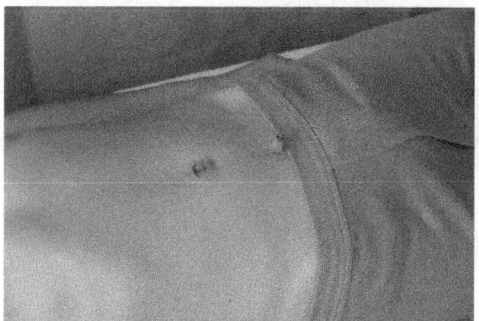

Figure 13.1.2 Non-scarring Moxa at Guan Yuan (RN-4)

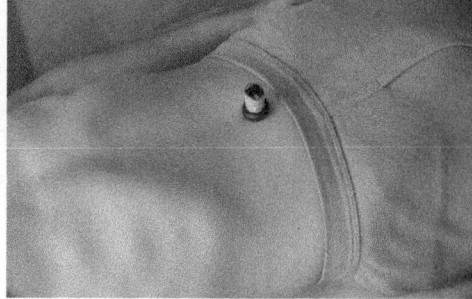

Figure 13.1.3 Moxa on Medicinal Cake at Shen Que (RN-8)

2. Sub-health State

Sub-health state is also referred to as latent illness or the third state, which is a intermediate physical state between health and illness. It refers to those who are not presenting with illness, but who have various predisposing factors of varying degrees and who have a high-risk tendency to develop a certain condition. The sub-health population is mostly over 40 years old and generally has a tendency of 'six highs and one low', namely high load (physical strength and mentality), hypertension, hyperlipemia, hyperglycaemia, high blood viscosity, high weight and low immune function. A sub-health state manifests as excessive fatigue and a decrease in energy, reaction ability and adaptability.

Main Symptoms: Low and irritable mood, depression, anxiety, chest discomfort and palpitations, wakefulness, morbid forgetfulness, fatigued, weakness, lumbar and general back pain and with a tendency for illness.

Acupoints: Da Zhui (DU-14), Zu San Li (ST-36), Ming Men (DU-4), Shen Que (RN-8), Guan Yuan (RN-4).

Moxibustion Method:

- Gentle Pole Moxa: Apply moxa to 3–4 points, for 20 minutes per point, once per day. Ten treatments comprise one course of treatment. (Figure 13.2.1)

- Moxa on Salt: Apply moxa to each point for 15–20 minutes. Perform treatment once per day. Ten treatments comprise one course of treatment. (Figure 13.2.2)

- Scarring Cone Moxa:* Put a 0.7cm moxa cone directly on points and light it. Tap around the points if the patient feels pain. Apply 7–9 cones to each acupoint. After moxibustion apply a sticking plaster to the area. Repeat the treatment when the blister heals. (Figure 13.2.3)

- Moxa on Ginger: Apply 5 cones per acupoint, once per day. Ten treatments comprise one course of treatment, with a 3–5 day interval between courses. (Figure 13.2.4)

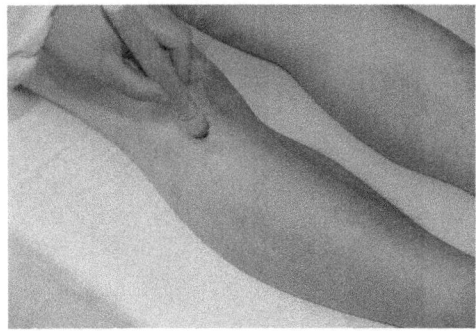

Figure 13.2.1 Gentle Pole Moxa at Zu San Li (ST-36)

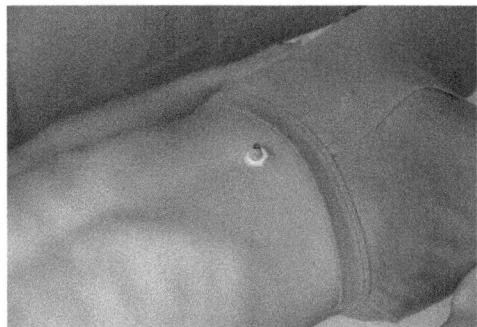

Figure 13.2.2 Moxa on Salt at Shen Que (RN-8)

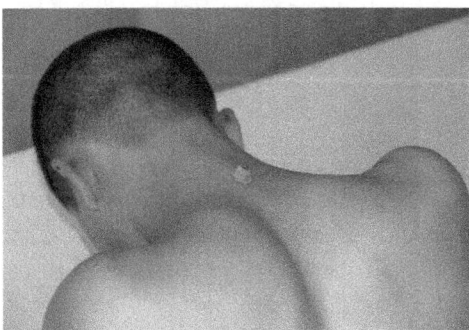

Figure 13.2.3 Scarring Cone Moxa at Da Zhui (DU-14)

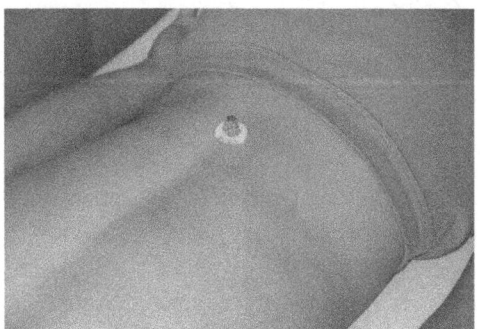

Figure 13.2.4 Moxa on Ginger at Ming Men (DU-4)

3. Anti-ageing

Ageing refers to a series of degradation processes of structural and physiological functionality. It is not considered a medical condition, but it may prevent sufferers from enjoying life to the full.

Main Symptoms: Sagging skin, wrinkles, age pigmentation, eye haustra, white hair, loss of hair, deafness and dim eyesight, aneuria, a decrease in memory, physical strength and sexual function.

Acupoints: Shen Que (RN-8), Guan Yuan (RN-4), Zu San Li (ST-36), Ming Men (DU-4), Qi Hai (RN-6), Shen Shu (BL-23).

Moxibustion Method:

- Gentle Pole Moxa: Apply moxa to each point for 6–15 minutes until reddening occurs. Perform treatment once per day continuously for 7 days at the beginning of every month. (Figure 13.3.1)

- Non-scarring Moxa: Apply 5–7 cones to each acupoint, perform treatment twice or three times a week; perform continuous treatment for 3 months each year. (Figure 13.3.2)

- Scarring Cone Moxa:* Apply 7–9 cones to each acupoint. Apply a sticking plaster to the area after moxibustion. Repeat the treatment when the blister heals. (Figure 13.3.3)

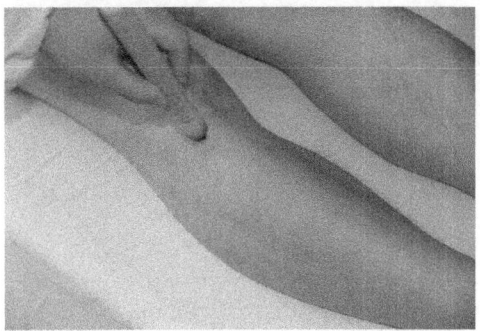 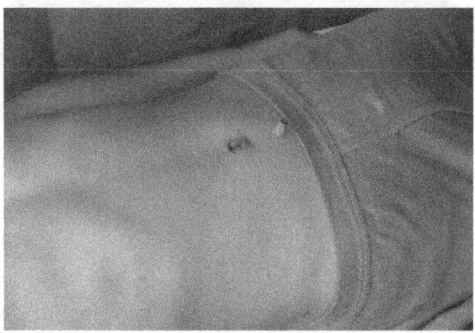

Figure 13.3.1 Gentle Pole Moxa at Zu San Li (ST-36)   *Figure 13.3.2 Non-scarring Moxa at Guan Yuan (RN-4)*

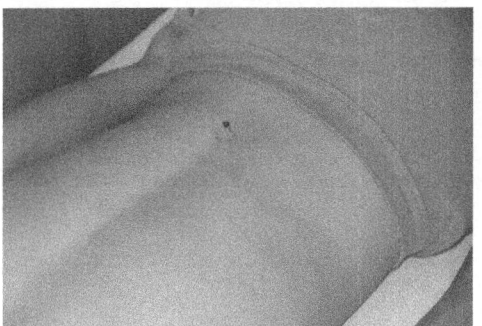 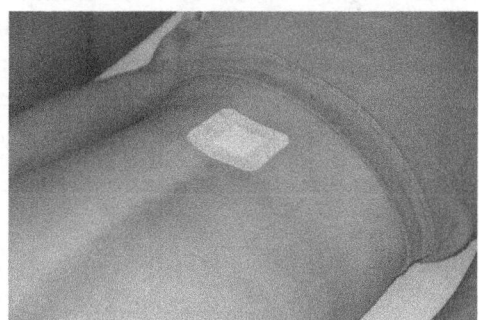

Figure 13.3.3 Scarring Cone Moxa at Ming Men (DU-4)

- Moxa on Medicinal Cake: Using a herbal concoction including Huang Qi (Astragali Radix), Dang Gui (Angelicae Sinensis Radix), Bu Gu Zhi (Psoraleae Fructus), Xian Ling Pi (Epimedii Herba), Da Huang (Rhei Radix et Rhizoma) and Dan Shen (Salviae Miltiorrhizae Radix), grind them into a fine powder, sieve, mix with 80% alcohol and form into a medicinal cake with a diameter of 3cm and thickness of

0.8cm. Apply 3 cones to each acupoint, perform treatment once every other day; 12 treatments comprise one course of treatment. (Figure 13.3.4)

- Moxa on Fu Zi Cake: Mix 2.5g of Fu Zi (Aconiti Radix Lateralis Praeparata) with yellow wine and form into a medicinal cake with a diameter of 2.5cm and thickness of 0.5cm. Apply 3 cones to each acupoint and perform treatment once every other day; 12 treatments comprise one course of treatment. (Figure 13.3.5)

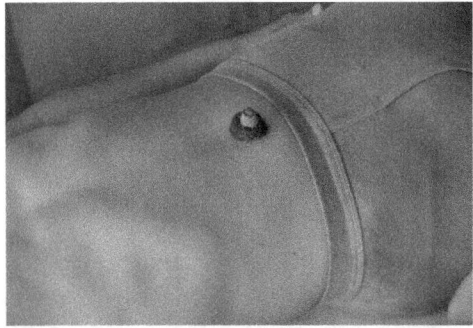
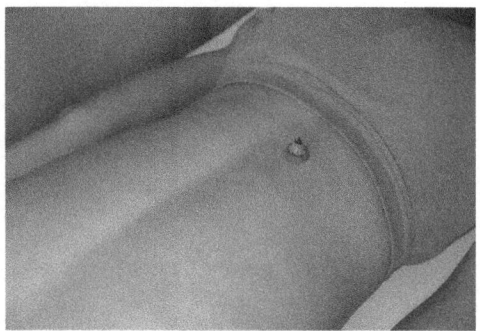

Figure 13.3.4 Moxa on Medicinal Cake at Shen Que (RN-8)

Figure 13.3.5 Moxa on Fu Zi Cake at Shen Shu (BL-23)

4. Obesity

Obesity refers to excessive adipose tissue caused by metabolic disorder. Simple obesity is mostly owing to an excessive intake of calories from food exceeding the required amount for activity, leading to accumulation of body fat. A body weight more than 20% above normal weight is considered to be obesity. It can occur at any age, but is most common in people over 40 years old and more often in females than males. People with long-term obesity often also suffer from diabetes, hypertension, hyperlipoidemia, atherosclerosis, CAD, RND, cholecystitis and gallstones. Female obesity may also be accompanied by irregular menses, amenorrhoea and infertility.

Main Symptoms: An overweight physique and body weight of more than 20% above normal weight.

Acupoints: Qu Chi (LI-11), Tian Shu (ST-25), Yin Ling Quan (SP-9), Feng Long (ST-40), Tai Chong (LR-3), Shang Ju Xu (ST-37).

Moxibustion Method:

- Gentle Moxa: Apply moxa to 3–5 points for 6–15 minutes, once per day or every other day, 20–30 times continuously. (Figure 13.4.1)

- Moxa on Ginger: Apply 5–7 cones per acupoint, once per day. One month comprises one course of treatment. (Figure 13.4.2)

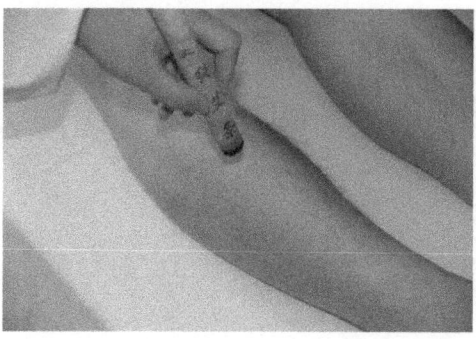
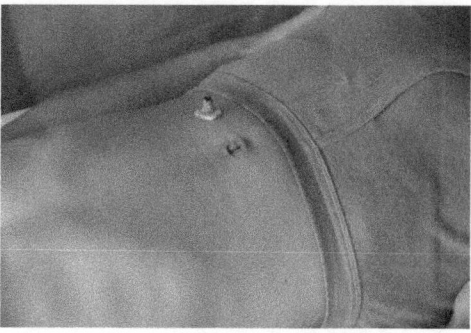

Figure 13.4.1 Gentle Moxa at Zu San Li (ST-36)   *Figure 13.4.2 Moxa on Ginger at Tian Shu (ST-25)*

5. Post Radiotherapy or Chemotherapy Side Effects

Side effects occurring after radiotherapy and chemotherapy can significantly affect the mental and physical strength of a patient. When digestive tract reactions and a poor appetite occur and are not treated appropriately, it can cause hypo-immunity, a decrease of white blood cells, the occurrence of a serious infection, and even a life threatening condition.

Main Symptoms: After radiotherapy and chemotherapy, anemia, a whitish complexion, lassitude of spirit, palpitations and shortness of breath, abdominal distension and sicchasia, a poor appetite, sweating and cold, myasthenia of the limbs, dizziness, agrypnia, emotional disturbances and a decrease of white blood cells can occur.

Acupoints: Da Zhui (DU-14), He Gu (LI-4), Ge Shu (BL-17), Pi Shu (BL-20), Wei Shu (BL-21), Shen Shu (BL-23), Qi Hai (RN-6), Xue Hai (P-10), Zu San Li (ST-36).

Moxibustion Method:

- Gentle Pole Moxa: Apply moxa to 3–4 points, 15–20 minutes per point, once per day; 5–10 days constitute one course of treatment. A blood test should be performed after each course. (Figure 13.5.1)

- Moxa on Bu Zhong Yi Qi Pill (or Gui Pi Pill): Slice the pill and put it on the points, place a moxa cone on the pill slice and light. Apply 3–5 cones per acupoint and perform once per day. Ten treatments comprise one course of treatment. (Figure 13.5.2)

- Moxa on Ginger: Apply 3 cones per acupoint, once per day for 7–10 days continuously. Conduct a blood test after each course and cease moxibustion when WBC levels increase to normal. (Figure 13.5.3)

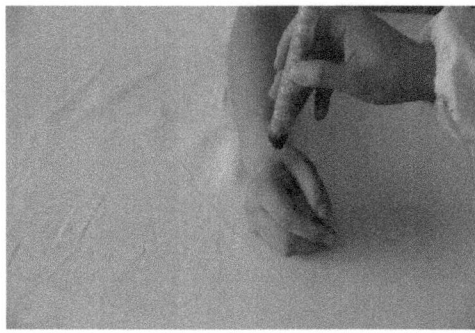

Figure 13.5.1 Gentle Pole Moxa at He Gu (LI-4)

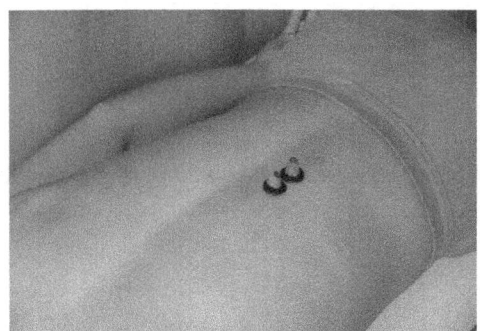

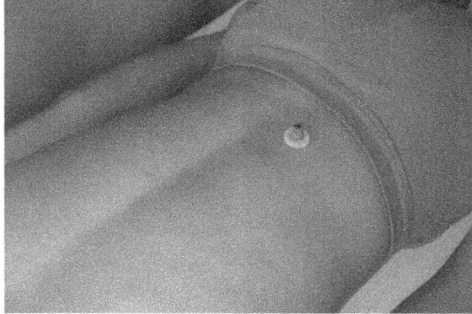

Figure 13.5.2 Moxa on Bu Zhong Yi Qi Pill at Pi Shu (BL-20) and Wei Shu (BL-21)   *Figure 13.5.3 Moxa on Ginger at Shen Shu (BL-23)*

6. Smoking Cessation

Smoking has many drawbacks and no advantages for the human body. It is an inducing factor for many diseases, such as respiratory system conditions, cardiovascular disease and some malignant tumours. Thus, smoking cessation is very important for achieving good health outcomes. In establishing the determination to stop smoking, moxibustion can help to alleviate nicotine addiction and obviate or relieve withdrawal symptoms after ceasing smoking.

Main Symptoms: Headache, somnolence, impaired concentration, anxiety and dysphoria appear during the process of smoking cessation.

Acupoints: Lie Que (LU-7), Jie Yan Xue (Quit Smoking Point; midway between Lie Que (LU-7) and Yang Xi (LU-5), Fei Shu (BL-13), Xin Shu (BL-15), Tong Li (HT-5).

Moxibustion Method:

- Gentle Moxa: Perform treatment once or twice per day. Ten treatments comprise one course of treatment, with a one-day interval between courses until withdrawal symptoms are alleviated. Apply moxa to Jie Yan Point during an addiction attack. (Figure 13.6.1)

- Moxa on Ginger: Perform treatment once or twice per day. Ten treatments comprise one course of treatment, with a one-day interval between the courses. (Figure 13.6.2)

- Scarring Moxa:* Apply moxa to Fei Shu (BL-13) and Xin Shu (BL-15). Perform treatment once or twice per day. Ten treatments comprise one course of treatment, with a one-day interval between courses. (Figure 13.6.3)

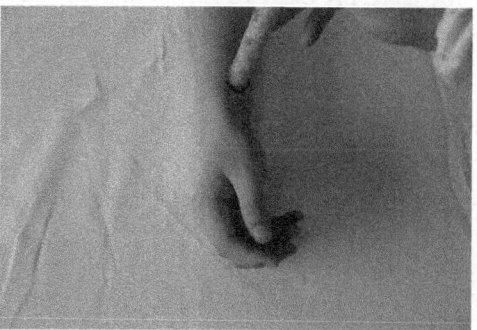

Figure 13.6.1 Gentle Moxa at Jie Yan Xue

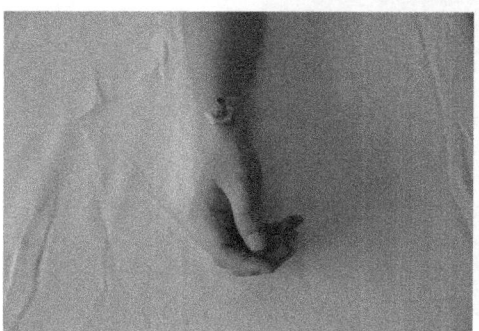

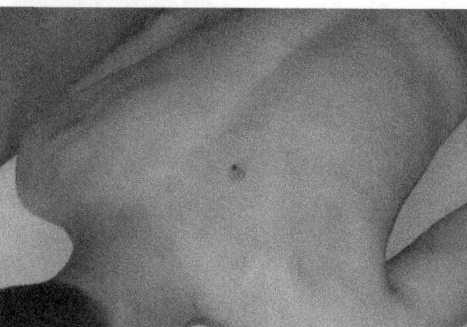

Figure 13.6.2 Moxa on Ginger at Lie Que (LU-7)   *Figure 13.6.3 Scarring Moxa at Xin Shu (BL-15)*

7. Drug Cessation

Heroin causes intractable and deep-rooted psychological and physiological dependence, leaving the body entirely dependent on the drug. Once the addiction has been established, withdrawal can cause severe symptoms and the addict will be unable to extricate himself or herself. This affects the physiological functioning of the body and can even be life-threatening.

Main Symptoms: Patients have a history of abusing heroin and have varying degrees of weeping, sneezing, yawning, coughing, accelerated breathing and chest distress, palpitations, abdominal pain, muscular soreness, general bone ache, a sensation like ants crawling on the skin, nephrasthenia asthma, sultriness, agrypnia, dysphoria, constipation and difficult urination.

Acupoints: Jia Ji (EX-B-2), Shen Shu (BL-23), Nei Guan (PC-6), Shen Men (HT-7), Zu San Li (ST-36), San Yin Jiao (SP-6).

Moxibustion Method:

- Gentle Moxa: Apply moxa to 2–4 points, 15–20 minutes per point, once per day; 6–15 treatments comprise one course of treatment. (Figure 13.7.1)

- Pecking Sparrow Moxa: Apply moxa to 2–4 points, 15–20 minutes per point, once per day. 6–15 treatments comprise one course of treatment. (Figure 13.7.2)

- Moxa on Garlic: Apply moxa to 2–4 points, 3–5 cones the size of a grain of wheat or soybean per point. Perform treatment once per day; 6–15 treatments comprise one course of treatment. (Figure 13.7.3)

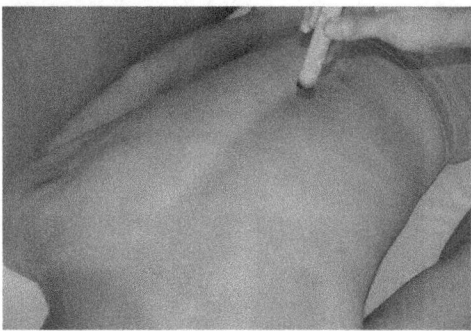

Figure 13.7.1 Gentle Moxa at Jia Ji (EX-B-2)

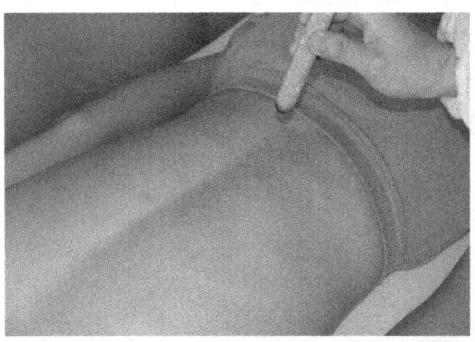 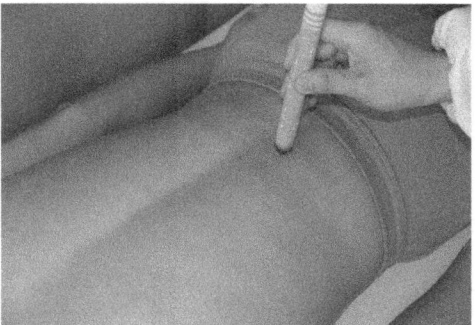

Figure 13.7.2 Pecking Sparrow Moxa at Shen Shu (BL-23)

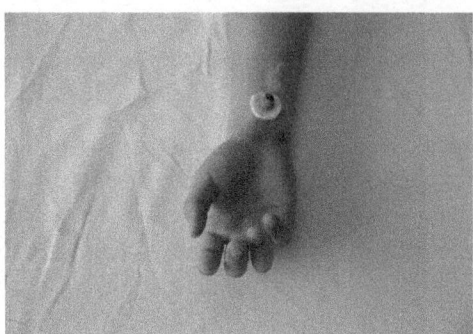

Figure 13.7.3 Moxa on Garlic at Nei Guan (PC-6)

- Moxa on Ginger: Apply moxa to 2–4 points, 3–5 cones the size of a grain of wheat or soybean per point. Perform treatment once per day; 6–15 treatments comprise one course of treatment. (Figure 13.7.4)

- Warm Needle Moxa: Apply moxa to 2–4 points, 3–5 cones the size of a grain of wheat or soybean per point. Perform treatment once per day or every other day. Ten treatments comprise one course of treatment. (Figure 13.7.5)

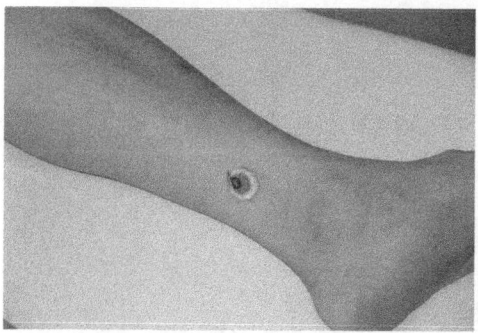 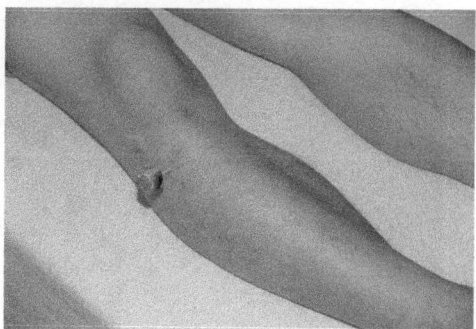

Figure 13.7.4 Moxa on Ginger at San Yin Jiao (SP-6)   *Figure 13.7.5 Warm Needle Moxa at Zu San Li (ST-36)*

8. Alcohol Cessation

Long-term excessive drinking can cause a variety of conditions. Alcohol stimulates the gastric mucosa making it prone to acute gastritis, induces angina cordis, myocardial infarct or arrhythmia, and damages hepatic cells causing adiposis hepatica or cirrhosis. Drinking makes individuals prone to brain haemorrhage, thus, alcohol cessation is very important.

Acupoints: Tong Li (HT-5), Ju Que (RN-14), Zhong Wan (RN-12), Feng Long (ST-40), Xin Shu (BL-15), Wei Shu (BL-21).

Moxibustion Method:

- Gentle Moxa: The patient drinks wine once a day, and performs treatment once per day. If the patient drinks wine twice a day, perform treatment twice per day. Ten treatments comprise one course of treatment, with a 1–3 day interval between courses. Moxibustion is more effective when carried out 0.5 to 1 hour before drinking. (Figure 13.8.1)

- Moxa on Ginger: Same as above. (Figure 13.8.2)

- Moxa on Garlic: Apply moxa to Xin Shu (BL-15) and Wei Shu (BL-21). The time and course are the same as above. (Figure 13.8.3)

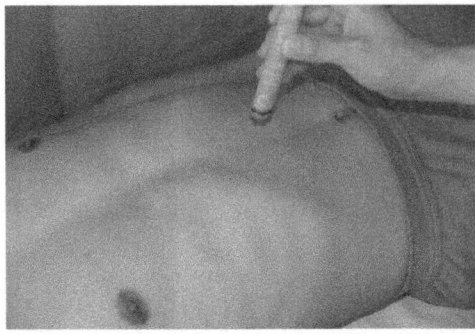

Figure 13.8.1 Gentle Moxa at Zhong Wan (RN-12)

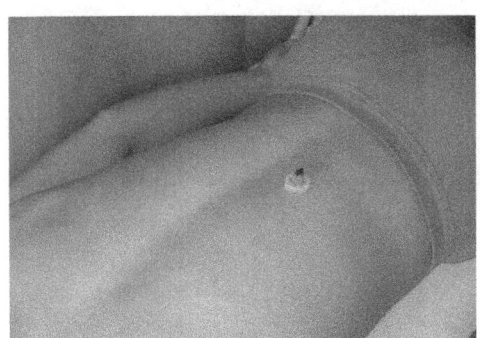

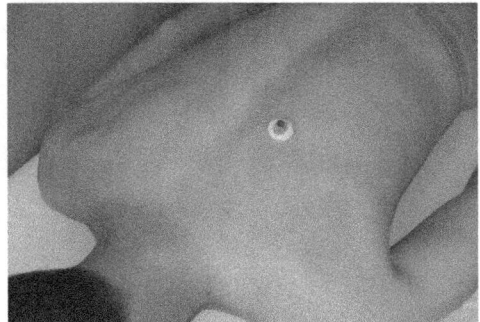

Figure 13.8.2 Moxa on Ginger at Wei Shu (BL-21)   *Figure 13.8.3 Moxa on Garlic at Xin Shu (BL-15)*

9. Poor Acclimatization

Poor acclimatization refers to uncomfortable symptoms that involve diarrhoea, abdominal pain, decreased appetite, a fatigued spirit and a lack of strength and poor sleep. These result from difficulty in adapting to a local climate, diet or living habit for a period of time when moving to a new living environment, this often occurs during a business trip, a move or while travelling.

Main Symptoms: Abdominal pain and distension, diarrhoea, decreased eating, poor sleeping, etc.

Acupoints: Tian Shu (ST-25), Zhong Wan (RN-12), Shen Que (RN-8), Pi Shu (BL-20), Zu San Li (ST-36), Shen Men (HT-7).

Moxibustion Method:

- Gentle Moxa: Apply moxa to each point for 6–20 minutes, once per day. Seven treatments comprise one course of treatment. (Figure 13.9.1)

- Moxa on Ginger: Apply 3–5 cones of moxa to each point. Seven treatments comprise one course of treatment. (Figure 13.9.2)

- Moxa on Salt: Use moxa cones the size of a jujube seed. Apply 5–7 cones to Shen Que (RN-8), once every other day. Ten treatments comprise one course of treatment. (Figure 13.9.3)

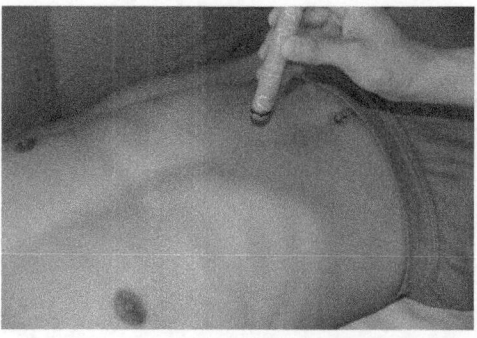

Figure 13.9.1 Gentle Moxa at Zhong Wan (RN-12)

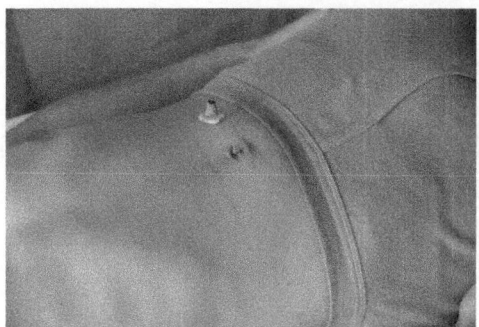

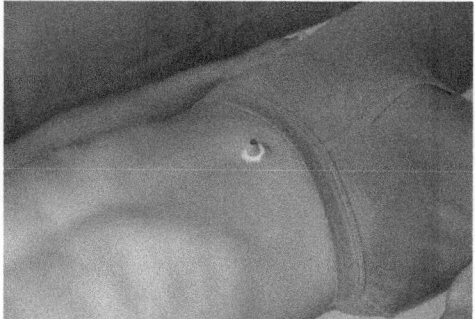

Figure 13.9.2 Moxa on Ginger at Tian Shu (ST-25)   *Figure 13.9.3 Moxa on Salt at Shen Que (RN-8)*

10. Motion Sickness

Motion sickness refers to a condition where patients feel dizzy or nauseous when travelling by car or ship.

Main Symptoms: Dizziness, dim eyesight, nausea, vomiting, debility, sweating and even symptoms of exhaustion that involve sudden fainting, a pale complexion, cold limbs and sweating.

Acupoints: Bai Hui (DU-20), Zhong Wan (RN-12), Nei Guan (PC-6), Zu San Li (ST-36), Shen Men (HT-7).

Moxibustion Method:

- Gentle Moxa: Apply moxa to each point for 6–20 minutes, once or twice when, or before, travelling by car or ship. (Figure 13.10.1)

- Moxa on Salt: Use moxa cones the size of a jujube seed. Apply to Shen Que (RN-8) for 20 minutes. Use this method as an emergency treatment in the case of fainting. (Figure 13.10.2)

- Special Treatment: Apply Shang Shi Zhi Tong Gao (Dampness Damage Pain-relieving Plaster) to Shen Que (RN-8) before travelling by car or a ship. (Figure 13.10.3)

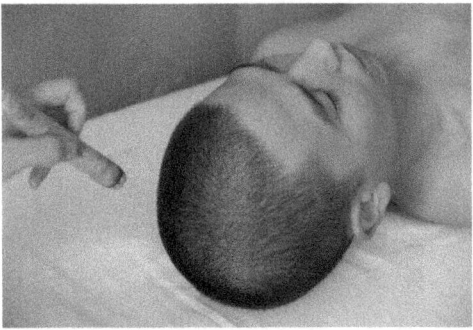

Figure 13.10.1 Gentle Moxa at Bai Hui (DU-20)

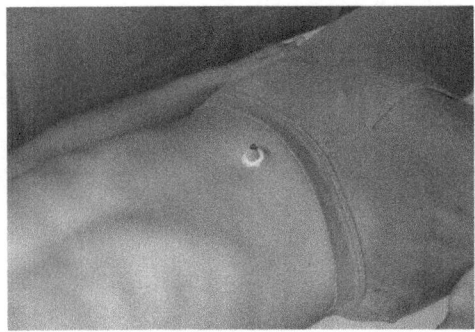
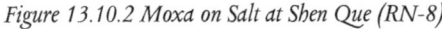

Figure 13.10.2 Moxa on Salt at Shen Que (RN-8)

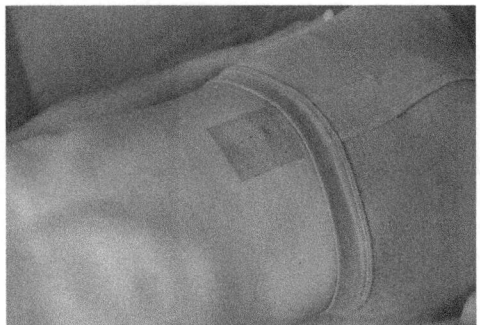

Figure 13.10.3 Special Treatment at Shen Que (RN-8)

11. Altitude Sickness

Altitude sickness affects individuals who live in low altitude areas whom experience uncomfortable symptoms such as dizziness, emotional upset, a poor spirit, fatigue, weakness, drowsiness, poor sleep, loose stools when entering high altitude areas.

Main Symptoms: Dizziness, emotional upset, a poor spirit, fatigue, weakness, poor sleep and a decreased appetite.

Acupoints: Pi Shu (BL-20), Ge Shu (BL-17), Zu San Li (ST-36), Qi Hai (RN-6), Shen Men (HT-7), Guan Yuan (RN-4).

Moxibustion Method:

- Gentle Moxa: Apply moxa to each point for 6–20 minutes, once per day. Ten treatments comprise one course of treatment. (Figure 13.11.1)

- Moxa on Garlic: Use moxa cones the size of a jujube seed. Apply 5–7 cones of moxa to each point once per day. Ten treatments comprise one course of treatment. (Figure 13.11.2)

- Cone Moxa: Use moxa cones the size of a grain of wheat. Apply 5–7 cones of moxa to each point once per day. Ten treatments comprise one course of treatment. (Figure 13.11.3)

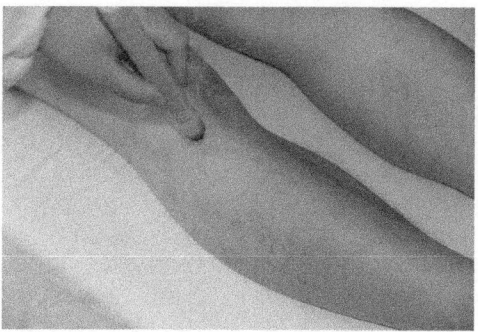

Figure 13.11.1 Gentle Moxa at Zu San Li (ST-36)

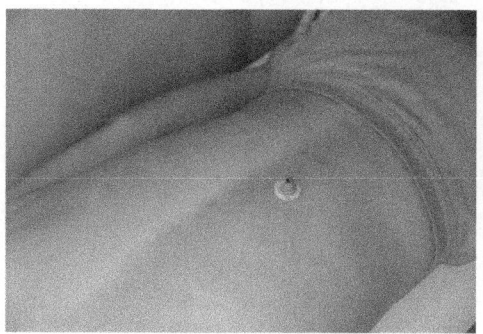

Figure 13.11.2 Moxa on Garlic at Pi Shu (BL-20)

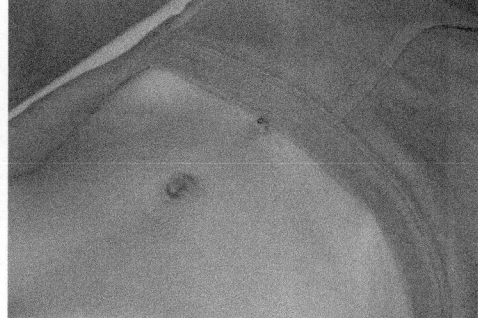

Figure 13.11.3 Cone Moxa at Qi Hai (RN-6)

Index